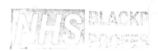 

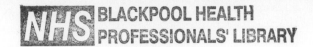

# Controversies in Total Knee Replacement

Edited by

## Richard S. Laskin MD

Professor of Clinical Orthopedic Surgery
*Weill Medical College of Cornell University*

Chairman of the Arthroplasty Council
and Attending Orthopedic Surgeon
*The Hospital for Special Surgery, New York*

# OXFORD

UNIVERSITY PRESS

Great Clarendon Street, Oxford OX2 6DP

Oxford University Press is a department of the University of Oxford.
It furthers the University's objective of excellence in research, scholarship,
and education by publishing worldwide in

Oxford New York

Athens Auckland Bangkok Bogotá Buenos Aires Cape Town
Chennai Dar es Salaam Delhi Florence Hong Kong Istanbul Karachi
Kolkata Kuala Lumpur Madrid Melbourne Mexico City Mumbai Nairobi
Paris São Paulo Shanghai Singapore Taipei Tokyo Toronto Warsaw

with associated companies in Berlin Ibadan

Oxford is a registered trade mark of Oxford University Press
in the UK and in certain other countries

Published in the United States
by Oxford University Press Inc., New York

© Oxford University Press, 2001

A catalogue record for this book is available from the British Library

Library of Congress Cataloging in Publication Data
(Data available)
ISBN 0 19 263072 5

1 3 5 7 9 10 8 6 4 2

Typeset by EXPO Holdings, Malaysia
Typeset in Plantin by 9/12 pt
Printed in Great Britain on acid-free paper
by T.J. International Ltd, Padstow, Cornwall

# Preface

It has been 35 years since pioneering surgeons in Europe and the United Kingdom began inserting metallic hinge prostheses in an attempt to alleviate the ravages of arthritis of the knee. Over the intervening years knee replacement has been refined to a point where it is the mainstay in treating advanced gonarthrosis and one of the two most successful orthopedic surgical procedures performed (the other, of interest, is total hip replacement). It is estimated that several hundred thousand knee replacements a year are performed worldwide.

The last 35 years have seen numerous changes in the way that knee prostheses are designed and the manner in which they are implanted. We have learned the hard and sad lessons of "strengthened" polyethylene, flat articular surfaces, rigid linked interfaces, and malpositioned components. Surgeons and scientists in the field of biomechanics have overcome these early problems and have perfected the procedure to a point where over 95% of patients have an extraordinary relief of pain and ability to return to an active productive life.

The field of total knee replacement, however, is not static. There remain areas of controversy: areas in which the knowledge of today can help further improve on the results of this surgery tomorrow. Some of these areas of controversy are in the arena of biomaterials and design, some in the control of potential medical complications of surgery, and some in improvement in accuracy of insertion of the implants.

This book examines many of the controversial areas of total knee replacement surgery. Each segment is presented as a debate with at least two authors responding to a basic controversy in total knee replacement. I then pose a series of questions to each of the authors, to help elucidate what they have said in their chapters. The questions are pointed and direct. I have encouraged each author to likewise be straightforward in replying.

I have tried, as much as I possibly can, to remain neutral in the debate. You must realize that no one is truly neutral; all of us come with some preconceived notions, which may be correct or incorrect. If in the debate questions my own feelings tend to show through, please accept the fact that I have tried to be equally challenging to both debaters, regardless of my opinions. As chairman of an annual Total Knee Course held in New York during the holiday season that is now approaching its twelfth year, I have found this debate-type format an excellent and enjoyable method for the dissemination of scientific information.

All the contributors are experts in their fields and have lectured and written extensively. Each author has graciously accepted the challenge not only of writing a chapter but also of being involved with the debate section that follows. I am proud to say that each of the authors is also a friend, for who else but a friend would allow someone to question him without the chance of being able to challenge back the questioner.

There are two non-debate chapters in the book as well. One is written by Professor Robert Bourne of London, Ontario, one of the leading orthopedic surgeons in the world in the field of knee replacement. He has written a review of several studies that he and his colleagues have performed on the value of knee replacement to both society and the patient. It should be the basis for our being able to show that "what we do" helps people and helps society. In a century where outcomes are becoming the benchmark for documenting the value of our "services", we must all graduate from the old ways of nondescript, poorly written chart notes (patient doing OK, satisfactory range of motion, etc.) into a precise methodology of collecting and expressing outcomes both as we and our patients see them. Mr. Jack Davis RN, a leading nurse educator with whom I have had the privilege of working for the past 7 years, has accepted the challenge to write a chapter on outcomes.

When traveling and lecturing I am always asked, "What do the doctors at HSS do in this particular situation?" Here at the onset I would like to tell you what we are doing *today* and how the majority of orthopedic surgeons at HSS would stand in the following debates. Realize, of course, that just because we do it, surely does not make it gospel, and likewise what we are doing today might just be modified tomorrow. Having said that, however, the majority of the arthroplasts at HSS use modular tibial components, resurface the patella, cement the implants in place and use CPM in the postoperative period. Most of us will do a two-stage exchange revision for infection, and when necessary, perform a proximal quadriceps release rather than a tibia tubercle osteotomy for exposure. Although HSS has traditionally been alluded to as the home of the PCL thrashers, there is a small, but enlightened group here who are making the decision whether to save or resect the PCL on an individual case. We still perform tibial osteotomies however the number is diminishing each year. The area where we have the most divergence is in the prophylaxis of DVT. Most of us have come to the conclusion that some form of mechanical compression device should be used. We have not, however, come to any conclusion as to which chemoprophylactic method is optimal. As such there are at least 10 anti-DVT protocols being followed each operative day. All of us use perioperative antibiotics for about 24 h, and, for the most part, all of our knee replacements are performed using epidural anesthesia that is continued postoperatively as PCA.

This book is intended for use by practicing orthopedic surgeons worldwide who are involved in the performance of total knee replacement, and for orthopedic residents and registrars in their training years. It likewise should be educational for those in the allied medical fields who help us care for our patients: nurses, physical therapists, and surgical operating theater staff.

I think that you will find the material timely, informative, at times provocative, and always relevant.

**Richard S. Laskin MD**
The Hospital for Special Surgery
Professor of Clinical Orthopedic Surgery, Weill Medical College of Cornell University

# Acknowledgements

I would like to thank my wonderful family for all their support and love: my wife and soul mate Judge Joyce Sparrow, our children Jonathan, Andrew and Nicole, Risa and Bruce and Doug and Beth, and the "big guys" Maxwell and Dylan.

I would like to take this opportunity to express my appreciation to my colleagues at the Hospital for Special Surgery for all their aid and assistance in the decade that I have had the privilege of working with them. They truly make going to work in the morning interesting, challenging, informative, and absolutely never dull. My hard working office staff, Ms. Lucinda Calandrella, Ms. Ting Miller, and Mr. Jack Davis always manage to keep everything running not only at a high level of efficiency, but always with compassion for our patients and their problems.

Working at HSS has been the highlight and the most exciting part of my career in orthopaedic surgery.

I would like to thank the members of the Knee Society for letting me join with them to commune, learn, teach, and drink fine wines. It is a fraternity in the best sense of the word composed of gentlemen (and ladies), scholars, and friends.

Finally I would like to thank three surgeons who I feel have made the greatest impression upon my in my years as an orthopaedic surgeon. They were always there for encouragement and to act as role models for me:

A. Graham Apley FRCS
John Insall MD
Richard Bryan MD.

# Contents

## 6

Two-stage exchange is the optimal treatment for an infected knee replacement

## 7

Acrylic cement is the method of choice for fixation of total knee implants

## 8

The patella need not be resurfaced during total knee replacement

## 9

The optimal way to balance the flexion space is to externally rotate the femoral component

## 10

Aspirin is sufficient prophylaxis for deep venous thrombosis for most total knee patients

# Abbreviations

| | | | |
|---|---|---|---|
| AAOS | American Academy for Orthopaedic Surgeons | OA | osteoarthritis |
| ACL | anterior cruciate ligament | PCA | Porous-Coated Anatomic (knee) |
| AEM | anteriorization of the extensor mechanism | PCA | patient-controlled anesthesia |
| AGC | Anatomical Graduated Components (knee) | PCL | posterior cruciate ligament |
| | | PE | pulmonary embolism |
| AORI | Anderson Orthopaedic Research Institute bone defect classification | PMMA | polymethylmethacrylate |
| | | PR | patellar resurfacing |
| | | PS | posterior stabilized |
| AP | anterior–posterior | QALY | quality-adjusted life years |
| CPM | continuous passive motion | QWBI | Quality of Well Being Index |
| CPN | common peroneal nerve | RA | rheumatoid arthritic |
| CVA | cerebrovascular accident | ROM | range of motion |
| DJD | degenerative joint disease | RSA | roentgenographic stereophotogrammetry |
| DVT | deep venous thrombosis | SBT | serum bactericidal titer |
| EMG | electromyelography | SF-36 | Medical Outcomes Study 36-item short-form health survey |
| HRQL | health-related quality of life | | |
| HSS | Hospital for Special Surgery | | |
| HTO | high tibial osteotomy | THA | total hip arthroplasty |
| IB | Insall–Burstein | TIA | transient ischaemic attack |
| LMWH | low molecular weight heparin | TKA | total knee arthroplasty |
| MI | myocardial infarct | UCA | unicompartmental arthroplasty |
| MIC | minimal inhibitory concentration | UHMWPE | ultra high molecular weight polyethylene |
| MODEMS | Musculoskeletal Outcomes Data Evaluation and Management System | V/Q | ventilation perfusion |
| | | WOMAC | Western Ontario and McMaster University Osteoarthritis Index |
| MRI | magnetic resonance imaging | | |

# Contributors

Eugene J. Alexander PHD

Thomas Andriacchi PHD

Johan Bellemans MD PHD

Robert B. Bourne MD

Scott A. Brumby MD PHD

Frederick F. Buechel MD FACS

Brian Crites MD

John P. Davis BS RN ONC

Lawrence D. Dorr MD

Chris O. Dyrby MS

Michael Freeman FRCS

Steven B. Haas MD MPH

Frank Hagena MD

John A. L. Hart MBBS FRACS FAOrthA FASMF FACSP(Hon.)

G. E. D. Howell FRCS ED (ORTH)

John Insall MD

Hiro Iwaki MD

Bertrand P. Kaper MD

Jonathan D. S. Klein

Kim M. Koffler MD

Kenneth Krackow MD

Donald B. Longjohn MD

Jess H. Lonner MD

Paul A. Lotke MD

William MacAuley MD

Alexander Miric MD

Sandeep Munjal MD

Jonathan Noble MB CHM FRCS FRCSE

Vera Pinskerova MD

James Rand MD

Michael Ries MD

Merrill Ritter MD

Cecil H. Rorabeck MD

Khalin Saleh MD MSC FRCS

Richard D. Scott MD

Giles Scuderi MD

Thomas P. Sculco

Klaus Steinbrink MD

James Stiehl MD

Thomas S. Thornhill MD

Jan Victor MD

Samuel R. Ward PT

Geoffrey H. Westrich MD

Leo Whiteside MD

Russell E. Windsor MD

Timothy Wright PHD

# 1

*In an era where monetary resources may often influence what type of care society can afford to give to its citizens, and how much, we are constantly asked to justify what we are doing. What are the results for the patient and for society as a whole? Should the procedure we are advocating have its funding increased or kept constant? These are questions that we rarely thought of during medical school. In this chapter, the authors describe their extensive research into the benefits of total knee replacement.*

# Total knee replacement is one of the most beneficial procedures both for patients and for society

Bertrand P. Kaper and Robert B. Bourne

During the second half of the twentieth century, advances in medicine progressed at an unprecedented rate. An aging population, new technologies, and progressive affluence have increased the demands for the newest, and often most expensive, medical services.

Yet, repeatedly, new technologies have been introduced before being properly and objectively assessed, often resulting in considerable patient morbidity—a few examples within orthopedics are surface-replacement total hip replacements, carbon-reinforced polyethylene, and silastic implants.[1–7] Total knee arthroplasty (TKA) has not been immune to this type of problem. In the mid-1980s, conventional wisdom might have suggested the use of a cementless TKA with a metal-backed patella, a round-on-flat articulation, and less than 5 mm of heat-pressed polyethylene. Less than 10 years later, these poorly assessed decisions have already produced inferior clinical results.[8] Revision rates of 10–12% for patella component failure, osteolysis, and/or tibial insert failure have been reported. Questions of quality assurance have arisen within the context of an emerging cost crisis, as various medical and surgical interventions compete for diminishing healthcare dollars. Reported differences in the use of hospital beds, expenditures, and operation rates *per capita*, without demonstrable improvement in the overall health of patient populations, have raised further questions about the application of medical technology and its relative cost-effectiveness.

From the viewpoint both of orthopedic surgeons and of their patients, TKA is an effective and successful procedure. The orthopedic literature abounds with numerous clinical studies documenting the excellent pain relief and return of near-normal function of joints replaced for debilitating knee arthritis.[9–12]

1

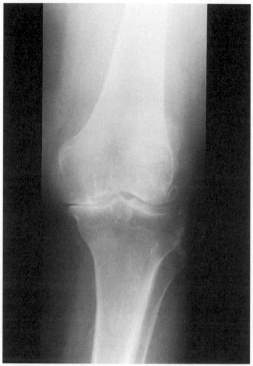

a

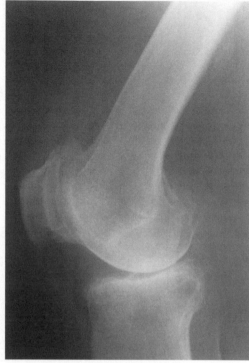

b

**Fig. 1.1**

Preoperative radiographs demonstrating end-stage arthritis of the knee: (a) AP; (b) lateral.

A recent meta-analysis of tricompartmental total knee replacement suggested that global rating scale scores were improved by 100% following TKA and that 89.3% of patients reported good or excellent outcomes.[13] At present, however, the burden rests with the orthopedic community to convince the payers of healthcare, ideally through prospective, randomized outcomes studies, that total joint arthroplasty is and will continue to be valuable to the patient and society, in a cost-effective manner. The issues of quality assurance and cost have, therefore, prompted the need to justify what we as orthopedic surgeons do.

Total joint replacement, of both the knee and hip, is considered by many to be a high-technology procedure that is expensive and used to treat a non-life-threatening disease. As third-party payers attempt to lower their costs, and thereby improve the overall cost-effectiveness of the interventions they cover, continued funding of total joint arthroplasty has come under considerable pressure. In the USA and other countries, the "graying" of society, especially the baby-boomer generation, will only serve to further increase the demand for total joint replacement. The magnitude and scope of the economics related to osteoarthritis and its global impact on society must be fully understood and appreciated. In 1997, an estimated 1–2.5% of the gross national product for the USA, Canada, the UK, France, and Australia was allocated for treatments of musculoskeletal conditions.[14] Of all afflictions of the musculoskeletal system, osteoarthritis

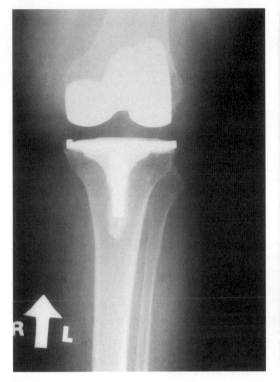

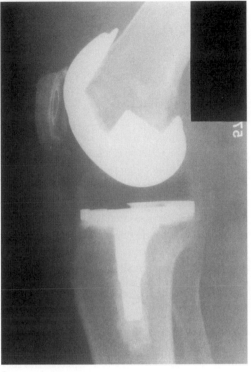

a                                                    b

**Fig. 1.2**

Postoperative radiographs showing excellent position and alignment of a TKA: (a) AP; (b) lateral.

is certainly the most common, accounting for significant economic, social, and psychological costs. The disability caused by arthritis in later life is compounded by the significant out-of-pocket expenses and loss of earnings due to changes in occupation and roles in domestic duties that are secondary consequences of osteoarthritis.

In order to firmly establish the efficacy and benefit of total knee replacement to both patients and society, and thereby justify the continued support for this procedure, four primary questions must be posed and answered.

- What are the costs associated with the continued nonoperative treatment of patients with end-stage arthritis, who are considered candidates for TKA?
- How does TKA benefit patients and society?
- What are the costs, direct and indirect, associated with TKA?
- How does the cost-effectiveness of TKA, in the form of cost per quality-adjusted life years (QALY), compare with other interventions that are competing for the limited healthcare dollar?

If the answers to these questions, as illustrated in the orthopedic literature, support the benefits of TKA, then we, as orthopedic surgeons, can continue to promote this procedure as one that benefits both our patients and society.

# Cost-effectiveness and value

Contemporary outcome studies assess the "value" of an intervention where:

$$\text{value} = \text{quality/cost}$$
$$\text{and}$$
$$\text{quality} = \text{outcome(s) and/or satisfaction.}$$

The instruments used to determine quality and cost therefore directly influence the parameters that are used to determine the ultimate "value" or cost-effectiveness of an intervention.[15] Careful reporting and accurate data collection are, therefore, of paramount importance in the process of standardization of outcome measures and cost-effectiveness analyses.[16,17] Direct costs related to an intervention such as total knee replacement are relatively easy to measure, but the direct and indirect costs of the alternatives to TKA often are not. Similarly, there exist significant challenges to the collection of accurate and objective data used to define the outcome and satisfaction of an intervention.

Traditional outcome measures have focused on physician-based scoring systems. Numerous orthopedic indices exist to assess the outcome of arthroplasty surgery.[18–26] The Knee Society clinical rating system and the Hospital for Special Surgery (HSS) knee rating system are often employed and reported in clinical studies. Despite the wide application of these and other instruments, rigorous validation is currently lacking. More recently introduced outcome instruments attempt to assess general, as well as specific, health-related perceptions of quality of life, as interpreted by the patients, not the providers. The most commonly employed health outcome instruments, including the global-health Short Form-36 (SF-36) and the disease-specific Western Ontario and McMaster University Osteoarthritis Index (WOMAC), are summarized in Table 1.1. Each of these instruments analyzes the health-related quality of life in a slightly different manner. Many of these systems have now been validated through prospective, randomized studies, and are therefore considered essential in the detailed analysis of cost-effectiveness data.[27,28]

The measurement of health-related quality of life (HRQoL) has gained significant recognition and acceptance during the past decade. In a review of previously published literature regarding "quality-of-life" studies, however, Gill and Feinstein found that, in general, the scientific basis used to determine QoL was poor.[29] The vast majority of studies defined QoL poorly, and little distinction was made between overall and health-related QoL. Accordingly, many of the conclusions drawn in the references reviewed do not reflect the type of accurate information that is necessary to support their conclusions. Two types of tools or instruments may be used to measure HRQoL[21]:

**Table 1.1** Scoring systems

CLINICAL SCORING SYSTEMS FOR JOINT REPLACEMENT

- Knee Society Score
- Hospital for Special Surgery Hip and Knee Scores
- Harris Hip Score
- Merle d'Aubigne Hip Score

OUTCOME-BASED SCORES FOR JOINT REPLACEMENT EVALUATION

- Western Ontario and McMaster University Osteoarthritis Index (WOMAC)
- Short Form(SF)-36 and SF-12
- Sickness Impact Profile (SP)
- Time Trade-off Technique
- McMaster–Toronto Arthritis Patient Preference Disability Questionnaire (MACTAR)
- Quality of Well Being Index
- Nottingham Health Profile (NHP)
- 15-Dimensional Profile

---

- discriminative or "utility" instruments, which allow differentiation between patients at a particular point in time
- evaluative instruments, which assess longitudinal changes within patient groups over a period of time.

Specifically defined, the "utility" measures are designed for individual decision-making under uncertainty, but, with additional assumptions, they can be aggregated across individuals to provide a group-utility function.[30] As such, the application of the "utility" instruments has been recommended for general clinical use in the assessment of health-related quality of life.[31] The goals of these HRQoL instruments are threefold:

- to assess important effects in clinical trials
- to measure the health of specific populations
- to provide information regarding policy decisions.

There is significant overlap of these three goals, especially in the setting of total joint arthroplasty, but the third goal is presenting receiving the most attention. Since the advent of the outcomes movement, the information generated by HRQoL data has given managed-care and other third-party payers the opportunity to dictate detailed policy decisions. This information now also includes QALY, a specific measure of cost-effectiveness, designed to aggregate in a single summary a measure of the total health improvement for a group of individuals, capturing improvements from impacts on both QoL and quantity of life. The net effect of the generation of this information is that the orthopedic surgery community, as well as the medical community in general, are now held much more accountable for their actions and the associated costs.

From the perspective of the third-party payers of medical and surgical interventions, gains in the relative "value" or cost-effectiveness of an intervention can only be achieved in one of two ways:

- improving the outcome or satisfaction of the intervention
- decreasing the cost of the intervention.

The "Oregon" solution, in which cost relative to QoL data was compiled, listed, and voted upon for funding, represents the clinical application of such a "value" assessment. In the Oregon plan, funding is provided for the most cost-effective interventions, but not for less cost-effective interventions falling below a certain threshold (e.g., liver transplantation, bone marrow transplantation, and spinal fusion).

Laupacis et al. attempted to place specific dollar values on interventions to categorize their relative cost-effectiveness.[6] The cost-outcome was divided into four groups (using 1989 Canadian dollars):

A: medical interventions costing less than $20 000 (very cost effective)
B: medical interventions costing $20 000–100 000 (moderately cost effective)
C: medical interventions costing over $100 000 (may be effective, but expensive)
D: noneffective medical interventions.

Items in group A were considered to be so cost-effective that they should be funded without question. Both total hip arthroplasty (THA)and TKA fall in this group. For comparison, Laupacis found the cost of renal transplantation to be $66 290 in the first year and $27,875 in the second year.[32] In relative terms, total joint arthroplasty

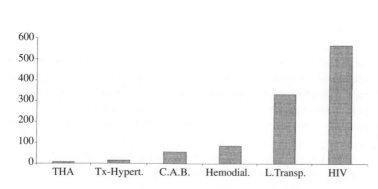

**Fig. 1.3**

Cost/utility data comparing total hip arthroplasty to other medical interventions. THA, total hip arthroplasty; Tx-Hypert., medical treatment of moderate hypertension; C.A.B., coronary artery bypass; Hemodial., hemodialysis; Liver Trans., liver transplantation; HIV, human immunodeficiency virus (cost per additional live saved); QALY, quality adjusted life years.

compares quite favorably with the medical treatment of hypertension, coronary artery bypass grafting, and even more favorably with renal and liver transplantation.[33]

## Cost-containment strategies

Cost-containment strategies related to total joint arthroplasty have been implemented to varying degrees over the past two decades. Numerous initiatives have been enacted in order to decrease the direct costs related to total joint arthroplasty.[34–45] These initiatives have included

* decreased length of hospital stay
* demand-matching of implants to patients
* reductions in implant costs
* reduction in surgical fees
* reduction in uses and costs of ancillary services.

Of these different measures, shorter length of acute hospital stay has been the most widely employed. As noted by Barber and Healy, average length of hospitalization was reduced from 17 days in 1980 to 9.3 days in 1991.[35] Further reductions have since been documented, with an average length of stay now typically between 4 and 6 days.

The cumulative result of cost-containment measures can be witnessed in the trends of total hospital cost for total joint arthroplasty. Healy and Finn compared costs related to TKA performed in 1983 and subsequently in 1991 at the Lahey-Hitchcock Clinic in Burlington, MA.[37]

Both the actual costs and the inflation-adjusted costs were determined for the various service centers within the hospital contributing to the overall hospital charge. With the implementation of various cost-saving measures, the average hospital cost decreased in inflation-adjusted dollars by 15% during this period. Iorio *et al.* used

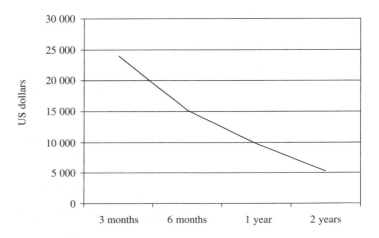

**Fig. 1.4**

Average cost per quality-adjusted life year (QALY) versus assessment interval. From Lavernia *et al.*[61]

data collected between October 1993 and September 1995 at the same institution, to analyze the costs of both total hip and TKA.[41] In this series 207 patients underwent primary TKA and 290 underwent THA. The average in-hospital cost incurred after a cost-saving program had been implemented was $10 421 for TKA and $11 104 for THA. The implementation of cost-saving measures was felt to have significantly decreased the overall costs incurred, allowing the authors to conclude that total joint arthroplasty can be delivered in a cost-effective manner, without compromising the benefits of this procedure.

The single largest unit cost in the hospital cost for TKA at present is the cost of the knee implants. Although most of the individual costs related to TKA have decreased, the inflation-adjusted cost of the implants has increased. Healy and Finn noted a 59% increase in the cost of the implant from 1983 to 1991.[37] The proportion of the total hospital costs dedicated to the cost of the implant increased from 13% in 1983 to 25% in 1991. Similarly, Lavernia *et al.* noted that more than 40% of the total charge for primary as well as revision THA and TKA was generated by the implant alone.[42] Obviously, and importantly in the era of cost-containment, reducing the overall and relative costs of knee implants could help achieve the goal of increased cost-effectiveness of this procedure. Knee implant standardization programs, competitive bidding programs, volume discounts, and hospital awareness programs are the primary strategies employed to contain the cost of the prostheses. As suggested by Iorio *et al.*, matching patients to one of five demand categories and then assigning specific implant designs to each demand category can offer savings anywhere from 8.4 to 27% of current costs.[40]

Several studies have demonstrated that a large proportion of the charges for total joint arthroplasty are generated in the immediate postoperative period. Using data from 50 primary total hip and 37 total knee arthroplasties, Meyers *et al.* determined that 76% of all costs are accounted for by the cost of the implant, anesthesia/operating room, and the nursing/hospital room costs.[43] Similarly, Healy *et al.* reviewed 391 joint replacement operations performed during 1996.[38] The average hospital cost was $10 231, and nearly 80% of this cost was generated during the first 48 h of hospitalization.

The charges of the operating room, nursing units, recovery room, and pharmacy accounted for a majority of the costs. Both these studies suggest that additional attempts to control or reduce the hospital cost of joint replacement should focus on these areas of opportunity.

There has also been a reduction in surgical fees for TKA. The mean fee for TKA was $2435 in 1992, but only $1825 in 1995. Additional cost-savings have been suggested through minimizing the use of postoperative radiographs, physical therapy, and other ancillary services.[44]

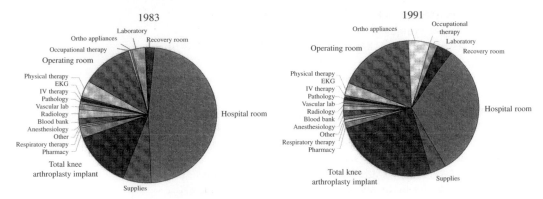

**Fig. 1.5**

In-hospital costs for total knee arthroplasty, 1983 versus 1991. From Ayers *et al.*[34]

The evolution and application of cost-containment strategies has raised several concerns:

- Will the measures employed to contain costs have a negative effect with respect outcomes and patient satisfaction with TKA?
- are the measures employed actually containing costs, or merely causing a shift from "direct" to "indirect" costs?
- How far do cost-containment strategies need to go, if total joint arthroplasty is already considered a highly cost-effective medical intervention?

Significant concerns have been raised about the possible negative repercussions of cost-savings measures. The challenge for the third-party payers for healthcare, therefore, is to insure that quality of care and outcome of a given procedure will not be adversely impacted by cost reduction measures. In a study analyzing the effects of a cost-savings program implemented for total hip replacement surgery, Meding *et al.* found that surgical results remained excellent, and the rate of perioperative complications, including infection, implant loosening, and revision hip surgery actually decreased.[26] The authors concluded that cost-effective programs could successfully be implemented without compromising results or increasing the complication rate. A similar conclusion may be inferred for TKA surgery.

Additional information has suggested that the reductions in length of stay may directly benefit patient outcomes. Rissanen *et al.* noted that the longest hospital stays were strongly related to postoperative complications encountered.[60] Shorter hospital stays certainly reduces the risk of subsequent nosocomial infections. Furthermore, early postoperative mobilization of patients has allowed for a decrease in the risk of deep venous thrombosis. Concurrent with the trend of shorter hospital stays has been the application of "critical-care pathways" in the setting of total joint arthroplasties. Such pathways were initially introduced in the busier arthroplasty centers, but are now also routinely found in smaller institutions. Typically, the busier arthroplasty centers have also been under the most pressure to reduce costs. Accordingly, it is not surprising that the number of arthroplasties performed in a given hospital has been shown to be inversely proportional to length of stay.

Cost shifting, rather than cost saving, is one of the problems arising from the pressure to decrease length of stay in hospital. From a hospital perspective, earlier discharge of patients to extended care facilities, rehabilitation centers, and nursing homes will reduce costs. This reduction in direct costs, however, results in an increase in indirect costs—costs that are still the responsibility of third-party payers. Killeen and Burt assessed this cost-shifting process in 1995.[49] The authors compared 1 week hospitalizations followed by discharge home, to early hospital discharges to extended care facilities. As could be expected, patients who were monitored in the hospital for 1 week and then discharged home generated a lower total cost for their total joint replacement than did those who were discharged early to an extended care facility. Early transfer to a rehabilitation setting, therefore, may result in apparent cost savings but, in actuality, merely represents a cost shifting.

To date, the cost-containing measures introduced for TKA surgery have seemingly not adversely affected surgical outcomes. Similarly, patient satisfaction with the procedure has not diminished. How much further the individual and total costs related to TKA could be reduced remains to be seen. As suggested by Meyers et al.[44] and Healy et al.[38], the largest percentage of costs are presently generated in the immediate postoperative period (Fig. 1.6). Attempts at further reductions in expenditures would most likely be directed to that area. This information confirms the widely held notion that further reduction in length of stay would not significantly reduce total hospital cost. Although current data suggests that total hip and TKA already is an extremely cost-effective procedure, the anticipated future increase

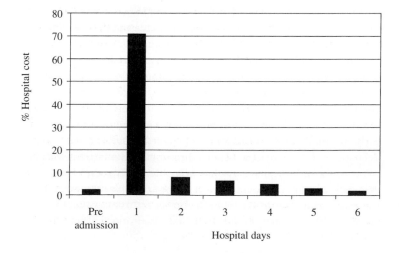

**Fig. 1.6**

Cost per day associated with hospitalization for total knee arthroplasty. From Healy et al.[38]

in the demand for these procedures will undoubtedly generate additional interest in further cost-containment measures.

## Total joint arthroplasty

The orthopedic literature currently contains only limited information regarding the true cost-effectiveness of THA or TKA, and more focus has been placed on hip arthroplasty than knee arthroplasty. The benefits of THA have been assessed in several studies.[17] [25,50–56] A multitude of outcome measures has been applied to this patient population, documenting consistent improvements in nearly all measures assessed, including pain, range of motion, energy, sleep, mood, social isolation, activities of daily living, social life, and family life. In the most thorough of these investigations, Laupacis *et al.*[57] reported marked improvement in physical function, social interaction, and overall health following hip replacement, as assessed by: the Sickness Impact Profile, the 6 minute walk test, the Harris Hip score, the Merle d'Aubigne score, the WOMAC, the McMaster–Toronto Arthritis Patient Preference Disability questionnaire, and the time trade-off score. The only factor that total hip replacement did not seem to improve was the work capacity. This finding was not surprising since the average age of patients in this study was 64 years. These health improvements noted postoperatively have been shown to persist for at least 5 years after surgery.[51]

Direct comparisons of the benefits of THA versus TKA have been made.[58] Ritter *et al.* used the SF-36 questionnaire to make a general health and QoL comparison of these two groups. Significant improvements in all QoL measures were noted at intervals of 6 months, 1 year, and 2 years after surgery for both groups. The data collected from patients undergoing TKA showed no significant differences in QoL measures when compared to the total hip group. The results, therefore, suggested that functional status and QoL data taken from one group could be equally applied to the other.

Additional comparisons between the patients undergoing THA and TKA data were made by Norman-Taylor *et al.*[48] Using data from the Harris Hip and the British Orthopaedic Association knee assessment scores, obtained preoperatively and 1 year postoperatively, the authors generated QoL scores from the Rosser Index Matrix. Preoperative QoL scores were noted to be significantly lower for patients awaiting TKA than THA. At 1 year after surgery, the QoL scores were high and nearly identical for both groups, suggesting that both TKA and THA are highly effective procedures. The relative gains for those patients undergoing knee replacement were significantly greater than in the total hip group, suggesting that these patients may actually have more to gain than those undergoing hip replacement.

Rissanen *et al.* performed one of the few prospective studies assessing the costs and cost-effectiveness of total hip and knee replacements.[60] Data collected from 276 THA and 176 TKA patients were assessed pre- and postoperatively using a general and health-related QoL measure (15-dimensional HRQoL and Nottingham Health Profile). Total costs (in 1991/2 dollars) were $10 500 for THA and $11 500 for TKA. Total hip arthroplasty procedures were felt to be more cost-effective and offer a greater gain in HRQoL than TKA, although the differences were not dramatic. Furthermore, the cost-effectiveness ratio for TKA patients less than 60 years old was noted to exceed that for patients greater than 60 years. This discrepancy, however, may be reflected in the gains in work potential that is not typically realized in those patients over the age of 60, the retirement group. In general, major improvements were observed to pain, sleep, and physical mobility. Those patients with the worst HRQoL preoperatively were noted to have gained most from the operation. Advanced age did not lessen the benefits of THA, but did seem to diminish that of TKA for the most elderly.

Liang *et al.* studied the cost-effectiveness of total joint arthroplasty, both of the hip and knee, for patients with the preoperative diagnosis of osteoarthritis.[14] Within 6 months of hip and knee replacement, significant improvements were seen in global health and in functional status, using the Index of Well-Being. A large effectiveness-to-cost differential was noted, confirming the high degree of cost-effectiveness of both these interventions. The highest cost-effectiveness was noted in those patients with the poorest health—those with the most to gain.

In 1994, the National Institutes of Health convened a panel of experts to review the current state of affairs in THA.[9] The consensus statement issued by the panel concluded that THA offers patients immediate and substantial improvement in pain, functional status, and overall HRQoL—results that were found to persist over the long term. The panel noted that fewer than 10% of all artificial joints are ever revised, and THA was deemed to be a highly successful treatment for pain and disability, with an excellent long-term prognosis. A similar consensus statement has yet to be issued with respect to TKA, but parallels in postoperative gains allow the extrapolation of similar conclusions from this data.

Rorabeck *et al.*[53,62] studied the cost-effectiveness and its impact on HRQoL within a group of hip arthroplasty patients, comparing patients who received a cemented prosthesis to those in whom an uncemented prosthesis was used. No significant differences were found in the two groups with respect to cost. Both groups were noted to be extremely effective in improving HRQoL. The cost-per-QALY, therefore, was also similar between the two groups. In 1988 Canadian dollars, the average cost per QALY was $27 139 during the first year and $8031 during the first 2 years. These figures confirm the high cost-effectiveness of hip replacement surgery, whether performed using cemented or uncemented prostheses.

The question of costs of related to continued nonoperative care of end-stage arthritis has been addressed in several studies.[63-66] From a societal standpoint, total joint replacement offers an opportunity to reduce the demand for community health and welfare services. Chang *et al.* performed a cost-effectiveness study to estimate the lifetime functional outcomes and costs of THA compared to nonoperative management of hip osteoarthritis.[65] Their results revealed that the cost-effectiveness ratio of THA increases with age and is higher for men than for women. Total hip arthroplasty is cost saving because of the high costs of custodial care associated with dependency due to worsening osteoarthritis. Quality-adjusted life expectancy is increased by approximately 6.9 years for a 60 year old white woman with advanced hip osteoarthritis.

Ritter *et al.* studied of the benefits of total joint arthroplasty from a different perspective.[67] These authors compared the life expectancy of patients undergoing THA to that of the general population. Using 3807 THA patients, the authors found that for the group of patients over the age of 60 there were significant differences, with those patients having undergone THA demonstrating high survival rates. This data would suggest that not only does total joint arthroplasty address the patients' physical function, but also it enhances their overall state of well-being and subsequent longevity.

As noted, the studies comparing the cost-per-outcome data for total knee replacement to that of THA show little difference between the two procedures. By inference, therefore, the data documenting the cost-effectiveness of THA can be used to corroborate similar conclusions for TKA.

## Cost-effectiveness of TKA

The extrapolation of data generated by the THA patient population provides insight into the cost-effectiveness of TKA. Ideally, studies focusing specifically on TKA are also necessary, but so far only a few studies specifically address the cost-effectiveness and QoL analysis for TKA.

Lavernia *et al.* performed the most current and thorough analysis of information regarding TKA.[68] The authors used the Quality of Well Being Index (QWBI) to calculate the cost per quality of well year in knee arthroplasty surgery. The difference in QWBI scores before and after TKA were calculated and then multiplied by the patient's life expectancy. The procedure cost was then divided by this figure, allowing a determination of the cost of a quality well year. These costs per quality well year were $30 695 at 3 months after surgery, $17 804 at 6 months, $11 560 at 1 year, and $6656 at 2 years. Health economists consider any intervention, medical or surgical, costing less than $30 000 per quality of well year to be a bargain to society. When compared to other interventions, such as coronary artery bypass surgery ($5000 per quality of well year) and renal dialysis ($50 000 per quality of well year), TKA is a cost-effective procedure and should be considered an appropriate investment by society.

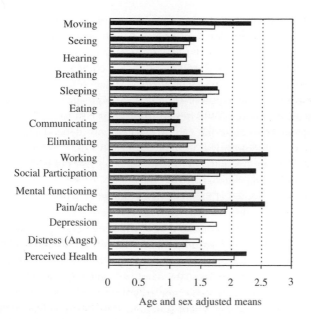

**Fig. 1.7**

Health-related quality of life (HRQoL) in pre- and postoperative total knee arthroplasty patients compared to the general population, using the 15-dimensional outcome measure. Black bars, before operation; white bars, after operation; grey bars, general population aged 64–70 years. From Rissanen et al.[58].

Kreibich et al. compared six different scoring systems in the postoperative assessment of TKA.[28] In an attempt to assess validity, reliability, and responsiveness, each system was applied to a cohort of 71 patients undergoing TKA. The highest value achieved was with the WOMAC osteoarthritis index and the Knee Society clinical rating scale. The worst scores were noted with the SF-36 and the time trade-off scores. This study elegantly addressed the question of the "ideal" outcome measure to assess total knee replacement surgery. Although each instrument offered a slightly different perspective and added elements of valuable information about the postoperative results, the results from the WOMAC and the Knee Society scales seemed to offer the most accurate measure of potential changes in a patient's clinical status, as influenced by their knee replacement.

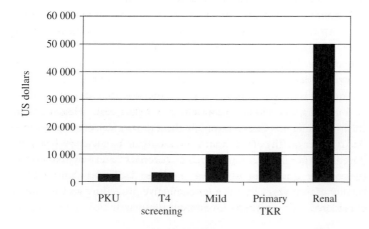

**Fig. 1.8**

Cost per quality adjusted life year for various medical interventions. PKU, phenylketonuria; TKR, total knee replacement; Renal, renal dialysis. From Lavernia et al.[61]

Drewett et al. applied several HRQoL measures to patients undergoing total knee replacement surgery.[20] A series of 26 patients were assessed using the Nottingham Health Profile for their global health status, the McGill Pain Questionnaire for pain assessment, and the Hospital Anxiety and Depression Scale for anxiety and depression. Substantial reductions were noted in pain, anxiety and depression, while a significant improvement was found in mobility. This data was used to generate a QALY figure. For knee replacement surgery, a gain of 0.42 QALY was noted. This figure was substantially lower (nearly 10-fold) than has previously been shown for hip replacement surgery. However, the authors felt that this difference was attributable not to differences in the success of the operation, but rather to the scope that QALY calculations give for allocating different QoL states to comparable patients. The authors recommended that tighter criteria are needed if QALY are to be applied to the setting of knee replacement surgery.

A moderate amount of attention has been given to the application of TKA to people aged over 75. In line with the notion that TKA addresses a non-life threatening disease, healthcare policy makers have suggested that this medical intervention be withheld because of limited cost-effectiveness in this elderly patient population. Studies by Anderson et al.[69] and Zicat et al.[70] assessed groups of patients over the age of 75 and 80, respectively, undergoing TKA. In 74 patients with 98 total knee arthroplasties, Anderson et al. noted a 90.8% improvement in self-reported pain, physical function, mental health, and satisfaction. Similarly, Zicat et al. analyzed two groups of patients undergoing TKA—those under or over 80 years of age. No significant differences were noted between the two groups with respect pain relief, functional level, strength, stability, or range of motion at 2 years' follow-up. More importantly, in an analysis of cost-effectiveness, in-hospital costs and length of stay were essentially the same for the two groups. There was a slightly greater cost-per-patient after discharge in the octogenarian group, mirroring the intensity of their co-morbidities. Both these studies concluded that TKA is a beneficial and cost-effective procedure, even in elderly patients.[55]

Attention has also been given to the influence of volume and location on the cost-effectiveness of TKA. Gutierrez et al. attempted to estimate the relationship between hospital procedure-specific volume and average hospital treatment costs.[71] They noted that the average costs associated with knee replacement surgery were inversely proportional to a hospital procedure-specific volume. Savings of up to 10% of hospital's average treatment cost were noted in the hospitals with the highest volume level. Although specific cost-savings programs were not identified, it was assumed that hospitals in which the largest number of knee replacement procedures are performed stood the most to gain from cost reduction measures. Culler et al. reviewed Medicare data regarding the location of service for patients undergoing TKA.[72] The predicted cost per case was found to be lower in rural hospitals than in urban hospitals, across all patients. No significant differences were found with respect to mortality rates or perisurgical complications between the two settings. Complication rates in the rural hospitals performing TKA correlated inversely with procedure volume—higher complication rates were noted in rural hospitals where fewer than nine total knee arthroplasties were performed annually. This data suggests that successful TKA can be delivered in both rural and urban settings, but that some rationalization of this procedure may offer the benefit of a decreased complication rate.

In 1994, Mushinski performed an analysis of charges related to knee replacement surgery.[45] In 1994 dollars, the average charge for this procedure was $28 340. Significant geographic differences were noted, with a range from 19.3% below the mean in Ohio and 27.1% above the national mean in both New York and California. Physician fees averaged $7150, and ranged from $11 930 in New York to $6290 in Colorado. Such geographic variation suggests that national standardization of fees and charges may lead to decreases in the overall costs associated with TKA surgery.

A prospective randomized study comparing the costs of operative versus nonoperative treatment of patients with severe, disabling arthritis has not so far been performed. Ethical considerations may preclude such a study. Gottlob *et al.* did, however, develop a sophisticated model to compare the cost-effectiveness of total knee replacement with nonoperative care of an elderly patient disabled with severe osteoarthritis (personal communication, HS Hirsch, 1998). Their study suggested that TKA was significantly cost-effective as measured by QALY gained for all patients, even up to the age of 85 years.

## Conclusion

Cost–benefit data have demonstrated that both total hip and total knee replacements are among the most cost-effective interventions known. Furthermore, studies have demonstrated that patients with severe osteoarthritis of the hip and knee have degrees of disability similar to those of patients who suffer from intractable angina, chronic renal failure, or metastatic malignancy. This is an important issue in the competition for healthcare dollars, because non-life-saving procedures often are not as well funded as their so-called life-saving counterparts. Well-done cost-effectiveness data will, it is hoped, force a rethinking of this approach. There are obviously many ethical ramifications of such endeavors. We would all hope that hemodialysis, coronary artery bypass, or liver transplantation would be available to us should the need arise. However, cost-to-utility data suggest that in an era of diminishing healthcare dollars, care should be taken before resources are diverted from very cost-effective procedures to those that are more expensive and less effective.

# References

1   Bartel DL, Bicknell VL, Wright TM: The effect of conformity, thickness, and material on stresses in ultra-high-molecular weight components for total joint replacement. *Journal of Bone and Joint Surgery* [Am] **68**:1041, 1986.

2   Bayley JC, Scott RD, Ewald FC, Holmes GB Jr: Failure of the metal-backed patellar component after total knee replacement. *Journal of Bone and Joint Surgery* [Am] **70**:668, 1988.

3   Bloebaum RD, Nelson K, Dorr LD *et al.*: Investigation of early surface delamination observed in retrieved heat pressed tibial inserts. *Clinical Orthopedics* **269**:120, 1991.

4   Gordon M, Bullough PG: Synovial and osseous inflammation in failed silicone-rubber prostheses. *Journal of Bone and Joint Surgery* [Am] **64**:574, 1982.

5   Hungerford DS, Kenna RV, Krackow K: The porous coated anatomic total knee. *Orthopedic Clinics of North America* **13**:103, 1982.

6   Laupacis A, Bourne RB, Rorabeck CH *et al.*: Costs of elective total hip arthroplasty during the first year. Cemented versus noncemented. *Journal of Arthroplasty* **9**:481, 1994.

7   Rorabeck CH, Bourne RB, Laupacis A *et al.*: A double-blind study of 250 cases comparing cemented with cementless total hip arthroplasty. Cost-effectiveness and its impact on health-related quality of life. *Clinical Orthopedics* **298**:156, 1994.

8   Blunn GW, Walker PS, Joshi A, and Hardinge K: The dominance of cyclic sliding in producing wear in total knee replacements. *Clinical Orthopedics* **273**:253, 1991.

9   NIH Consensus Statement: Total Hip Replacement, 1994.

10  Harris W, Sledge CB: Total hip and total knee replacement (first of two parts). *New England Journal of Medicine* **323**:725, 1990.

11  Harris WH, Sledge CB: Total hip and total knee replacement (second of two parts). *New England Journal of Medicine* **323**:801, 1990.

12  Hirsch HS: Total joint replacement: a cost effective procedure for the 1990's. *Medicine and Health, Rhode Island* **81**:162, 1998.

13  Callahan CM, Drake BG, Heck DA, Dittus RS: Patient outcomes following tricompartmental total knee replacement. A meta-analysis. *JAMA* **271**:1349, 1994.

14  Liang MH, Cullen KE, Larson MG *et al.*: Cost-effectiveness of total joint arthroplasty in osteoarthritis. *Arthritis and Rheumatism* **29**:937, 1986.

15  Bourne RB: The cost effectiveness of total knee arthroplasty. In *Current concepts in primary and revision total knee arthroplasty*, ed. JN Insall, WN Scott, GR Scuderi, p. 269. Lippincott-Raven, Philadelphia, 1996.

16  Drake BG, Callahan CM, Dittus RS, Wright JG: Global rating systems used in assessing knee arthroplasty outcomes. *Journal of Arthroplasty* **9**:409, 1994.

17  Rorabeck CH, Murray P: Cost effectiveness of revision total knee replacement. *Instructional Course Lectures* **46**:237, 1997.

18  Bennett KJ, Torrance GW, Moran LA *et al.*: Health state utilities in knee replacement surgery: the development and evaluation of McKnee. *Journal of Rheumatology* **24**:1796, 1997.

19  Bergner M, Bobbitt RA, Carter WB, Gilson BS: The sickness impact profile: Development and final revision of a health status measure. *Medical Care* **19**:787, 1981.

20  Drewett RF, Minns RJ, Sibly TF: Measuring outcome of total knee replacement using quality of life indices. *Annals of the Royal College of Surgeons of England* **74**:286, 1992.

21  Guyatt GH, Feeny DH, Patrick DL: Measuring health-related quality
    of life. *Annals of Internal Medicine* **118**:622, 1993.
22  Hilding MB, Backbro B, Ryd L: Quality of life after knee arthroplasty.
    A randomized study of 3 designs in 42 patients, compared after 4
    years. *Acta Orthopaedica Scandinavica* **68**:156, 1997.
23  Hornberger JC, Redelmeier DA, Peterson J: Variability among methods
    to assess patients' well-being and consequent effect on a cost-
    effectiveness analysis. *Journal of Clinical Epidemiology* **45**:505, 1992.
24  Kaplan RM and Bush JW: Health-related quality of life measurement
    for evaluation research and policy analysis. *Health Psychology* **1**:61,
    1982.
25  March LM and Bachmeier CJ: Economics of osteoarthritis: a global
    perspective. *Baillière's Clinical Rheumatology* **11**:817, 1997.
26  Meding JB, Keating EM, Faris PM, Ritter MA: Maximizing cost-
    effectiveness while minimizing complications in total hip
    replacement. *American Journal of Orthopedics* **27**:295, 1998.
27  Bellamy N, Buchanan WW, Goldsmith CH *et al.*: Validation study of the
    WOMAC: A health status instrument for measuring clinically
    important patient relevant outcomes to antirheumatic drug therapy
    in patients with osteoarthritis of the hip or knee. *Journal of
    Rheumatology* **15**:1833, 1988.
28  Kreibich DN, Vaz M, Bourne RB *et al.*: What is the best way of
    assessing outcome after total knee replacement. *Clinical Orthopedics*
    **331**:221, 1996.
29  Gill TM, Feinstein AR: A critical appraisal of the quality of quality-of-
    life measurements. *JAMA* **272**:619, 1994.
30  Torrance GW: Utility approach to measuring health-related quality of
    life. *Journal of Chronic Diseases* **40**:593, 1987.
31  Siegel JE, Weinstein MC, Russell LB, Gold MR: Recommendations for
    reporting cost-effectiveness analyses. Panel on cost-effectiveness in
    health and medicine. *JAMA* **276**:1339, 1996.
32  Laupacis A, Feeny D, Detsky AS, Tugwell PX: How attractive does a
    new technology have to be to warrant adoption and utilization?
    Tentative guidelines for using clinical and economic evaluation.
    *Canadian Medical Association Journal* **146**:473, 1992.
33  Evans RW, Manninen DL, and Maier A: The quality of life of kidney and
    heart transplant recipients. *Transplantation Proceedings* **17**:1579, 1985.
34  Ayers DC, Berman AT, Duncan CP *et al.*: Economic aspects of total
    joint replacement: AAOS Committee on Hip and Knee Arthritis.
    AAOS Meeting, Anaheim 1999.
35  Barber TC, Healy WL: The hospital cost of total hip arthroplasty: a
    comparison between 1981 and 1990. *Journal of Bone and Joint
    Surgery* [Am] **75**:321, 1993.
36  Healy WL: Economic considerations in total hip arthroplasty and
    implant standardization. *Clinical Orthopedics* **311**:102, 1995.
37  Healy WL, Finn D: The hospital cost and the cost of the implant for
    total knee arthroplasty. *Journal of Bone and Joint Surgery* [Am]
    **76**:801, 1994.
38  Healy WL, Iorio R, Richards JA: Opportunities for control of hospital
    cost for total knee arthroplasty. *Clinical Orthopedics* **345**:140, 1997.
39  Healy WL, Iorio R, Richards JA, Lucchesi C: Opportunities for control
    of hospital costs for total joint arthroplasty after initial cost
    containment. *Journal of Arthroplasty* **13**:504, 1998.
40  Iorio R, Healy WL, Kirven FM, Patch DA, Pfeifer BA: Knee implant
    standardarization: an implant selection and cost reduction program.
    *American Journal of Knee Surgery* **11**:73, 1998.

41  Iorio R, Healy WL, Richards JA: Comparison of the hospital cost of primary and revision total knee arthroplasty after cost containment. *Orthopedics* **22**:195, 1999.

42  Laupacis A, Keown P, Pus N *et al.*: A study of the quality of life and cost-utility of renal transplantation. *Kidney International* **50**:235, 1996.

43  Merle d'Aubigne R, Postel M: Functional results of hip arthroplasty with acrylic prosthesis. *Journal of Bone and Joint Surgery* [Am] **36**:451, 1954.

44  Meyers SJ, Reuben JD, Cox DD, Watson M: Inpatient cost of primary total joint arthroplasty. *Journal of Arthroplasty* **11**:281, 1996.

45  Moskal JT, Diduch DR: Postoperative radiographs after total knee arthroplasty: a cost-containment strategy. *American Journal of Knee Surgery* **11**:89, 1998.

46  Rorabeck CH, Murray P: The cost benefit of total knee arthroplasty. *Orthopedics* **19**:777, 1996.

47  McGuigan FX, Hozack WJ, Moriarty L *et al.*: Predicting quality-of-life outcomes following total joint arthroplasty. Limitations of the SF-36 health status questionnaire. *Journal of Arthroplasty* **10**:742, 1995.

48  Norman-Taylor FH, Palmer CR, Villar RN: Quality-of-life improvement compared after hip and knee replacement. *Journal of Bone and Joint Surgery* [Br] **78**:74, 1996.

49  Killeen K, Bert J. Does early hospital discharge versus early transfer to a transitional care unit or nursing home result in a decrease in the total direct cost of total joint arthroplasty? 244, AAOS, Orlando 1995.

50  Borstlap M, Zant JL, Van Soesbergen M, Van der Korst JK: Effects of total hip replacement on quality of life in patients with osteoarthritis and in patients with rheumatoid arthritis. *Clinical Rheumatology* **13**:45, 1994.

51  Rissanen P, Aro S, Sintonen H *et al.*: Costs and cost-effectiveness in hip and knee replacements. A prospective study. *International Journal of Technology Assessment in Health Care* **13**:575, 1997.

52  Rissanen P, Aro S, Sintonen H *et al.* Quality of life and functional ability in hip and knee replacements: a prospective study. *Quality of Life Research* **5**:56, 1996.

53  Ritter MA, Albohm MJ, Keating EM *et al.*: Life expectancy after total hip arthroplasty. *Journal of Arthroplasty* **13**:874, 1998.

54  Torrance GW, Feeny D: Utilities and quality-adjusted life years. *International Journal of Technology Assessment in Health Care* **5**:559, 1989.

55  Wiklund I, Romanus B: A comparison of quality of life before and after arthroplasty in patients who had arthrosis of the hip joint. *Journal of Bone and Joint Surgery* [Am] **73**:765, 1991.

56  Wilcock GK: Benefits of total hip replacement to older patients and the community. *BMJ* **2**:37, 1978.

57  Laskin RS: Total knee replacement in patients older than 85. *Clinical Orthopedics*, **367**:43–9, 1999.

58  Rissanen P, Aro S, Slatis P *et al.*: Health and quality of life before and after hip or knee arthroplasty. *Journal of Arthroplasty* **10**:169, 1995.

59  Mushinski M: Average charges for a total knee replacement: United States 1994. *Statistical Bulletin/Metropolitan Insurance Companies* **77**:24, 1996.

60  Rissanen P, Aro S, Paavolainen P: Hospital- and patient-related characteristics determining length of hospital stay for hip and knee replacements. *International Journal of Technology Assessment in Health Care* **12**:325, 1996.

61 Lavernia CJ, Guzman JF, Gachupin-Garcia A: Cost effectiveness and quality of life in knee arthroplasty. *Clinical Orthopedics* **345**:134, 1997.

62 Laupacis A, Bourne RB, Rorabeck CH *et al.*: The effect of elective total hip replacement on health-related quality of life. *Journal of Bone and Joint Surgery* [Am] **75**:1619, 1993.

63 Boettcher W: Total hip arthroplasties in the elderly: morbidity, mortality, and cost-effectiveness. *Clinical Orthopedics* **274**:30, 1992.

64 Bourne RB and Kim PR: Cost effectiveness of total hip arthroplasty. In *The adult hip.* ed. JJ Callaghan, AG Rosenberg, HE Rubash, p. 839. Lippincott-Raven, Philadelphia, 1998.

65 Chang RW, Pellisier JM, Hazen GB: A cost-effectiveness analysis of total hip arthroplasty for osteoarthritis of the hip. *JAMA* **275**:858, 1996.

66 Hughes SL, Dunlop D, Edelman P *et al.*: Impact of joint impairment on longitudinal disability in elderly persons. *Journal of Gerontology* **49**:S291, 1994.

67 Ritter MA, Albohm MJ, Keating EM *et al.*: Comparitive outcomes of total joint arthroplasty. *Journal of Arthroplasty* **10**:737, 1995.

68 Lavernia CJ, Drakeford MK, Tsao AK *et al.*: Revision and primary hip and knee arthroplasty. A cost analysis. *Clinical Orthopedics* **311**:136, 1995.

69 Anderson JG, Wixson RL, Tsai D *et al.*: Functional outcome and patient satisfaction in total knee patients over the age of 75. *Journal of Arthroplasty* **11**:831, 1996.

70 Zicat B, Rorabeck CH, Bourne RB *et al.*: Total knee arthroplasty in the octogenarian. *Journal of Arthroplasty* **8**:395, 1993.

71 Gutierrez B, Culler SD, Freund DA: Does hospital procedure-specific volume affect treatment costs? A national study of knee replacement surgery. *Health Services Research* **33**:489, 1998.

72 Culler SD, Holmes AM, Gutierrez B: Expected hospital costs of knee replacement for rural residents by location of service. *Medical Care* **33**:1188, 1995.

73 Gottlob C, Pellissier J, Wixson RL. The long-term cost-effectiveness of total knee arthroplasty for the treatment of osteoarthritis. Hirsch HS. 1998. Personal Communication.

# 2

*The initial tibial components used in total knee replacement were nonmodular and made either entirely of polyethyelene or of polyethylene molded directly on to a metal base. In the late 1980s designers began to fabricate tibial components with a metal baseplate into which a modular polyethylene bearing surface could be inserted. The use of such a modular system was purported to increase the facility with which the surgeon could perform the knee replacement, and to decrease the inventory of components in the operating room. Is modularity really helpful, however, or should we consider returning to one-piece tibial components?*

# The tibial component should routinely be modular and metal-backed rather than all polyethylene

## Pro: Jan Victor

In the process of its development over the past 30 years, total knee arthroplasty (TKA) has experienced its share of problems and inherent flaws. The advent of metal backing was a step in the perpetual attempt to improve the performance of the operation in terms of functional predictability and survival of the implant. It was noticed that tibial components acted as surface replacements and, as such, transferred loads directly to the underlying trabecular bone. Failure of this underlying bone under excessive stress was suspected to be the prime mover in loosening of the tibial component. Implant designers looked at a method of improving load transfer across the proximal tibia. Metal backing was added to the tibial component of several knee prostheses in the early 1980s, on the basis of finite-element analysis[1] and *in vitro* biomechanical studies.[2-4] This was not a new idea, as metal backing of polyethylene already had a history of use in hip prostheses. Clinically, the metal-backed design proved to have a better long-term outcome in survivorship analysis for a posterior stabilized prosthetic design.[5,6]

Three more opportunities boosted the interest for metal-backed tibial implants: the introduction of cementless fixation, the popularization of mobile bearing designs, and modularity. The option of adding modular extensions to the system was attractive as this satisfied the need for more versatile and comprehensive total knee systems. It was now possible to add wedges, blocks, and extension stems and use different levels of constraint within a single total knee system.

The scope of this contribution is to highlight the advantages of this approach. Unfortunately, the evolution that led to reliable modular metal-backed systems was not devoid of poor engineering and misconceptions. In order to make a clear judgement, these errors demand further analysis.

## Metal backing

A scientifically sound argument to justify the use of metal backing as an improvement in the survival of the prosthesis can only be provided by a long-term prospective study comparing an identical prosthetic device with and without metal backing. To our knowledge, such a study is not available at present. Comparison of results from different total knee designs to analyze the value of metal backing should be approached with great care. Most of the early full polyethylene tibial components were thick and highly conforming, in contrast to many of the early metal-backed tibial components. However, long-term follow-up on identical systems with and without metal backing is available for the Total Condylar prosthesis, the Insall–Burstein posterior stabilized prosthesis and the Anatomical Graduated Components (AGC) knee.

Survivorship of the original posterior stabilized prosthesis with an all-polyethylene tibial component was reported as 94% at 12 years (annual failure rate 0.4%).[7] Another analysis on 1430 cemented primary posterior stabilized total knee arthroplasties operated in the same institution yielded no aseptic loosening of the tibial component in the subgroup of 917 knees with a metal-backed tibial component.[6] This trend was confirmed in a later survivorship analysis. The prosthesis with an all-polyethylene tibia had an average annual rate of failure of 0.38% and a 16 year success rate of 94.10% versus an annual rate of failure of 0.14% and a 14 year success rate of 98.10% for the metal-backed version.[8] Nafei et al.[9] reported a cumulative survival rate of 92.3% at 12 years with the same prosthesis including an all-polyethylene tibial component.

Apel et al.[10] compared the results of the total condylar prosthesis with and without metal backing. They compared nonrandomized but matched groups of 131 knees with an all-polyethylene component and 69 knees with a metal-backed component. They reported no difference in clinical and roentgenographic assessment at an average follow-up of 6.5 years.

A third design that is available for longer-term follow-up in both a metal-backed and all-polyethylene version is the AGC knee. Ritter et al. reported on a multi-center follow-up of 2001 metal-backed AGC knees. A subgroup of 71 knees had a minimum follow-up of 10 years. Only 5 tibial failures were noted.[11] A later report with an average follow-up of 4.19 years on 538 knees on the same prosthesis with an all-polyethylene tibial component showed clearly different figures: in this group 50 tibial component revisions are reported, and in addition 45 knees display medial tibial plateau collapse and 155 knees have a medial plateau radiolucency of 1 mm or more. The authors conclude that the "failure rates for the flat all-polyethylene tibial component are exceedingly high."[12]

## Modularity

The clinical rationale for the use of a metal-backed modular system includes bone loss (on tibia, femur, or patella), deficient bone quality, and instability. Other indications include fractures or simultaneous osteotomies. Some of these technical challenges can be addressed by using custom-made devices. As compared to these custom-made knees, modular systems have the advantage of offering better intra-operative flexibility, size interchangeability between tibial insert and femoral component, and instant availability of all needed equipment. Other advantages include the option of standard instrumentation systems and a lower overall cost. Disadvantages to the use of a modular system include possible intraoperative mistakes, and fretting, corrosion, or breakage at the connecting metal interfaces. It is also clear that a comprehensive modular system will generate a large inventory.

Bone defects are frequently encountered in TKA, in both primary and revision procedures.[13] In primary total knee replacement, bone defects are most often seen in patients with angular deformities, rheumatoid arthritis, or hemophilic arthropathy. The optimum way to deal with these bone defects remains a matter of controversy. The available options include a deeper proximal tibial resection, shifting the component away from the defect, the use of methylmethacry-late—either plain[14-17] or reinforced with screws,[18] the use of bone autografts or allografts, modular metal wedges or blocks,[19-21] and custom-made devices.

The use of modular wedges or blocks attached to the tibial component is a well-established way of dealing with moderate to large bone defects, especially if they are noncontained (Fig. 2.1). These

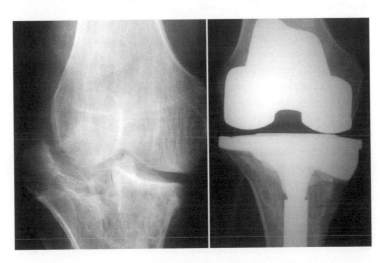

**Fig. 2.1**

Arthritic knee with sever varus deformity and instability, treated with a posterior stabilized TKA, including a modular wedge and stem extension.

metal augments are available in different sizes and shapes and can easily be assembled intraoperatively. Likewise, the construct can be further stabilized by using stems that are fixed to the tibial trays. There is biomechanical evidence that these constructs optimize stress distribution and provide sufficient resistance to the loads that are transmitted to the proximal tibia. In an *in vitro* study Brooks et al.[22] measured the tray-bone deflections that occur on loading the tibial tray in the presence of a wedge-shaped defect that was filled in. The highest tray-bone deflections were recorded when the defect was filled in with cement only. Stiffness improved after the cement was reinforced with screws. The best results were obtained with metal wedges and custom-made devices. A central stem 70 mm long carried 23–38% of the axial load and was considered useful when the proximal bone was deficient. As far as the shape of the metal augments is concerned, there seems to be no significant difference in the maximum strains that are generated across the bone–prosthesis construct. Either blocks or wedges can be used, and the choice can be guided by the geometry of the defect.[21]

The clinical outcome of bone grafts is unpredictable for larger peripheral defects. Problems, in the form of fragmentation of the graft and subsidence of the tibial component, have been reported.[19,23,24] Laskin reported an overall success rate of only 67%, 5 years after grafting tibial defects with bone removed from the posterior femur.[24]

It has been shown in clinical follow-up studies that the use of cement alone is not feasible for the management of larger defects.[14–16]

Initial good clinical results with modular augments have been reported, although frequently noted radiolucent lines cautioned against undue optimism.[19,20] A later follow-up at 5 years[13] confirmed radiolucent lines at the cement–bone interface beneath the metal wedge in 13 out of 28 knees. None of these lines proved to be progressive. The authors concluded that "No deterioration of the wedge–prosthesis or wedge–cement–bone interface was seen at mid-term follow-up." Several studies report on the outcome of modular systems with the use of a metal-backed tibial tray in revision TKA. In a series of 76 revisions using a modular system with press-fit stems, 84% good or excellent results were achieved at 3 years.[25] In a review of 41 revision TKAs using a modular system, Rand[26] reported good or excellent results in 98% of the cases at 3 years. No complications relating to the modular system were reported. Similar results were reported in a study of 39 revision TKAs using a modular system at mean follow-up of 20 months. Nonprogressive radiolucent lines were seen in 72% of the knees.[27]

## Technical issues

The use of a metal-backed modular tibial component offers distinct technical benefits for the surgical procedure.

- First, the surgeon is allowed to fix the tibial tray, either cemented or cementless, without having to make the final decision on the thickness of the polyethylene insert. The insert can eventually be chosen after a final trial with all components fixed. This feature might not be necessary for all uncomplicated primary TKAs, but it can be of value in knees with significant bone loss where correct evaluation of the flexion and extension gap tension can only accurately be determined after fixation of the femoral and tibial component.[28]

- A second surgical bonus is the removal of excessive cement posterior to the tibial component after application of the cement and insertion of the tibial tray, hence reducing the chance of three-body wear.[29] This removal of cement is technically more demanding when an all-polyethylene component is used as the "full thickness" of the device is already in place, blocking access to the posterior part of the knee. Again, this might not concern all primary knees, but for the patient with a tight knee joint it is an undeniable advantage.

Having stated this, one has to recognize a potential hazard. During the manipulation of the knee in the process of removing trial inserts and introducing final inserts one has to be very careful in avoiding contact between the metal tibial tray and the femoral component. Scratches on the femoral bearing surface have to be avoided by all means, as they have an ominous effect on the development of polyethylene wear.[30]

When modular tibial components were first introduced it was perceived that the system would allow for exchange of the modular polyethylene insert, without removal of the components, in case of progressing polyethylene wear. Few reports on this technique are found in the literature.[28,31] Bert et al.[28] gathered data from five different institutions in North America. Out of 62 revision cases, exchange of the insert without revising the tibial or femoral component was performed in 7 knees only, the reason being "significant scoring, burnishing or damage to the tibial component." It should be stressed, however, that the implants that were revised had a tibial component thickness of 6–7 mm in 80% of the cases, which explains the accelerated failure rate, and metal-to-metal contact at the time of revision. To take advantage of the exchange of the insert, the thinning of the polyethylene has to be recognized early on. As there is no clinical follow-up of any significant length on this technique it should be looked at critically and used with great caution.

## Caution: backside wear and stiffness

A particular concern with metal-backed tibial trays is increased polyethylene wear. This may be due to decreased polyethylene thickness, stiffer polyethylene, and backside wear.

Polyethylene wear limits the lifespan of the prosthetic device by its mechanical, clinical and biological consequences. The biological response to loose foreign particles outweighs the mechanical problems in most cases. However, progressive thinning of the polyethylene can finally lead to metal-on-metal contact in metal backed tibial trays, thereby further enhancing the release of small particles that are phagocytosed in large amounts and contribute to massive osteolysis, the so-called mode-2 wear,[32] defined as a primary bearing surface moving against a secondary surface that it is not intended to move against.[29] Such reports are numerous for certain designs of metal-backed tibial trays.[33-38] Engh et al.[32] observed severe wear in 51% of metal-backed tibial components representing 16 different implant designs after an average of 39 months in situ. In another study Bugbee et al.[31] report on 186 consecutive modular knees, followed for 4–6 years. Seven patients were revised for polyethylene wear (5) and tibial osteolysis (2). Interestingly the revisions were carried out by exchange of the failed polyethylene insert alone.

Another type of wear that can occur with metal-backed tibial trays is the so-called mode-4 wear, characterized by two secondary surfaces rubbing together.[29] This type of wear is mostly abrasive. The undersurface of the polyethylene rubs against the metal tray as micromotion occurs under loading conditions.[31,39,40]

In contrast to mode-1 wear, which occurs between two primary bearing surfaces of the prosthesis and is inherent to its function, mode-2 and mode-4 wear are characteristic of the construction of the modular metal-backed tibial tray. They can completely be avoided by the use of an all-polyethylene tibial component. It is clear that, in order to take advantage of the positive features of the metal backing, it is of utmost importance to avoid additional wear. This can only be achieved if certain criteria are fulfilled:

- The minimum thickness of the polyethylene should be respected. This eliminates the problem of increased mode-1 wear because of excessive polyethylene stiffness and protects against wear-through over time. It is generally accepted that the minimum thickness for polyethylene in total knee arthroplasty is 6–8 mm.[33,34,37,41,42] Given the knowledge that most metal trays have a thickness of 2.5–3 mm, a minimum thickness for the metal-polyethylene unit of 9.5–10 mm is recommended. Unfortunately, many manufacturers have sinned against this prerequisite,[33] mostly for marketing reasons.

- One has to realize, however, that metal backing takes space and that sufficient bone has to be removed from the proximal tibia to accommodate the metal–polyethylene construct. Sufficient resection of the proximal tibia should not concern the surgeon as the strength of the proximal tibia remains fairly constant in the area of 4–10 mm below the articular surface.[43] Only the sub-chondral plate displays a higher strength but this amount of bone has always to be removed, even if extremely thin tibial components were to be used.

- The polyethylene should be rigidly fixed on the metal tray to reduce micromotion between the tray and the insert. The tray should be polished and flat as any irregularities may act as a rasp if micromotion occurs.[31] Screw holes should be avoided because polyethylene will enter the hole as a result of cold flow and can be damaged when micromotion occurs.[37,44]

## Conclusion

Metal backing of the tibial component improves the stress distribution across the proximal tibia, as proven in biomechanical studies and clinical investigation. It allows for intraoperative flexibility if modular attachments are provided. Modularity offers distinct technical advantages during surgery. Two specific characteristics call for special attention: sufficient polyethylene thickness (minimum 7 mm) and rigid fixation of the polyethylene on a flat and polished tray are mandatory to avoid the mistakes of the past.

# References

1    Bartel DL, Burstein AH, Santavicca EA, Insall JN: Performance of the tibial component in total knee replacement—conventional and revision designs. *Journal of Bone and Joint Surgery* [Am] **64**:1026–1033, 1982.

2    Askew MJ, Lewis JL, Jaycox D *et al.*: Interface stresses in a prosthesis-tibia structure with varying bone properties. *Transactions of the Orthopaedic Research Society* **3**:17–21, 1978.

3    Walker PS, Greene D, Reilly D *et al.*: Fixation of tibial components of knee prostheses. *Journal of Bone and Joint Surgery* [Am] **63**:258–267, 1981.

4    Murase K, Crowninshield RD, Pedersen DR, Chang TS: An analysis of tibial component design in total knee arthroplasty. *Journal of Biomechanics* **16**:13–22, 1983.

5    Scuderi GR, Insall JN, Windsor RE, Moran MC: Survivorship of cemented knee replacement. *Journal of Bone and Joint Surgery* [Br] **71**:798–803, 1989.

6    Windsor RE, Scuderi GR, Moran MC, Insall JN: Mechanisms of failure of the femoral and tibial components in total knee arthroplasty. *Clinical Orthopaedics and Related Research* **248**:15–20, 1989.

7    Stern SH, Insall JN: Total knee arthroplasty with posterior cruciate ligament substitution designs. In *Surgery of the Knee*, ed. JN Insall, p. 861. Churchill Livingstone, New York, 1993.

8    Font-Rodriguez DE, Scuderi GR, Insall JN: Survivorship of cemented total knee arthroplasty. *Clinical Orthopaedics and Related Research* **345**:79–86, 1997.

9    Nafei A, Kristensen O, Knudsen HM *et al.*: Survivorship analysis of cemented total condylar knee arthroplasty. *Journal of Arthroplasty* **11**:7–10, 1996.

10   Apel DM, Tozzi JM, Dorr LD: Clinical comparison of all-polyethylene and metal backed tibial components in total knee arthroplasty. *Clinical Orthopaedics and Related Research* **273**:243–52, 1991.

11  Ritter MA, Worland R, Saliski J *et al.*: Flat-on-flat, nonconstrained, compression molded polyethylene total knee replacement. *Clinical Orthopaedics and Related Research* **321**:79–85, 1995.

12  Faris PM, Ritter MA, Keating EM, Meding JB: Mid term follow-up of all-poly tibial component in flat-on-flat design. *Journal of Arthroplasty* **14**:245, 1999.

13  Pagano MW, Trousdale RT, Rand JA: Tibial wedge augmentation for bone deficiency in total knee arthroplasty. *Clinical Orthopaedics and Related Research* **321**:151–155, 1995.

14  Insall JN, Lachiewicz PF, Burstein AH: The posterior stabilised condylar prosthesis: A modification of the total condylar design. Two to four year clinical experience. *Journal of Bone and Joint Surgery* [Am] **64**:1317–1323, 1982.

15  Ewald FC, Jacobs MA, Miegel RE *et al.*: Kinematic total knee replacement. *Journal of Bone and Joint Surgery* [Am] **66**:1032–40, 1984.

16  Cornell CN, Ranawat CS, Burstein AH: A clinical and radiographic analysis of loosening of total knee arthroplasty using a bilateral model. *Journal of Arthroplasty* **1**:157–163, 1986.

17  Lotke PA, Wong RY, Ecker ML: The use of methylmethacrylate in primary total knee replacements with large tibial defects. *Clinical Orthopaedics and Related Research* **270**:288–294, 1991.

18  Ritter MA: Screw and cement fixation of large defects in total knee arthroplasty. *Journal of Arthroplasty* **1**:125–129, 1986.

19  Brand MG, Daley RJ, Ewald FC, Scott RD: Tibial tray augmentation with modular metal wedges for tibial bone stock deficiency. *Clinical Orthopaedics and Related Research* **248**:71–79, 1989.

20  Rand JA: Bone deficiency in total knee arthroplasty: use of metal wedge augmentation. *Clinical Orthopaedics and Related Research* **271**:63–71, 1991.

21  Fehring TK, Peindl RD, Humble RS *et al.*: Modular tibial augmentations in total knee arthroplasty. *Clinical Orthopaedics and Related Research* **327**:207–217, 1996.

22  Brooks PJ, Walker PS, Scott RD: Tibial component fixation in deficient tibial bone stock. *Clinical Orthopaedics and Related Research* **184**:302–309, 1984.

23  Rand JA: Modular augments in revision total knee arthroplasty. *Orthopedic Clinics of North America* **29**:347–353, 1998.

24  Laskin RS: Total knee arthroplasty in the presence of large bony defects of the tibia and marked knee instability. *Clinical Orthopaedics and Related Research* **248**:66–70, 1989.

25  Haas S, Insall JN, Montgomery W. *et al.*: Modular tibial augmentations in total knee arthroplasty with use of modular components with stems inserted without cement. *Journal of Bone and Joint Surgery* [Am] 77, 1700–1707, 1995.

26  Rand JA: Modularity in total knee arthroplasty. *Acta Orthopaedica Belgica* **62**:180–185, 1996.

27  Takahashi I Gustilo R: Nonconstrained implants in revision total knee arthroplasty. *Clinical Orthopaedics and Related Research* **309**:156–162, 1994.

28  Bert JM, Reuben J, Kelly F *et al.*: The incidence of modular tibial polyethylene insert exchange in total knee arthroplasty when polyethylene failure occurs. *Journal of Arthroplasty* **13**:609–614, 1998.

29  Schmalzried TP, Callaghan JJ: Wear in total hip and knee replacements. *Journal of Bone and Joint Surgery* [Am] **81**:115–113, 1999.

30  Gabriel SM, Dennis DA, Honey MJ, Scott RD: Polyethylene wear on the distal tibial insert surface in total knee arthroplasty. *The Knee* **5**:221–228, 1998.

31 Bugbee WD, Ammeen DJ, Parks NL, Engh GA: 4- to 10-Year results with the anatomic modular total knee. *Clinical Orthopaedics and Related Research* **348**:158–165, 1998.

31 Parks NL, Engh GA, Topoleski LDT, Emperado JBS: Modular tibial insert micromotion. . *Clinical Orthopaedics and Related Research* **356**:10–15, 1998.

32 Engh GA, Dwyer KA, Hanes CK: Polyethylene wear of metal backed tibial components in total and unicompartmental knee prostheses. *Journal of Bone and Joint Surgery* [Br] **74**:9–17, 1992.

33 Chillag KJ, Barth E: An analysis of polyethylene thickness in modular total knee components. *Clinical Orthopaedics and Related Research* **273**:261–63, 1991.

34 Collier JP, Mayor MB, McNamara JL *et al.*: Analysis of the failure of 122 polyethylene inserts from uncemented tibial knee components. *Clinical Orthopaedics and Related Research* **273**:232–242, 1991.

35 Jones SMG, Pinder IM, Moran CG, Malcolm AJ: Polyethylene wear in uncemented knee replacements. *Journal of Bone and Joint Surgery* [Br] **74**:18–22, 1992.

36 Kim YH, Oh JH, Oh SH: Osteolysis around cementless porous-coated anatomic knee prostheses. *Journal of Bone and Joint Surgery* [Am] **77**:236–241, 1995.

37 Kilgus DJ, Moreland JR, Finerman GA *et al.*: Catastrophic wear of tibial polyethylene inserts. *Clinical Orthopaedics and Related Research* **273**:223–231, 1991.

38 Tsao A, Mintz L, McRae CR *et al.*: Failure of the porous-coated anatomic prosthesis in total knee arthroplasty due to severe polyethylene wear. *Journal of Bone and Joint Surgery* [Am] **75**:19–26, 1993.

39 Fisher J, Firkins P, Reeves EA *et al.*: The influence of scratches to metallic counterfaces on the wear of ultra-high molecular weight polyethylene. *Proceedings of the Institution of Mechanical Engineers. Part H, Journal of Engineering in Medicine* **209**:263–264, 1995.

40 Wasielewski RC, Parks NN, Williams I *et al.*: The tibial undersurface as a contributing source of polyethylene wear debris. *Clinical Orthopaedics and Related Research* **345**:53–59, 1997.

41 Bartel DL, Bicknell VL, Ithaca MS, Wright TM: The effect of conformity, thickness and material on stresses in ultra-high molecular weight components for total joint replacement. *Journal of Bone and Joint Surgery* [Am] **68**:1041–51, 1986.

42 Wright TM, Bartel DL: The problem of surface damage in polyethylene total knee components. *Clinical Orthopaedics and Related Research* **205**:67–74, 1986.

43 Dequeker J, Mokassa L, Aerssens J, Boonen S: Bone density and local growth factors in generalized osteoarthritis. *Microscopic Research Techniques* **37**:358–371, 1997.

44 Lewis PL, Rorabeck CH, Bourne RB: Screw osteolysis after cementless total knee replacement. *Clinical Orthopaedics and Related Research* **321**:173–177, 1995.

## Con: Brian Crites and Merrill Ritter

There are many factors that influence polyethylene wear in total knee replacements. This chapter addresses only one—implant design. Many total knee designs are modular. This modularity can come in two forms:

- In some designs a modular polyethylene liner is inserted on to a metal tibial tray.
- Some tibial component designs have modular metal parts in which the post or fin is separate from the tray portion and requires assembly before insertion. This form of modularity is most common with implants designed for revisions, but is available in some primary implants also.

The advantages and disadvantages of modularity are discussed below. It must be understood that all current implant designs wear over time and thus produce wear debris. It is up to the surgeon to choose a design that produces the least amount of wear and thus offers the best chance for good, long-term function.

## Osteolysis

Total knee replacement utilizing modern techniques and systems has led to very good clinical results (Ritter unpublished data 1999).[1] so many more patients now request or seek total knee replacements at earlier ages than in the past. As the average age decreases, the useful lifetime of a knee replacement becomes more important. Recently, osteolysis has been recognized as a major factor in loosening of cemented and uncemented total knee replacements.[2-13] Figure 2.2

**Fig. 2.2**

Loose total knees with osteolysis.

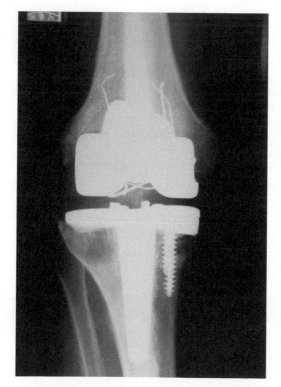

a

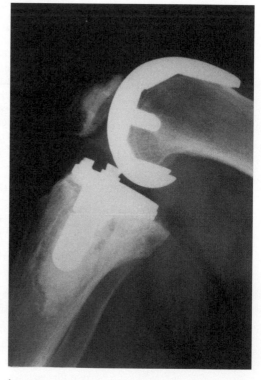

b

demonstrates two cases that show loosening and osteolysis. Both knees were painful and underwent revision.

Osteolysis was first recognized in total hip arthroplasties. It has since been shown that osteolysis is secondary to wear debris; specifically, polyethylene particles generated from wear.[2,14,15] The polyethylene particles have been shown to induce bone resorption through a macrophage-mediated mechanism.[2,10,17–19] It is also known that the size of the particles is important in whether or not they induce an osteolytic response.[20] The size range of biologically active wear debris particles appears to be 0.2–7 μm.[21] This becomes relevant when one considers the difference in polyethylene wear characteristics in total knee replacements compared to total hip replacements. Polyethylene wear in total knees commonly results in articular surface delamination and the production of larger, less biologically active, particles.[22] In a study comparing the sizes of polyethylene particles generated in total knees compared to total hips, it was found that larger and biologically inactive particles were more common in total knees.[23] However, this study also demonstrated that the majority of the polyethylene particles found in knees were in the submicron size range. Thus, the production of the smaller, biologically active polyethylene wear debris is an important consideration in total knee replacement.

## Aspects of tibial modularity

There are advantages to tibial modularity. Modularity enables the surgeon to achieve optimal fit intraoperatively, minimizes device inventory, and allows for polyethylene exchange in revisions. However, it is the opinion of the authors that the advantages of tibial modularity do not outweigh the disadvantages.

### Backside wear

There are several disadvantages to tibial modularity. Chief among these is polyethylene wear. In a case report, Rise et al.[12] felt that the interface between a polyethylene liner and the tibial baseplate may have been the source of polyethylene wear leading to osteolysis and loosening. Subsequently, Lewis et al.[24] theorized that polyethylene wear debris came from undersurface wear secondary to the locking mechanism of the polyethylene tray to the baseplate.[23] In addition, undersurface deformation and cold flow was demonstrated in areas of screw holes in tibial trays in one study.[25] It has been shown that backside wear does occur in modular acetabular components in total hips.[26,27] Nonetheless, these observations and theories were not confirmed for total knees until recently. In a retrieval study involving a wide variety of cementless total knee implants, Wasielewski et al.[28] found a significant correlation between nonarticular, backside wear and osteolysis of the tibial metaphysis. The presence of severe articular surface wear did not correlate with osteolysis. They felt that micromotion between the polyethylene insert and the metal tibial tray should be reduced with an adequate locking mechanism. However, in a follow-up study, Parks *et al.*[29] investigated the micromotion between the polyethylene liner and the tibial baseplate in nine different modern total knee designs. They found that in all nine designs, sufficient motion occurs at the polyethylene baseplate interface to create backside fretting of the polyethylene regardless of the type of locking mechanism. Although particle size was not assessed, they felt that this backside wear does create the size of particles sufficient to induce an osteolytic response. On the basis of this recent evidence appears, with current technology, that the only way to completely eliminate backside polyethylene wear and subsequent osteolysis is to eliminate the interface between the metal tray and the liner. Nonmodular, compression-molded, metal-backed polyethylene tibial components do in fact eliminate this source of particulate debris.

*Polyethylene liner exchange*

The ability to exchange a worn polyethylene liner during a revision is often cited as an advantage for tibial modularity. However, as discussed above, the wear of polyethylene generates particles that induce osteolysis. It has been our experience that in revisions for aseptic loosening the tibial baseplate is more often than not loose and is not amenable to simple polyethylene exchange. This was also demonstrated in a recent study by Bert *et al.*[30] in which the incidence of polyethylene liner exchange was investigated. This series showed that polyethylene exchange is not common at revision surgeries. Almost 89% of the revisions for polyethylene failure required more than just a new liner. This may be because the extent of osteolysis is often difficult to assess on routine radiographs. In a series of 17 cases of total knee revisions for osteolysis, the amount of osteolysis was consistently underappreciated based on preoperative radiographs.[13] As a result, the surgeon may find more extensive osteolysis and component loosening than expected at the time of revision for simple polyethylene liner exchange requiring full component revision.

Another distinct disadvantage to modular polyethylene tibial components is that the polyethylene can dissociate from the metal tray *in vivo*. This is a rare complication but it has been reported in the literature.[31]

## Intraoperative fit

The capacity to achieve optimal fit by utilizing insert trials of varying sizes after insertion of the tibial component is only an apparent advantage of modular tibial systems. It has been our experience, after 15 years of utilizing a nonmodular tibial component, that proper intraoperative trialing prior to insertion of the final component leads to the same soft tissue tension and range of motion as that achieved after the final component is inserted. In addition, proper adjustment of the flexion and extension gaps should be done prior to implantation because just changing the thickness of the insert could possibly produce laxity in either flexion or extension.

## Metal corrosion

The second type of tibial component modularity (that of modular metal tray and stem) also has the disadvantage of yet another source of particulate debris. Modular Morse taper junctions are routinely used in the design of modern total hip arthroplasties. However, these junctions have been shown to create metal debris from corrosion and fretting which may contribute to third body wear at the articular surface.[13,14] In addition, another study investigated the tissue found near the junction of fixation screws and the acetabular cup in total hip arthroplasties and found metal debris.[32] The presence of osteolysis around fixation screws in metal tibial baseplates has also been seen.[6] Although modular metallic junctions may provide the best option for the surgeon during revisions, they should be avoided in primary TKA because of the potential for the production of metal debris.

## Metal backing

If modularity is not recommended, then should metal backing be used at all? The answer to this question is yes. There are many factors which can lead to loosening of a total knee implant. One such factor is abnormally high stresses at the interface between the tibial component and the metaphyseal bone.[33] Metal backing has been shown to improve the distribution of load in the proximal tibia.[34–36] This may explain the results of a study of over 9000 TKAs in which a better survival rate was found in tibial components which were metal-backed.[37]

Surgeons who do not favor metal-backed tibial components often cite the fact that the metal backing leads to a thinner polyethylene component. With most designs, in order to have a minimum of 6–8 mm thickness of polyethylene proximal metaphyseal bone must be sacrificed. However, with the best available polyethylene (compression molded), proximal bone need not be sacrificed. The wear characteristics are so superior to other types of polyethylene[36] (W. L. Rohr Jr, personal communication, May 1999) that the minimum thickness of polyethylene may indeed be less than the accepted 6–8 mm. Data from our institution has shown a 95% survival and superb clinical scores at an average of 10 years of follow-up in 387 total knees which were implanted with a compression molded polyethylene thickness of 4.4 mm (M. A. Ritter, E. M. Keating, P. M. Faris and J. B. Meading, unpublished data). No loose tibial components were identified and there was no evidence of osteolytic lesions. The thickness of the metal backing was 3.6 mm, giving a total thickness of 8 mm for the tibial component which does not sacrifice too much proximal bone.

The improved wear characteristics of the compression molded polyethylene coupled with the improved load distribution in the proximal tibia make a nonmodular, metal-backed tibial component the best choice for TKAs.

## Summary

We do not recommend modular tibial components because they can contribute to loosening through osteolysis from backside polyethylene wear and potentially from metal debris. In addition, the need to exchange polyethylene liners is small and intraoperative trialing after baseplate implantation is unnecessary. Nonmodular tibial components can eliminate the concern for backside polyethylene wear. When coupled with compression molded polyethylene and metal backing, nonmodular tibias have excellent clinical results. With this type of tibial component 10 year results from our institution have been superb;[1] recently the series of over 4000 knees was re-analyzed and showed a 98.86% survival at 15 years (MA Ritter, unpublished data, 1999). There was only a 0.4% incidence of tibial loosening. The good clinical results of nonmodular, compression-molded tibial components has not been limited to our clinic. The Insall–Burstein I tibial component was manufactured with and without metal backing and has also shown excellent results clinically.[38] On the basis of these clinical results we recommend the use of nonmodular, metal-backed tibial components which consist of compression molded polyethylene for routine primary TKAs.

## References

1   Ritter MA, Worland R, Saliski J *et al.*: Flat-on-flat, nonconstrained, compression molded polyethylene total knee replacement. *Clinical Orthopedics* **321**:79–85, 1995.

2   Amstutz HC, Campbell P, Kossovsky N, Clarke IC: Mechanism and clinical significance of wear debris-induced osteolysis. *Clinical Orthopedics* **276**:7–18, 1992.

3   Berry DJ, Wold LE, Rand JA: Extensive osteolysis around an aseptic, stable, uncemented total knee replacement. *Clinical Orthopedics* **293**:204–207, 1993.

4   Cadambi A, Engh GA, Dwyer KA, Vinh TN: Osteolysis of the distal femur after total knee arthroplasty. *Journal of Arthroplasty* **9**:579–594, 1994.

5   Dannenmaier WC, Haynes DW, Nelson CL: Granulomatous reaction and cystic bony destruction associated with high wear rate in a total knee prosthesis. *Clinical Orthopedics* **198**:224–230, 1985.

6   Ezzet DA, Garcia R, Barrack RL: Effect of component fixation method on osteolysis in total knee arthroplasty. *Clinical Orthopedics* **321**:86–91, 1995.

7   Kilgus DJ, Moreland JR, Finerman GA *et al.*: Catastrophic wear of tibial polyethylene inserts. *Clinical Orthopedics* **273**:223–231, 1991.

8   Kilgus DJ, Funahashi TT, Campbell PA: Massive femoral osteolysis and early disintegration of a polyethylene-bearing surface of a total knee replacement. A case report. *Journal of Bone and Joint Surgery* [Am] **74**:770–774, 1992.

9   Kim YH, Oh JH, Oh SH: Osteolysis around cementless porous-coated anatomic knee prostheses. *Journal of Bone and Joint Surgery* [Br] **77**(2):236–241, 1995.

10  Nolan JF, Bucknill TM: Aggressive granulomatosis from polyethylene failure in a uncemented knee replacement. *Journal of Bone and Joint Surgery* [Br] **74**(1):23–24, 1992.

11  Peters PC, Engh GA, Dwyer KA, Vinh TN: Osteolysis after total knee arthroplasty without cement. *Journal of Bone and Joint Surgery* [Am] **74**:864–876, 1992

12  Rise MD, Guiney W Jr., Lynch F: Osteolysis associated with cemented total knee arthroplasty. A case report. *Journal of Arthroplasty* **9**:555–558, 1994.

13  Robinson EJ, Mulliken BD, Bourne RB *et al.*: Catastrophic osteolysis in total knee replacement. A report of 17 cases. *Clinical Orthopedics*, **321**:98–105, 1995.

14  Jasty M, Bragdon C, Jiranek W *et al.*: Etiology of osteolysis around porous-coated cementless total hip arthroplasties. *Clinical Orthopedics* **308**:111–126, 1994.

15  Willert HG, Bertram H, Buchhorn GH: Osteolysis in alloarthroplasty of the hip. The role of ultra high molecular weight polyethylene wear particles. *Clinical Orthopedics* **258**:95–107, 1990.

16  Athanasou NA, Quinn J, Bulstrode CJK: Resorption of bone by inflammatory cells derived from the joint capsule of hip arthroplasties. *Journal of Bone and Joint Surgery* [Br] **74**(1):57–62, 1992.

17  Jiranek WA, Machado M, Jasty M *et al.*: Production of cytokines around loosened cemented acetabular components. Analysis with immuno-histochemical techniques and in situ hybridization. *Journal of Bone and Joint Surgery* [Am] **75**:863–879, 1993.

18  Mundy CR, Altman AJ, Gondek MD, Bandelin JG: Direct resorption of bone by human monocytes. *Science* **196**:1109–1111, 1977.

19  Murray DW, Rushton N: Macrophages stimulate bone resorption when they phagocytose particles. *Journal of Bone and Joint Surgery* [Br] **72**(6):988–992, 1990.

20  Horowitz SM, Doty SB, Lane JM, Burstein AH: Studies of the mechanism by which the mechanical failure of polymethylmethacrylate leads to bone resorption. *Journal of Bone and Joint Surgery* [Am] **75**:802–813, 1993.

21  Green T, Fisher J, Ingham E: Polyethylene particles of a critical size are necessary for the induction of IL-6 by macrophages in vitro. *Transactions of the Orthopedics Research Society* **22**:733, 1997.

22  Schmalzried TP, Jasty M, Rosenberg A, Harris WH: Polyethylene wear debris and tissue-reactions in knee as compared to hip-replacement prostheses. *Journal of Applied Biomaterials* **5**:185–190, 1994.

23  Schmalzried TP, Campbell P, Schmitt AK *et al.*: Shapes and dimensional characteristics of polyethylene wear particles generated in vivo by total knee replacements compared to total hip replacements. *Journal of Biomedical Materials Research* **38**(3):203–210, 1997.

24  Lewis PL, Rorabeck CH, Bourne RB: Screw osteolysis after cementless total knee replacement. *Clinical Orthopedics* **321**:173–177, 1995.

25  Engh GA, Dwyer KA, Hanes CK: Polyethylene wear of metal-backed tibial components in total and unicompartmental knee prostheses. *Journal of Bone and Joint Surgery* [Br] **74**(1):9–17, 1992.

26  Guttmann D, Schmalzried TP, Kabo JM, Amstutz HC: Characterization of back-side wear in modular polyethylene liners. *Orthopedics Transactions* **18**:418–419, 1994.

27  Rosner BI, Postak PD, Greenwald AS: Cup/Liner incongruity of two piece acetabular designs: Implications in the generation of polyethylene debris. *Orthopedics Transactions* **18**:1143, 1994–1995.

28 Wasielewski RC, Parks NL, Williams I *et al.*: Tibial Insert undersurface as a contributing source of polyethylene wear debris. *Clinical Orthopedics* **345**:53–59, 1997.

29 Parks NL, Engh GA, Topoleski LDT, Emperado J: Modular tibial insert micromotion. A concern with contemporary knee implants. *Clinical Orthopedics* **356**:10–15, 1998.

30 Bert JM, Reuben J, Kelly F, Gross M, Elting J: The incidence of modular tibial polyethylene insert exchange in total knee arthroplasty when polyethylene failure occurs. *Journal of Arthroplasty* 13(6):609–614, 1998.

31 Davis PF, Bocell JR Jr, Tullos HS: Dissociation of the tibial component in total knee replacements. *Clinical Orthopedics* **272**:199–204, 1991

32 Huk OL, Bansal M, Betts F *et al.*: Polyethylene and metal debris generated by non-articulating surfaces of modular acetabular components. Journal of Bone and Joint Surgery [Br] **76**(4):568–574, 1994.

33 Burstein AH, Wright TM: Biomechanics. In *Surgery of the knee*, 2nd edn, ed. JN Insall, p. 58. Churchill Livingstone, New York, 1993.

34 Bartel DL, Burstein AH, Santavicca EA, Insall JN: Performance of the tibial component in total knee replacement. Conventional and revision designs. *Journal of Bone and Joint Surgery* [Am] **64**:1026, 1982.

35 Murase K, Crowninshield RD, Pedersen DR, Chang TS: An analysis of tibial component design in total knee arthroplasty. *Journal of Biomechanics* **16**:13, 1983.

36 Walker PS, Greene D, Reilly DT *et al.*: Fixation of tibial components of knee prostheses. *Journal of Bone and Joint Surgery* [Am] **63**:258–267, 1981.

37 Rand JA, Ilstrup DA: Survivorship analysis of total knee arthroplasty: Cumulative rates of survival of 9200 total knee arthroplasties. *Journal of Bone and Joint Surgery* [Am] **73**:397–409, 1991.

38 Colizza WA, Insall JN, Scuderi GR: The posterior stabilized total knee prosthesis: Assessment of polyethylene damage and osteolysis after a ten-year-minimum follow-up. *Journal of Bone and Joint Surgery* [Am] **77**:1713–1720, 1995.

## Questions and answers

*Moderator:* Dr. Ritter, for the surgeon in a smaller hospital doesn't the increased inventory necessitated by a nonmodular component outweigh its benefits?

*Dr. Ritter:* In the past, inventory was a major concern, as hospitals were required by the implant companies to purchase their inventory. However, in today's competitive business environment, hospitals are no longer buying the inventory but have it in stock on a consignment basis. Thus the costs of holding a large inventory are not an issue. In addition, nonmodular components do not necessarily translate into a large inventory. Let's look at just one size, for example: a 70 mm wide tibial component with four different thicknesses. A modular system would require one baseplate and four different polyethylene inserts for a total inventory volume of five pieces. A nonmodular system would require only four inventory pieces consisting of the baseplate with four different thicknesses attached. Thus, the total number of stock items can be less. If cost is not an issue, in that the hospital does not have to buy the implants up front, then inventory size is not really an issue.

*Moderator:* Let me ask that question in a slightly different way to you, Dr. Victor. In this area of cost-containing do you think that a metal-backed modular component adds enough to justify its extra cost?

*Dr. Victor:* The question refers to the issues of quality *and* cost. Both items are expressed in different units and are consequently difficult to link in comparison. We could refer to Albert Einstein, who said "Not everything that counts can be counted and not everything that can be counted counts." Unfortunately the latter is not true for money, and there is no escape for cost-containment and "more value for the money." However, cost measurement implies all costs—direct and indirect, early and late. The cost of the implant is easily calculated but represents only approximately one-third of the total price of the procedure. Provided that both metal-backed and all-poly implants yield the same cost in surgical time and hospital stay, the overall price for the all-poly implant procedure will be approximately 2% cheaper. Given the slightly higher revision rate for the all-poly tibial component this is not sufficient to cover the cost of the revision surgery. Consequently, without even taking the quality issue and patient-related factors into account, the cost argument is pointless!

*Moderator:* Dr. Ritter, you have used molded polyethylene now for almost 20 years and are obviously pleased by your results. Do you think that these results could be bettered using cross-linked polyethylene?

*Dr. Ritter:* Quite frankly, we do not believe that our results can be improved. Our 15 and 20 year survival rate nears 99%. The six failures that occurred were secondary to surgical errors. In addition we have recently looked up our results of some of our earliest total knees with compression-molded polyethylene that had a thickness of 4 mm and we have not had a single failure. We do not believe that cross-linked polyethylene could improve on these results.

*Moderator:* Dr. Victor, you have stated that screw holes should be avoided as a possible initiator of cold flow. Do you feel that one can perform an uncemented tibial component without screws, and if not, how to you trade off the value of screws against the possibility of cold flow?

*Dr. Victor:* Screw holes do indeed initiate cold flow. This cold flow is relatively harmless as long as the polyethylene is rigidly fixed to the baseplate. Micromotion *in combination* with irregularities in the undersurfaces of the construct is the main inductor of backside polyethylene wear. Engineering of cementless devices has to rule out either micromotion of the polyethylene insert or irregularities like screw holes in the baseplate. The problem with cementless fixation is the need for perfect fixation of the baseplate to the bone. Initial fixation is the key factor in success of cementless devices and screw fixation clearly helps to achieve this, especially by its unique capacity to exert compressive forces. If we give up the use of screws, we raise the need for other adjustments to the baseplate, like bigger stems and peripheral spikes. It is highly questionable whether they can achieve the same high degree of initial fixation that screws do. A possible solution to this dilemma is the use of screws that leave a perfectly flat upper surface with a flat and nearly seamless fill-in of the screw hole, combined with rigid fixation of the polyethylene to the baseplate.

*Moderator:* I can assume from what you have said that you would not recommend the use of an uncemented tibial component that was one piece, that is polyethylene molded to the baseplate?

*Dr. Victor:* That is correct.

*Moderator:* Dr. Victor, since you feel so strongly about rigid fixation between the polyethylene and the baseplate, and since absolute engineering rigid fixation between two dissimilar materials is, in theory, impossible, do you feel that the material of the tibial baseplate is important or not in reducing wear with the polyethylene? Do you feel that there is a place for a ceramic baseplate?

*Dr. Victor:* The material of the base is important. As long as engineering techniques do not allow us to fix the polyethylene perfectly to the baseplate, this interface has to be considered as a "bearing surface." Wear performance is better for ceramic–polyethylene than for cobalt-chrome alloy–polyethylene, and this is better than that for titanium alloy–polyethylene. From a theoretical wear standpoint, the ceramic baseplate ought to yield the least wear particles. A word of caution , however: ceramic baseplates have a different modulus of elasticity than cobalt-chrome baseplates. The effect of differential stiffness of the baseplate on the long-term fixation of the latter to the proximal tibial bone is unknown. Taking a significant risk for an optional minor improvement is hard for me to justify. Long-term behavior in terms of fixation of cemented cobalt-chrome baseplates is well documented. With its acceptable performance as a bearing surface, it seems the best trade-off for construction of the baseplate.

*Moderator:* Have you, Dr. Ritter, ever had a situation in which the permanent component had been cemented in and for some reason you felt you needed a thicker implant or a more stabilized one? Let me modify that questions by asking not how often this happens to a surgeon who has been doing several hundred knee replacements a year, but rather the average surgeon who, we have been told, does only 10–20 knee replacements yearly?

*Dr. Ritter:* We have never had that situation in our 15–20 year experience with nonmodular tibial components. In the system that we use, the trials are the exact same size as the nonmodular component of the corresponding size. Thus, if the trial is the appropriate size, then the final component will fit the same way. This means that you have to pay careful attention during the trial process. As far as needing a stabilized component, the surgeon must assess soft tissue balance and ensure that the posterior cruciate ligament has been spared prior to and during trailing thus eliminating any surprises once the final component is in place. The average surgeon should be able to avoid problems by paying attention to simple details of sparing the posterior cruciate ligament and careful analysis of the trial fit.

# 3

*Bone loss from the proximal tibia or distal femur is a common finding in the patient with advanced degenerative arthritis. For small defects, merely lowering the resection line on the tibia, or raising the resecting line on the femur may be sufficient. For larger defects, however, one must often resort to other methods of treatment. Two options are the use of prosthetic augments or bone grafts.*

# The use of prosthetic augments is the optimal way to correct for bone defects during total knee replacement

## Pro: James Rand

Bone loss is a frequent problem in primary and revision total knee arthroplasty (TKA). In primary arthroplasty, bone defects are primarily encountered in association with large angular deformities, prior surgery, or post-traumatic arthritis. An understanding of the types of bone defects and options for management is essential to achieve a durable result from a TKA. Modular metal augments are the optimal mode of management of midsize defects of the tibia and femur. Metal augments may be utilized to fill bone defects, assist with soft tissue balancing, and allow joint line restoration. Modular augments do not restore lost bone as can bone graft but do not depend upon healing to sclerotic poorly vascularized host bone.

### Classification of bone loss

A variety of classification techniques can be utilized for the description of bone loss, but no single classification system has been universally accepted and applied in the literature. The simplest classification system is that of a contained or uncontained bone defect. A contained defect has a supporting rim of intact host bone, whereas an uncontained defect has a deficient peripheral rim of host bone. An example of an uncontained bone defect would be loss of medial tibial bone in a long-standing varus deformity (Fig. 3.1). An example of a contained defect would be a bone cyst in an arthritic knee or concavity of the lateral tibial plateau in a valgus knee. Another method of classifying defects is that of being either central or peripheral in location.[1] A peripheral defect is often uncontained but a central defect is usually contained. These vague descriptions of bone loss complicate

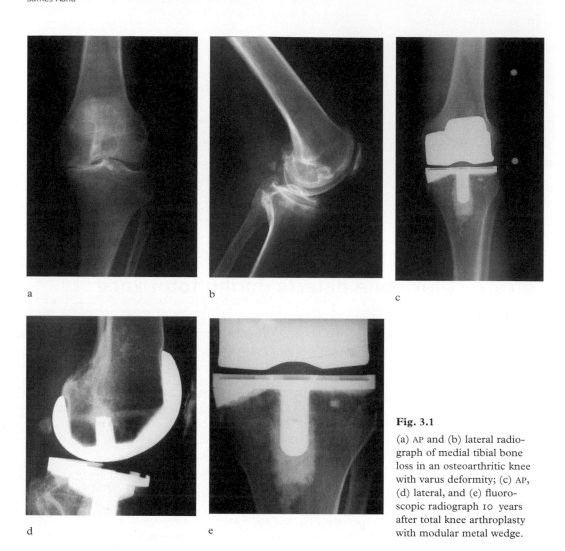

**Fig. 3.1**

(a) AP and (b) lateral radiograph of medial tibial bone loss in an osteoarthritic knee with varus deformity; (c) AP, (d) lateral, and (e) fluoroscopic radiograph 10 years after total knee arthroplasty with modular metal wedge.

attempts to compare various authors' publications on bone defect management and especially revision TKA.

The recent classification of bone loss by G. Engh has gained increasing acceptance as a technique for bone defect classification that is easily applied but its prognostic significance will require a

**Table 3.1** Bone defect classification (Engh[2])

| Type | Metaphyseal bone | Treatment |
| --- | --- | --- |
| Type I | Intact | Primary component |
| Type II | Damaged | Augments; revision implant |
| Type III | Deficient | Bulk allograft; long stems |

large prospective series[2] (Table 3.1). The classification system describes three types of defects.

- A type 1 defect has intact metaphyseal bone. On the femoral side, bone is present distal to the epicondyles. On the tibial side, bone is present above the tibial tubercle. In the case of a revision, there is no component subsidence or osteolysis.
- A type 2 defect has damaged metaphyseal bone, which on radiographs appears as a shortened metaphyseal flare. On the femoral side, there is component subsidence or joint line elevation or osteolytic defects distal to the epicondyles. On the tibial side, there is component subsidence to or below the tip of the fibular head or a shortened metaphyseal flare.
- A type 3 defect has a deficient metaphyseal segment. On the femoral side, bone loss extends to or is proximal to the epicondyles, or there is component subsidence to the epicondyles. On the tibial side, there is bone loss or component subsidence to the tibial tubercle.

The use of modular bone augments is primarily for type 2 defects or selected type 1 defects. Type 3 defects should be managed by bone graft or custom augmented implants, not modular bone augments, except for patients with low demand or short life expectancy. The remainder of this discussion focuses on the use of modular augments for these moderate size peripheral bone defects.

## Options for bone defect management

Options for management of bone defects in TKA include

- translating the component away from the defect
- increased bone resection
- cement filling with or without reinforcing screws
- bone graft either morselized or structural
- modular bone augments
- custom augmented implants.

An intramedullary stem is an important adjunct to bone defect management. In an *in vitro* study using strain gauges, loss of tibial component–tibial bone contact decreased strain in the proximal tibia by 33–60%.[3] A cemented tibial stem was found to relieve stress on the cortex for the entire length of the stem. An extended intramedullary stem can improve fixation by fixing the implant to intact bone. Whether a press-fit or cemented stem is preferable has been controversial. Advantages of cement fixation include initial fixation, fixation in osteopenic bone, and the ability to position the implant independent of the stem position. Disadvantages of cement fixation are related to difficulty in removal. Advantages of press-fit stems include the ease of subsequent revision and the preservation of bone. Disadvantages of press-fit stems include less secure initial fixation than cement, and the stem determines the position of the implant.

Translating the component away from the defect results in a smaller tibial component that does not cover the tibia. This technique should be reserved for small peripheral defects in older patients with limited demands. Increased bone resection in primary arthroplasty may be utilized for small deficiencies when bone resection does not result in removal of more than 1 cm of bone from the proximal tibia or distal femur.[4] In a recent series of primary total knees using a posterior cruciate retaining total condylar design, with the numbers available, there was no significant correlation between the level of proximal tibial bone resection and the loosening or revision rate at 8 years.[5,6] Excess tibial bone resection below the tip of the fibular head results in fixation in weaker bone and a smaller tibial component size which can be problematic in total knee systems that do not allow mismatch in sizes between the femur and tibia, and may result in medial overhang of a long-stemmed tibial component with impingement on the medial collateral ligament. Increased femoral bone resection results in elevation of the joint line with the potential for altered kinematics in the posterior cruciate retained knee, impingement of the patella against the tibial component, or mismatches in the flexion and extension spaces with soft tissue imbalance. Increased bone resection is not an option in most revision operations as bone is already deficient.

Cement filling can be used successfully for central defects and small peripheral defects but is mechanically inferior to other options. In a study of peripheral wedge-shaped bone defects in the tibia *in vitro*, axial loads of 1780 N and varus loads of 1340 N at 28 N m were

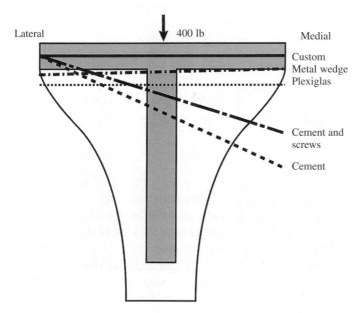

**Fig. 3.2**

*In vitro* loading across a peripheral bone defect (least deflective upon eccentric loading) is best with a custom implant or modular metal augment (Reprinted with permission from Brooks *et al.*[18])

assessed[7] (Fig. 3.2). The vertical deflections on the medial and lateral sides of the tibial component were measured. The greatest deflections occurred when cement or cement and screws were utilized to fill the defect. The least deflections, amounting to 9% of the value for cement alone, occurred when a custom-augmented tibial component was used to fill the defect. A modular metal wedge for filling of the defect provided a deflection of 17% of the value for cement alone. A cemented central stem of 70 mm in length carried 28–38% of the axial load in the presence of a bone defect. In an *in vitro* study of bone defects in a bovine model, the least stiffness was found when the defect was filled with a cement wedge compared to converting the defect to a step shape[8] (Fig. 3.3). A metal wedge or block provided similar stiffness when treating a 20° peripheral wedge-shaped defect. In another *in vitro* study of peripheral wedge-shaped tibial defects, the lowest strains were present when the defect was filled with a rectangular block compared to cement[9] (Figs 3.4, 3.5). Filling of the defect with a metal wedge was intermediate in strain compared to cement or a metal block.

In a series of 57 primary total knees followed at 6 years treated by cement and screw filling of a bone defect, there were no failures but radiolucent lines were present adjacent to 27% of the defects.[5] In a series of 54 primary total knees treated with cement filling of a peripheral tibial bone defect and followed for 7 years, there was only one loosening.[10] Radiolucent lines were identified adjacent to 70% of knees in which the preoperative bone defect was 10–20 mm in depth compared to 83% of knees in which the defect was greater than 20 mm in depth. The use of cement filling in revision surgery should

**Fig. 3.3**

A step-shape cement wedge provides better loading (stiffness) than an angled cement wedge. Grey bars, no augmentation; white bars, wedge augmentation; black bars, block augmentation (Reprinted with permission from Chen *et al.*[8])

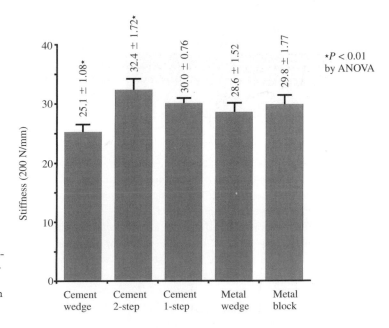

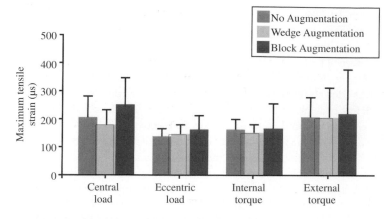

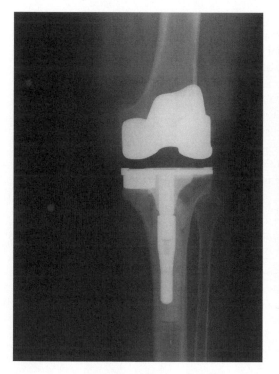

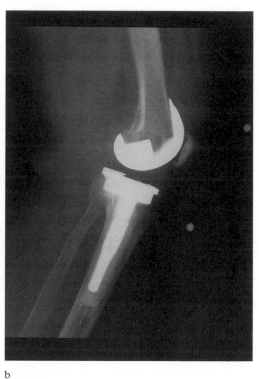

**Fig. 3.4**

A rectangular metal block provides better *in vitro* loading (maximum tensile strain) than cement or an angled wedge (Reprinted with permission from Fehring *et al.*[9]).

a             b

**Fig. 3.5**

(a) AP and (b) lateral radiograph of a rectangular modular metal augment used in an osteoarthritic knee with preoperative varus deformity.

be limited to contained defects with an intact peripheral rim of bone upon which to seat the implant. The results of cement filling of bone defects in revision have not been reported.

The results of use of a modular metal wedge for treatment of peripheral tibial bone defects in primary arthroplasty have been reported. A review of 22 knees in 20 patients in which a modular metal wedge had been utilized to fill a peripheral bone defect was performed at a mean of 37 months.[11] There were 17 primary and 5 revision knees. Incomplete radiolucent lines that were nonprogressive were identified in 6 (27%) at the wedge–cement interface. There were neither mechanical failures nor loosening. In another study of 28 knees in 25 patients followed for 2–3.5 years, a metal wedge was utilized on the medial side in 24 and lateral side in 4 knees.[12] Radiolucent lines at the bone–cement interface beneath the wedge were present in 13 knees but were nonprogressive. There were no mechanical failures. In a subsequent study of the same group of patients, 24 knees were evaluated at a mean follow-up of 5 years.[13] There were no mechanical failures of the wedges but nonprogressive radiolucent lines were identified at the bone cement interface beneath the wedge in 13 knees. A retrieval of a tibial component with a modular metal wedge was subjected to biomechanical testing.[14] The shear strength of the modular metal wedge after 6.5 years *in vivo* was 77% that of a freshly cemented wedge (Fig. 3.6). The author has not encountered mechanical failure between the augment and the tibial or femoral component of any of the modular augments utilized for bone defect management in either primary or revision arthroplasty.

The results of modular metal wedges in revision surgery have not been reported as an isolated series. The results of modular augmented implants in revision surgery have been reported with excellent results. The results of 41 consecutive revisions using a modular Genesis TKA were reported at a follow-up of 3 years.[15] The results were good or excellent in 98% of the knees with a 7% complication rate. Femoral wedge augments were required distally in 2 knees, posteriorly in 16 knees, and combined in 12 knees. Tibial wedge augments were required medially in 6 knees, combined medial and lateral in 4 knees, and as a custom augmented tray in 3 knees (Fig. 3.7). Intramedullary stems were cemented on the femoral side in 14 knees and press-fit in 17 knees. Intramedullary stems were cemented on the tibial side in 14 knees and press-fit in 16 knees. A posterior stabilized design was utilized in 24 knees and a posterior cruciate retaining design in 17 knees. The Hospital for Special

**Fig. 3.6**

The shear strength of attachment of a modular metal wedge after 5 years *in vivo* was 77% that of a freshly cemented wedge.

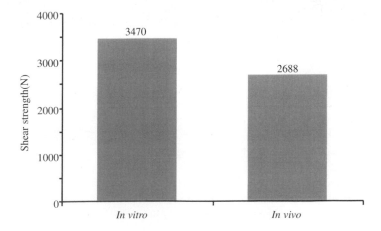

Surgery mean knee score was 80 in the posterior stabilized and 85 in the posterior cruciate retaining knees at last evaluation. The Knee Society pain score improved from a mean of 38 prior to revision to 91 at last evaluation. The Knee Society function score improved from a mean of 40 prior to revision to 68 at last evaluation. There were no mechanical failures of any knees and, with the numbers available, no differences in the results between press-fit or cemented stems, or posterior cruciate retaining or substituting knees. In another study of 39 knees in 36 patients, the results of revision were reported at a mean

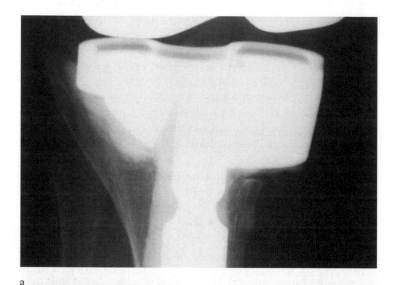

a

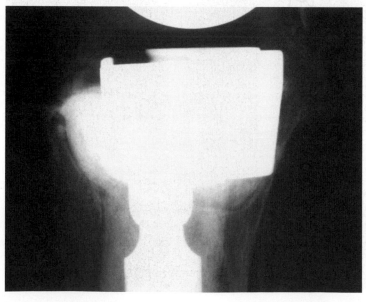

b

**Fig. 3.7**

(a) AP and (b) lateral radiograph of custom medial and modular lateral wedge augmented tibial component 5 years following revision.

of 24 months.[16] A posterior stabilized design was utilized in 31 and a posterior cruciate retaining design in 8 knees. The Knee Society pain score improved from 50 to 83 and the function score from 36 to 56 points. A residual patella infera was present in 21% and correlated with a lower knee score ($p < 0.01$). The importance of joint line restoration at the time of revision TKA has been controversial. In a recent report of 107 knees followed for 3.7 years, Rorabeck *et al.* found a higher knee score of 149 in those knees with less than compared to a score of 130 in those knees with greater than 5 mm of joint line elevation[17] (Fig. 3.8).

The results of 76 revisions using a modular constrained condylar or posterior stabilized design was reported at a follow-up of 3.5 years.[18] A posterior stabilized design was used in 57 knees and a constrained condylar design in 19 knees. Modular augments were utilized on the tibia in 25 knees and on the femur in 23 either distally, posteriorly, or in both locations. An intramedulllary stem was press-fit in both the tibia and femur. A good or excellent result was achieved in 56 (83%) of 67 knees that were followed. Radiolucent lines were identified at the bone–cement interface adjacent to 22 (33%) of the femoral components, and 43 (64%) of the tibial components. The radiolucent lines were complete adjacent to three tibial components and were progressive in one femoral and two tibial

**Fig. 3.8**

(a) AP and (b) lateral radiograph 5 years after use of a modular femoral augment for joint line restoration in a revision total knee.

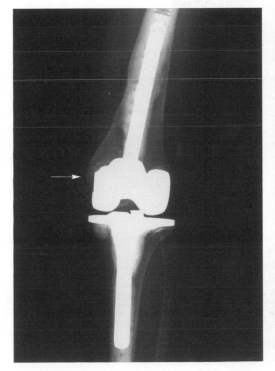
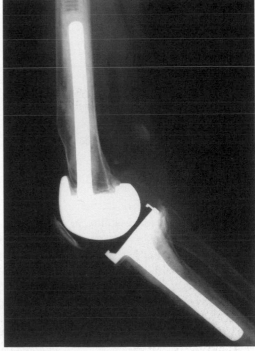

a

b

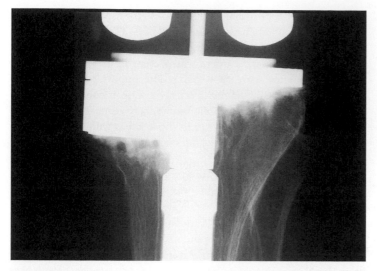

a

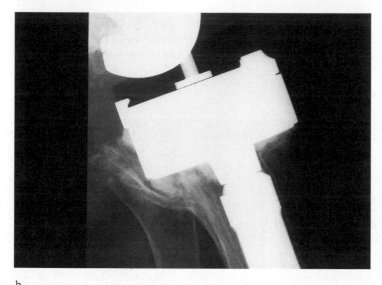

b

**Fig. 3.9**

(a) AP and (b) lateral radiograph 5 years after revision total knee with modular stems, and medial tibial rectangular modular augment.

components. There were six failures, due to infection in 3, aseptic loosening in 2, and instability in 1 knee. Using an end-point of revision, survivorship was predicted at 83 per cent at 8 years (Fig. 3.9). In another series of 57 revision knees using a posterior stabilized or constrained condylar prosthesis, the results were good or excellent in 45 (79%) knees at a mean of 5 years.[19] An intramedullary stem was used on 57 femoral components of which 23 were cemented and 11 press-fit. An intramedullary stem was used on 18 tibial components of which 9 were cemented and 9 press-fit. Bone defects were managed by cancellous allograft for contained and cortical allograft for noncontained defects. Five knees utilized an allograft–prosthetic composite. Four knees failed due to loosening in 1, and instability in 3. Radiolucent lines were identified adjacent to 6 of 7 press-fit compared to 3 of 19 cemented femoral stems ($p < 0.02$). Radiolucent lines were identified adjacent to 4 of 7 press-fit compared to 2 of 6 cemented tibial stems (n.s.). There were no failures of the allograft–prosthetic composite grafts. In yet another study of the constrained condylar design followed for 5 years, good or excellent results were achieved in 13 of 16 knees.[20] There were 3 failures due to loosening in 1, supracondylar fracture with loosening in 1, and infection in 1. In yet another study of 44 revisions followed for 2–6 years, 3 of 13 constrained condylar knees compared to none of 31 posterior stabilized designs had radiographic evidence of loosening of a press-fit stem (Fig. 3.10).[21] The mean Knee Society scores at last evaluation were 84 for pain and 83 for function. The use of nonmodular cemented long stems has been satisfactory. In a series of 40 cemented long stem kinematic total knees, there was only 1 femoral loosening at a mean of 5 years.[22]

Bone graft is an alternative to metal augments for the management of bone defects, and has the potential to restore bone stock for subsequent revisions. Options for bone graft include autograft or allograft. Autograft is available in primary TKA but is not available locally in most revisions. Iliac crest bone can be considered for contained defects but is not adequate for structural grafts to replace a deficient

**Fig. 3.10**

(a) AP radiograph of femoral and (b) lateral radiograph of tibial stem demonstrating radiolucency adjacent to press-fit stems of a revision total knee.

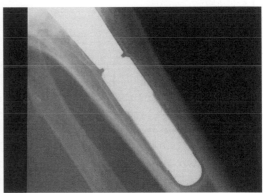

b

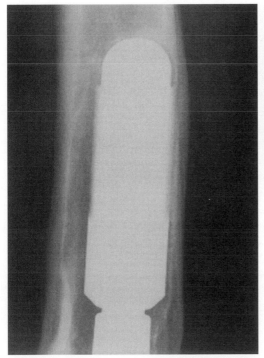

a

condyle. Allograft of either a femoral head or massive graft of the distal femur or proximal tibia may be utilized as structural or morselized graft. Structural grafts heal to host bone but are not revascularized nor remodeled.[23] Morselized graft can be revascularized and remodeled but provides limited structural support during healing. The results of bone grafts in TKA have been variable. In a series of 24 total knees of which 10 were primary and 14 revisions, local autograft was utilized in 10 primary and 9 revisions; iliac crest in 4; and an allograft femoral head in 1.[1] Nonunion of the graft occurred in 2 knees and was attributed to varus malalignment in 1 and a poorly vascularized bone bed in the other knee. Biopsy of 3 knees revealed viable bone in 2. In a series of 26 primary TKAs with large angular deformities resulting in tibial bone loss, local bone was used in 22 and iliac crest bone in 4 knees.[24] At 5 years following TKA, 4 bone grafts had fragmented and failed. Needle biopsy of 9 knees with surviving bone grafts revealed viable bone in 4 knees. In contrast, a study of 35 allografts in 30 patients, found good or excellent results in 26 knees:[2] 29 femoral heads, 5 distal femoral allografts, and 1 proximal tibial allograft were used. All 4 primary arthroplasties and 22 of the 26 revisions had good or excellent knee scores at a mean of 50 months. Incorporation of the graft was demonstrated in 20 of 30 patients at a mean of 7 months. Three components seated on structural grafts subsided, 2 were press-fit femoral and 1 a press-fit tibial component. In a series of 63 knees in which morselized bone graft was utilized to treat bone defects at the time of revision, 2 knees developed loosening and required another revision.[25] Biopsy of the graft obtained at the time of reoperation in 14 knees found evidence of revascularization and remodeling.

## Summary

Management of bone defects at the time of primary and revision arthroplasty is often difficult. A variety of options may be considered. Bone grafting is an option that should be reserved for the massive type 3 bone defect that would otherwise require a custom implant. For the type 1 and 2 bone defects, modular metal augments provide a simple, rapid and dependable technique that provides predictable results for at least 5–10 years. Modular augments allow joint line restoration and facilitate soft tissue balancing by selective augmentation of the femoral component. Mechanical failure has not been a frequent problem to date with any of the various attachment mechanisms utilized for the modular augments.

## References

1   Dorr L, Ranawat C, Sculco T, McKaskill B, Orisek B: Bone graft for tibial defects in total knee arthroplasty. *Clinical Orthopedics* **205**:153–165, 1986.

2   Engh G, Herzwurm P, Parks N: Treatment of major defects of bone with bulk allografts and stemmed components during total knee

arthroplasty. *Journal of Bone and Joint Surgery* [Am] **79**:1030–1039, 1997.

3   Bourne R, Finlay J: The Influence of tibial component intramedullary stems and implant–cortex contact on the strain distribution of the proximal tibia following total knee arthroplasty. *Clinical Orthopedics* **208**:95–99, 1986.

4   Garg A, Walker P: The effect of the interface on the bone stresses beneath tibial components. *Journal of Biomechanics.* **19**(12):957–967, 1986.

5   Ritter M, Keating M, Faris P: screw and cement fixation of large defects in total knee arthroplasty. *Journal of Arthroplasty* **8**(1):63–65, 1993.

6   Ritter M, Montgomery T, Zhou H *et al.*: The clinical significance of proximal tibial resection level in total knee arthroplasty. *Clinical Orthopedics* **360**:174–181, 1999.

7   Brooks PJ, Walker PS, Scott RD: Tibial component fixation in deficient tibial bone stock. *Clinical Orthopedics* **184**:302–308, 1984.

8   Chen F, Krackow KA Management of tibial defects in total knee arthroplasty. *Clinical Orthopedics.* **305**:249–257, 1994.

9   Fehring TK, Peindl RD, Humble RS *et al.* Modular tibial augmentations in total knee arthroplasty. *Clinical Orthopedics* **327**:207–217, 1996.

10  Lotke P, Wong R, Ecker M: The use of methylmethacrylate in primary total knee replacements with large tibial defects. *Clinical Orthopedics* **270**:288–294, 1991.

11  Brand M, Daley R, Frederick, C *et al.*: Tibial tray augmentation with modular metal wedges for tibial bone stock deficiency. *Clinical Orthopedics* **248**:71–79, 1989.

12  Rand J: Bone deficiency in total knee arthroplasty. Use of metal wedge augmentation. *Clinical Orthopedics* **271**:63–71, 1991.

13  Pagnano M, Trousdale R, Rand J: Tibial wedge augmentation for bone deficiency in total knee arthroplasty. *Clinical Orthopedics* **321**:151–155, 1995.

14  Rand J: Augmentation of a total knee arthroplasty with modular metal wedge. *Journal of Bone and Joint Surgery* [Am] **77**:266–268, 1995.

15  Rand J: Modularity in total knee arthroplasty. *Acta Orthopaedica Belgica* **62**:Suppl I, 1996.

16  Takahashi Y, Gustilo R: Nonconstrained implants in revision total knee arthroplasty. *Clinical Orthopedics* **309**:156–162, 1994.

17  Parthington, P, Sawhney, J, Rorabeck C *et al.*: Joint line restoration after revision total knee arthroplasty: clinical significance and accuracy. Presented at The Knee Society, Anaheim, California, 7 February 1999.

18  Haas S, Insall J, Montgomery W, Windsor R: Revision total knee arthroplasty with use of modular components with stems inserted without cement. *Journal of Bone and Joint Surgery* [Am] **77**:**11**:1700–1707, 1995.

19  Peters C, Hennessey R, Barden R *et al.*: Revision total knee arthroplasty with a cemented posterior-stabilized or constrained condylar prosthesis. *Journal of Arthroplasty* **12**(8):896–903, 1997.

20  Hartford J, Goodman S, Schurman D, Knoblick G: Complex primary and revision total knee arthroplasty using the condylar constrained prosthesis. *Journal of Arthroplasty* **13**(4):380–387, 1998.

21  Vince K, Long W: Revision knee arthroplasty. the limited press fit medullary fixation. *Clinical Orthopedics* **317**:172–177, 1995.

22  Murray P, Rand J, Hanssen A: Cemented long-stem revision total knee arthroplasty. *Clinical Orthopedics* **309**:116–123, 1994.

23  Parks N, Engh, G: Histology of nine structural bone grafts used in total knee arthroplasty. *Clinical Orthopedics* **345**:17–23, 1997.

24  Laskin, R: Total knee arthroplasty in the presence of large bony defects of the tibia and marked knee instability. *Clinical Orthopedics* **248**:66–70, 1989.

25  Whiteside L, Bicalho P: Radiologic and histologic analysis of morselized allograft in revision total knee replacement. *Clinical Orthopedics* **357**:149–156, 1998.

# Con: Thomas P. Sculco, Alexander Miric, Jonathan D.S. Klein, and William MacAulay

Over the past two decades, total knee replacement has evolved into one of the most successful of orthopedic procedures. The quality of the clinical results has become predictable and reproducible, pain is relieved, and function is improved. With excellent results in the less complex cases and increased surgical experience, more severely damaged knees have been addressed. It is in these more complex knees that combinations of soft tissue and bone deficiency exist and these present challenging reconstructive dilemmas to the operating surgeon. In an effort to address these reconstructive dilemmas, a myriad of surgical techniques have been proposed as possible solutions.

This contribution focuses on the alternatives available to the surgeon when performing a TKA in a knee with bone deficiency. We first define the problem by reviewing the typical locations of these deficiencies and the classification schemes used to describe them. Second, we review the surgical options that have been proposed to deal with these situations, along with the problems and benefits with each. Special attention is given to bone grafting of these defects. In addition to benefits and problems posed by this alternative, we discuss the principles, methodology, and results of this technique. Furthermore, we contrast bone grafting of defects to the option of using prosthetic augmentation. It is our contention that in most cases the use of bone graft represents the most versatile solution and produces a construct that is more biologically and biomechanically sound.

## Bone deficiency

Bone loss in knees with angular deformity occurs most frequently on the tibial side of the joint. The defects are usually localized posteriorly on the tibial plateau due to the frequently associated flexion deformity in these knees. In osteoarthritis (OA), for example, bone defects are most frequently located on the posteromedial tibia and are associated with a varus deformity.[1] There may be associated fragmentation of the tibial surface, but as a rule the tibial surface is concave, extremely sclerotic, and completely devoid of cartilage (Fig. 3.11). Because there is often frank subluxation of the femur on the tibia, there tends to be little, if any, peripheral tibial rim remaining. The deficiency occurs as a result of the progression of the deformity and the forces driving the femur into the tibial surface.

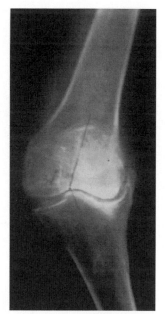

**Fig. 3.11**

Severe tibial bone loss in a valgus knee with marked sclerosis on the lateral tibial plateau surface (Reprinted with permission from Sculco 1994).

Consequently there is a steep descent from the middle of the tibial surface to the periphery.

Femoral bone loss on the concave side of an angular deformity occurs with much less frequency than does tibial bone loss. An exception to this is the valgus knee, where combinations of both tibial and femoral bone loss are seen. The sclerotic quality of the femoral subchondral bone and the ram's-horn configuration of the distal femoral condyle favor the tibia collapsing rather than the femur. When femoral condylar collapse does occur there may be an element of osteonecrosis present which facilitates this destruction.

If severe degrees of bone loss are associated with marked fragmentation and disorganization of the joint, one must suspect an underlying neuropathic process. In this instance, severe degrees of deformity with marked loss of joint stability and bone destruction are present which are out of proportion to the mild degree of pain perceived by the patient. A careful history and neurological examination is important in these patients. The most common cause of a neuropathic joint is diabetes mellitus and, although more distal lower extremity joints are affected, the knee may be involved in some patients. Successful TKA in the neuropathic knee is unlikely. The underlying pathological environment for knee joint destruction remains, and therefore this entity should be viewed as a relative contraindication to total knee replacement.

## Classification schemes

Systematic classification of bony deficiency in TKA can be a useful tool when evaluating techniques of managing bone deficiencies. The first classification of bone defects in TKA was proposed by Dorr in

**Table 3.2** Classifications of bone deficiency in TKA

| | |
|---|---|
| Dorr (1989)[2] | Primary TKA |
| | Central |
| | Peripheral |
| | Revision TKA |
| | Central |
| | Peripheral |
| Rand (1991)[3] | Minimal (<50%,<5 mm) |
| | Moderate (50–70%, 5–10 mm) |
| | Extensive (70–90%, >10 mm) |
| | Cavitary (>90%) |
| | (a) Intact peripheral rim |
| | (b) Deficient peripheral rim |
| Ghazavi (1997)[4] | Contained |
| | Uncontained |
| | Noncircumferential (<3 cm or > 3 cm) |
| | Circumferential (<3 cm or > 3 cm) |
| AORI (Engh 1998)[5] | F, femur; T, tibia |
| | 1, minor defect; 2, significant defect; 3, major defect |

1989[2] (Table 3.2). This scheme distinguished between central and peripheral defects in primary and revision TKA. This represents a significant contribution in the analysis of bone defects as it highlights the importance of peripheral support, in particular for the tibial component. While reporting his early experience with metal wedge augmentation in 1991, Rand[3] provided a new classification of bone defects in TKA (Table 3.2) which placed an emphasis on the extent of condylar involvement. Gross[4] has described a classification of bone defects in a review of medium-term results with allografts for the reconstruction of massive bone defects in revision TKA (Table 3.2). In this system, defects are classified as contained or uncontained. Uncontained defects are then subclassified as circumferential or noncircumferential and further as either greater or less than 3 cm in size. The most recent contribution is the classification of bone defects (Anderson Orthopaedic Research Institute Bone Defect Classification: AORI) proposed by Engh and Ammeen in 1998[5] (Table 3.2). This system, which distinguishes between femoral (F) and tibial (T) defects and grades them according to severity (1 = minor, 2 = significant, 3 = major), essentially involves six subtypes: F1, T1, F2, T2, F3, and T3. Although each classification scheme is slightly different, as a group they focus on important concepts that are similar (containment and severity of the defect). Despite this, however, these classifications remain unvalidated.

It is important to recognize that the nature of bone defects encountered during primary TKA is very different from that of the bone deficiencies encountered during revision TKA. We have had success in addressing these two different situations with two separate classification schemes, which we address later in this chapter.[6,7]

## Treatment options

The basic goal in treating bone defects during TKA is to provide adequate support to the implant. This can be achieved in numerous ways, including avoiding the defect, removing the defect at tibial resection, filling the defect with cement, filling the defect with bone graft, and using prosthetic wedges or custom components. Each treatment option offers advantages that make it an attractive alternative. However, each alternative also harbors a host of potential problems and the surgeon must be aware of these when considering the best course of action.

### Avoiding the defect

This method is rarely used and is applicable only for very small defects that encompass less than 5% of the resected surface.[8] Windsor et al.[1] discussed the surgical technique of shifting the position of the tibial component away from the defect. This technique, however, often requires downsizing of the tibial component and has the potential to alter the force transmission across the implant to the host bone with the chance of early loosening.[3] Use of a smaller tibial tray results in higher unit force transmission across the tray to the underlying bone. Additionally the percentage of the tray supported by cancellous bone, as opposed to cortical bone, increases and may lead to component subsidence.[9] Such downsizing is especially problematic if the component is inserted without cement, as Laskin[10] demonstrated a statistical increase in the rate of component subsidence when uncemented components do not include cortical rim contact.

Despite all the potential problems with this technique, Lotke et al.[11] published 3–8 year results using this method to avoid tibial defects and reported no mechanical failures. This technique of avoiding the defect by shifting the component is not typically applicable to femoral bone loss. Downsizing in the medial to lateral plane usually requires downsizing in the anteroposterior plane, which can lead to either notching of the femoral cortex or laxity of the flexion space. Downsizing the femoral component to accommodate posterior bone loss will result in an increased flexion gap and subsequent instability in flexion or elevation of the joint line.[3,12]

### Resection of the defect

On the surface, this would appear to represent the most expeditious and cost-effective method of treating bone defects during TKA. It is important to realize, however, that the greatest strength and quantity of bone is usually found adjacent to the joint surface. Both Hvid[13] and Sneppen et al.,[14] through the use of cadaveric studies, have demonstrated that the strength of trabecular bone decreases with distance from the articular surface. Overzealous resection can result in an implant seated on a shell of cortical bone with little cancellous support. This method of dealing with bone defects has also raised some concerns about the resulting stress exerted on the bone–cement interface. Dorr et al.[15] reported an increase in the rate of tibial radiolucencies when greater than 5 mm of bone was removed.

In addition to its affects on the biomechanics of the resultant construct, too low a resection of tibia can adversely influence the characteristics of the tibial component. A low resection will greatly reduce the cross-sectional area of tibial bone able to support the prosthesis, and often requires that a smaller tibial component be used. This can cause problems with matching the size of the femoral component if the knee arthroplasty system employed is not very versatile. In addition, a low resection will also mandate the use of a very thick polyethylene component. This can lead to impingement of the tibial polyethylene implant and patella.[8]

Increasing the amount of femur resected leads to an abnormal elevation of the joint line. Proximal elevation diminishes the amount of posterior condylar bone available to support the implant, and, consequently restricts the size of the implant that can be used. In addition, elevation of the joint line raises multiple biomechanical concerns and may adversely affect the lifespan of the arthroplasty.

## Filling the defect with cement

The use of polymethylmethacrylate (PMMA) as fill with screw augmentation in the management of bone defects in TKA was originally advocated by Ritter[16] Support for this technique has been offered in the form of 10 year results in 47 patients with no failures.[17] Biomechanical studies of the proximal tibia have shown that cement possesses poor mechanical properties when used unsupported.[18] For this reason authors such as Ritter[16,17] and Freeman et al.[19] have suggested the use of screw or wire mesh reinforcement of the cement construct. Although satisfactory results using this technique have been reported by both authors, the reported rates of radiolucency may be cause for some concern.

The method of failure when using cement to fill a defect may include cement shrinkage and the development of laminations leading to fragmentation. Simplex-P cement has been shown to lose 2% of its volume when it sets. The effect of this on the bone–cement or prosthesis–cement interface is unknown.[18] Modern cement techniques depend on sustained pressurizing of the cement into the bony interstices. The shrinkage volume will have the opposite effect of pressurizing the cement. Insufficient pressurization of the cement compromises the intratrabecular bone penetration.[20]

Although cement can be used to fill small, contained defects, its use in dealing with larger or peripheral defects has been discouraged.[8] Thermal necrosis has also long been considered to be a major reason for loosening of a knee prosthesis. The larger the defect, the greater the volume of cement used and the greater the temperature becomes when the cement sets. The risk of thermal necrosis becomes more significant with a large defect.[20]

## Augments, wedges, and custom prostheses

Uncontained bone defects of the proximal and distal femur are frequently managed with prosthetic modularity and custom implants. Proposed advantages of this technique include: predictable early results,[21] satisfactory load transfer,[22] intraoperative flexibility,[5,21,23] and the elimination of risk of disease transmission, malunion, nonunion, or resorption.[22] One of advantages often cited is the strength of the construct produced when metal is used to fill the defect. Brooks et al.[18] reported on a cadaveric study in which defects were filled using a variety of materials and the constructs were then tested under axial and varus loads. The least deflection of the tibial tray was seen when a custom tibial component was used; metal wedge augmentation provided almost equivalent support. Cement, either alone or with screws, gave poor results, and leaving the tray without support was least effective. It should be noted, however, that bone graft constructs were not tested in this study.

At this point, it appears that these findings have translated into good clinical results. Brand et al.[23] reviewed the 3 year follow-up results of 20 TKAs performed using modular wedges. No failures were reported and the incidence of nonprogressive radiolucencies was only 27%. Similar results were described by Rand[3] who reported no failures and 100% excellent or good results among 28 TKAs performed using modular metal wedges. Even the most ardent proponent of prosthetic augmentation must concede, however, that these studies have relatively short-term follow-up. Furthermore, when evaluating the effectiveness of this technique, one finds only a handful of studies with short-term follow-up and a conspicuous lack of studies with long-term follow-up.

The relative paucity of studies, however, is not the only concern when evaluating the use of this surgical strategy. The use of a custom prosthesis greatly increases the cost of the procedure and results in a delay due to the time required for design and production.[1,23–27] Moreover, although the size and shape of these devices are determined through preoperative radiographic studies, the defects found at the time of surgery often do not exactly match the implant,[1,23–28] thus rendering the component relatively useless. The use of modular wedge augmentation eliminates the delay introduced by production and provides the surgeon a great deal of flexibility by allowing component "customization" during the procedure. This ability to customize the component, however, is determined by the size of the augments themselves, and use of prosthetic augmentation is often limited by the size and shape of the bone defect.[22,29,30] Augments may not be able to approximate larger defects, thus limiting the ability of the surgeon to restore an appropriate joint line.[30] Furthermore, this method continues to result in increased costs. These costs are realized as both the charge for the augments themselves and the required increase in inventory.

There is another issue presented by the use of additional components when augmenting the prosthesis. This concerns the possibility of augment loosening and subsequent generation of wear debris.[21,22] The use of augments potentially allows for an additional moveable component within the prosthesis and introduces a new interface that could possibly generate additional wear debris.[24] Furthermore, the method of fixation between an augment and the prosthesis may also provide additional problems.

Modular metal augmentation wedges and blocks are affixed to the undersurface of the implantable tibial tray with cement, screws, or snap-lock mechanisms. The durability of the cement interface between the prosthetic tray and the modular augment has been the subject of considerable speculation.[9] The extent of *in vivo* biomechanical analysis consists of a single case of cemented wedge retrieval reported by Rand.[31] Following 5 years of use, the interface between the modular metal wedge and the tibial tray remained well fixed. No data are available for assessment of screw or snap-fit modular junctions at this time. Micromotion and debris generation at the screw–augment or augment–tray interface remain of theoretical concern.

The last concern raised by prosthetic augmentation is largely a philosophical one and centers around the fact that this technique often results in additional bone loss.[9,24,28] A basic tenet of reconstructive joint surgery is to preserve bone stock at all time.[6] The use of wedge and block prosthetic augmentation almost always requires that additional bone be removed to ensure that the construct seat appropriately on the bone bed. Should a revision procedure be warranted in the future, retaining as much bone stock as possible will become a critical consideration. It is probably for this reason that Mason and Scott[9] recommend that the use of prosthetic augmentation be limited to "less active, older patients."

Most of the surgical techniques discussed to this point have an adverse affect on the amount of bone stock. Resection of the defect and preparation of the bone bed for either cement-fill or prosthetic augmentation require the removal of additional bone. In effect, these methods treat bone loss by first increasing the amount of bone loss present. Only one method reverses this trend and increases the amount of bone stock available: bone grafting.

## Bone grafting

As stated previously, it is important to recognize that the nature of bone defects encountered during primary TKA is very different from that of the bone deficiencies encountered during revision TKA. We have had success in addressing these two different situations with two separate classification schemes. Primary bone defects can be simply divided into femoral defects, tibial defects less than 12 mm in depth, and tibial defects greater than 12 mm in depth.[6] Bone deficiencies encountered during revision TKA may be classified into three major categories: cystic; plateau or condylar defects of femur and tibia; and central cavitary defects.[6,7]

### Autogenous bone grafting in primary total knee arthroplasty

In patients with less than 6 mm of deficiency on the medial side of the tibia, the tibial osteotomy can be performed at the base of the defect. If there is a slightly greater deficit, a small defect may remain after tibial resection. In these cases, the remaining sclerotic bed can be fenestrated with an 3 mm drill to allow penetration of bone cement, and the 2–3 mm remaining void can be filled with PMMA. Larger defects, and those defects encountered with deficiencies greater than 12 mm are best treated with autogenous bone graft.

Autogenous bone is readily available at the time of primary TKA and can be harvested from a number of areas. Laskin[32] has reported on bone utilized from the posterior femoral condyle to fill these tibial defects. Although this is a useful technique, the bone is often insufficient if reconstruction of large defects is needed. The bone is also primarily cortical and subchondral and the cancellous substrate is quite meager. The following technique has been developed by the senior author (TPS), and utilizes bone resected from the distal femur.[1,28]

The initial tibial proximal osteotomy is performed perpendicular to the long axis of a line drawn from the midpoint of the tibial surface to the midpoint of the ankle joint. This proximal tibial cut should be conservative, resecting no more than 8 mm of bone. An oscillating saw is then used to create an oblique osteotomy on the side of the tibial defect. The concave surface of the defect should be resected, as it will be filled with sclerotic, arthritic bone. The deep surface of the bed, once the osteotomy has been performed through the bed of the defect, should be 80–90% cancellous. There may be cystic areas in this bed once the sclerotic surface has been removed, and these may be curetted and filled with cancellous bone. It is important to adequately remove this sclerotic bed, as consolidation of the graft will be greatly impeded if there is not a cancellous bed onto which to place the donor bone. The cut should be planar and smooth so that a flattened graft will fit intimately with the bed (Fig. 3.12).

The tibial surface should then be gauged and prepared for the tibial component. Peg, keel, or other fixation surfaces should be made to ensure that the pin and screw stabilization of the bone graft do not compromise tibial component seating.

Attention is then drawn to the femur where distal femoral bone is resected in the standard manner. The resected distal medial femoral condyle is larger than the lateral condyle and therefore tends to be better graft material. Having resected the distal femoral condyle, this segment of bone is then rotated so that its cancellous surface fills the defect on the upper tibia and there is intimate coaptation between graft and underlying bed (Fig. 3.13). The defect should be completely filled with the graft. There will often be an overhanging segment of bone, which protrudes above the surface of the tibia. If there is any rocking of the graft or irregular surfaces on the tibial bed, these must be shaved until the surface is planar. Once coaptation is precise, two

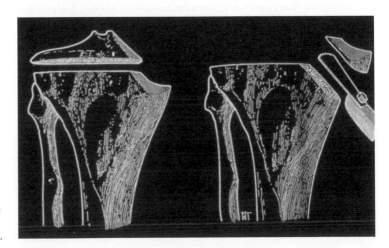

**Fig. 3.12**

Upper tibial osteotomy has been made with planar excision of the sclerotic bed of the bone defect (Reprinted with permission from Sculco 1994).

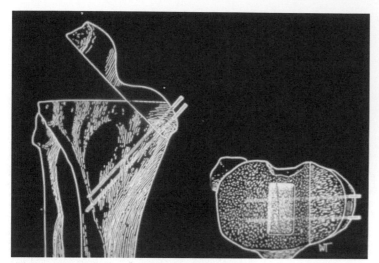

**Fig. 3.13**

Femoral condyle is used to fill the defect with cancellous-to-cancellous coaptation. Note reconstitution of the tibial peripheral rim on the view of the top surface of the tibia (right) (Reprinted with permission from Sculco 1994).

Kirschner wires may be used to stabilize the graft to the proximal tibia. The wires should be inserted peripherally so that when the overhanging portion of the bone graft is resected these pins do not prevent a complete osteotomy. Once this graft has been fixed, the excess graft bone is resected using the tibial cut of the opposite of the tibial plateau as a guide. At this point the proximal tibia will be reconstituted. On looking at the upper surface of the tibia the subchondral bone of the femoral condylar bone when resected will act as the peripheral tibial rim of the upper tibia.

The Kirschner wires are then individually removed and replaced with screws. Cancellous malleolar screws may be used for fixation. As an alternative, cortical screws can be used and the screw hole can be overdrilled at its entrance point to allow compression of the graft. The fixation hole of the prosthesis should be examined when the holes are being drilled and the screw length determined with a gauge to avoid inserting a screw that will contact the tibial prosthesis. This is particularly important if stainless steel screws are used, therefore vitallium or titanium screws are preferable (Fig. 3.14).

It is important that cement not be allowed to enter the interval between the graft and the recipient bed. This can be prevented by cementing the femoral and patellar components first. A small portion of cement can be used to caulk the interface between the graft and the underlying tibia by applying it to the upper surface of the tibia at the graft–tibia interface. This will harden so that when the lower-viscosity tibial cement is inserted it will not penetrate into the graft interface. Initially this was not appreciated and in the first patient undergoing this technique the graft became sclerotic. However, in follow-up at 13 years the graft had not resorbed or collapsed and there has been no shift in implant position (Fig. 3.15).

Postoperative rehabilitation for these patients is the same as for patients without bone grafting. Because the tibial implant support is

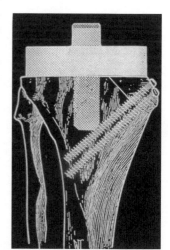

**Fig. 3.14**

Bone graft is fixed with cortical screws and the implant is seated (Reprinted with permission from Sculco 1994).

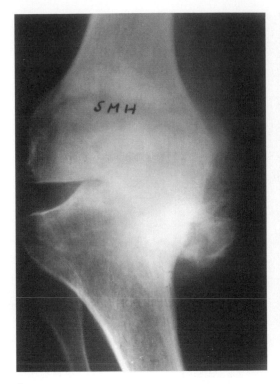

a

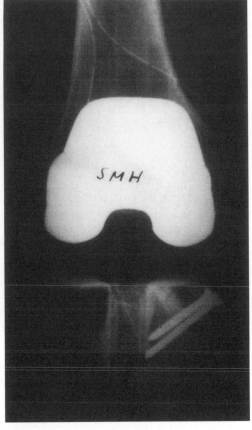

b

**Fig. 3.15**

(a) A 70 year old patient presented with varus deformity
and tibial bone loss. (b) This
represents the first autogenous
bone graft performed by the
senior author (TPS) using the
method he currently employs.
Note polymethylmethacrylate
in the graft-tibial interface.
(c) At 13 year follow-up, sclerosis of the graft is noted, but
there is no evidence of resorption or collapse (Reprinted
with permission from Sculco
1994).

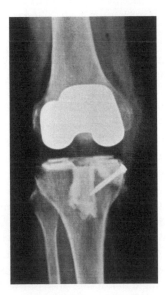

c

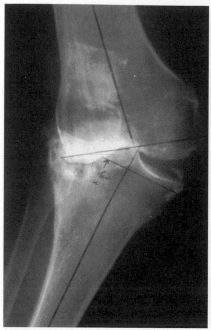
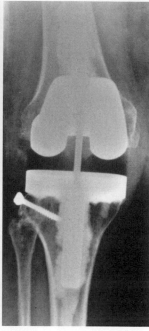

a
b

**Fig. 3.16**

(a) A severe valgus deformity with a severe lateral bone deficit. (b) Radiograph showing graft incorporation without evidence of resorption or collapse 8 years after the procedure (Reprinted with permission from Sculco 1994).

maintained on the more normal side of the tibia and because of the excellent fixation of the graft, modification of weightbearing has not been necessary. Continuous passive motion is employed on the first postoperative day and most patients are discharged with a cane.

This use of this technique has been reported in 35 patients over the last 14 years.[1,28] The results to date have been excellent with radiographic evidence of graft consolidation and no patient experiencing collapse of the graft (Fig. 3.16). In two patients reoperation has been necessary (one patient for infection, one for ligamentous instability after a fall). Examination of the graft site in both patients revealed evidence of trabecular incorporation at the graft–tibia interface.

### Femoral bone loss in primary total knee arthroplasty

Femoral bone loss occurs less commonly than tibial bone loss. It is typically seen in post-traumatic or inflammatory arthritis associated with osteonecrosis, occurs most frequently in the valgus knee, and is almost always associated with bone loss on the tibial side as well. The concepts of management of femoral bone loss are similar to those for tibial bone loss, and include developing a suitable cancellous bed for the graft, achieving optimal coaptation of the graft to the bed, maintaining position of the graft with internal fixation devices, and re-establishing the joint line to its proper height.

The surgeon must adequately expose the distal femoral condyles in order to visualize the anterior and posterior margins of the femoral bone. All soft tissue at the interface between the collapsed and normal bone must be debrided from the bony surface of the femur to allow thorough evaluation of the defect. In many instances the femoral bone loss may be cystic, especially in inflammatory arthritis, and these are easily grafted using bone from the intercondylar area or from the tibia during preparation of the tibial implant seating hole. This cancellous bone can be impacted into these cystic areas and a deficient surface can be completely filled with this bone.

For extensive defects where there has been complete loss of the condylar surface, more formal grafting will be necessary. Bone can be used from the intercondylar area and fixation screws can be inserted directly into the graft and advanced into the underlying femoral bone along the longitudinal axis of the femur. As with tibial grafts, screws must be composed of compatible metals, and precise coaptation must be achieved.

When grafting the distal femur it is important to re-establish the joint line at the location close to its anatomic origin. The distal articular surface of the femoral condyle was measured in a series of 30 knees at surgical reconstruction. Its location was determined by using the anterior margin of the collateral ligament at its origin from the femur. This is a constant landmark and is generally present except in the most severe cases of femoral condylar bone loss. The distance from the anterior margin of the ligament to the articular surface was 17–20 mm in this series of knees evaluated. Therefore the articular surface of the femoral component should be placed at this distance from the collateral ligament origin to approximate the normal location of the joint line. The graft must allow seating of the femoral component to reproduce this measurement if the joint line is to be maintained in the replaced knee.

## Bone grafting in revision total knee arthroplasty

Bone deficiency is a common finding in revision knee replacement surgery. Bone loss may at times be the cause of the total knee replacement failure, but more commonly it is produced when the implants themselves loosen. The inflammatory environment produced by PMMA fragmentation, wear debris, and other factors is not fully understood, but it is known that it can produce a progressive and injurious loss of bone support to the implant. Additionally, levering the component from the underlying bone at the time of revision surgery may cause further bone collapse and fracture.

In the revision knee replacement three major types of bone defects may be present, and each is managed in a different manner. There may be variations or combinations of these three general types of bone loss, but cystic deficiencies, central medullary deficiencies, and peripheral plateau or condylar bone loss remain the generic categories of bone loss in revision knee replacement.

### CYSTIC DEFICIENCIES

Cystic deficiencies are generally encountered on the surfaces of the tibia and femur after removal of the total knee implant. They may be the result of cement which has penetrated into the subchondral bone and produced a punctate crater. They also may occur when the implant itself is removed from the bone and portions of the bone adhere to the implant. If the femoral component has condylar fixation pegs, these may produce cystic areas of bone loss in the underlying bone. Usually these cystic areas are associated with larger plateau or condylar deficiencies and, therefore, combined techniques to handle both problems must be employed.

Cystic defects are easily filled with cancellous bone available locally at the time of the revision. The base of the deficiency should be cleared of any adherent cement and soft tissue. The cancellous bone should be driven deep into the depression with an impactor. The bone will usually compress without problem into these areas and a significantly improved surface will be available to the implant. If sufficient bone is not available from local bone removed at revision surgery, iliac crest bone can be used.

CENTRAL MEDULLARY DEFICIENCIES

Central medullary bone deficiencies may be present on the femur or tibia during revision surgery. These most often occur if the primary implants used had central intramedullary stems. The deficiency on the tibial surface is funnel-shaped and can be quite large. Often only the cortical rim is left without any cancellous plateau support on the medial or lateral side.

Because of the poor quality of supporting bone of the surface faces of the femur and tibia in these cases, the surgeon must add bone to the deficient areas and then transfer load and stress distal to the defect by utilizing an intramedullary stem. Usually autogenous bone is inadequate to deal with these larger defects even if the entire iliac crest is used. Femoral head allograft bone is often needed. The femoral head can be shaped to fill these large cavitary defects and a hole placed through the graft once the head has been impacted into place. The stem can then be passed through this fenestration and gain fixation beyond it (Fig. 3.17). Autogenous bone, when it is available, can be placed around the allograft in an attempt to augment incorporation of the periphery of the graft. There is concern that in using these large allografts resorption may occur with time, but this tendency may be lessened by unloading the graft with the use of intramedullary stems.

The availability of modular revision systems allows for variation in the length and thickness of the tibial and femoral stems. The length of the stem is determined by the quality of the proximal femoral and tibial bone. Currently the stems are not being cemented but rather are fluted rods, which are sized to gain purchase on the cortical bone of the femur and tibia. The stems are press-fitted into the canals, and the upper portion of the stem and implant are cemented in place. Careful preoperative planing is mandatory in these cases so that implants of the proper length and diameter are available.

**Fig. 3.17**

(a) A 70 year old patient with rheumatoid arthritis and loosening of the tibial component. (b) At time of revision, there is marked central cavitary bone loss (see also colour plate section). (c) Revision radiograph demonstrates a femoral head allograft in place to fill the defect, using a modular stemmed implant with wedge (Reprinted with permission from Sculco 1994).

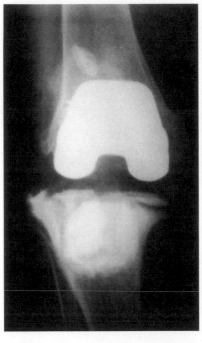

a

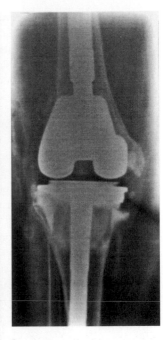

c

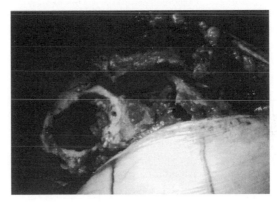

b

PERIPHERAL TIBIAL PLATEAU OR CONDYLAR BONE LOSS

Peripheral rather than intramedullary loss can occur in those cases in which the previous implant has been malaligned or where there has been an overload of once femoral condyle or tibial plateau. Bone collapse occurs on the overloaded side of the implant with tension forces on the opposite side causing liftoff of the implant from the bone. At times the entire plateau or condyle may collapse.

The tendency to resect further bone to get below the base of the defect must be avoided. These defects can be handled with either autogenous bone graft harvested from the iliac crest or bone allograft. Bone loss on the tibial side can be replaced by taking an iliac crest graft and using the cancellous surface against the cancellous bone and allowing the cortical surface to provide support to the implant. A stemmed component must be used in these cases to transfer load to the more distal tibia.

## Discussion

A number of potential concerns regarding the use of bone grafting techniques during TKA have been raised. Criticisms of the use of autograft bone are few and focus primarily on the finite supply available[22,27] and the degree of carpentry necessary to shape grafts for certain defects, specifically posterior femoral condylar defects.[33,34] Additional concerns have been raised regarding the use of bone allograft in conjunction with TKA. Some authors have questioned the biological capacity of this construct, pointing out the potential for delayed[21,23,28] or unpredictable[22,28,34,35] graft incorporation. Other authors have focused on the strength of the construct and the possibility for subsequent resorption[25-27,29,30] and late collapse.[22,23,30,35] Increased risk of infection, with the allograft acting as a source of viral transmission[22,29,30] or as a nidus for late infection,[4,30] represents the third category of concerns. The majority of these concerns can be addressed by reviewing the benefits of this surgical technique.

The advantages of bone grafting can be broadly divided into four categories: intraoperative, economic, biomechanical, and biological. Intraoperative advantages include bone availability,[26,27,30,35] graft versatility,[5,23,26,33] and the relative technical ease of the procedure.[28,35] Concerns about potentially prohibitive technical requirements appear to be unfounded in most situations. Economic advantages include the decreased cost of bone graft (particularly of autograft),[27,29,30] and the decreased need for the use of custom prostheses to address particularly large defects for which prosthetic augmentation may be insufficient.[1,26] Biomechanical advantages include better load transfer,[15,22,23] and uniform cement thickness and decreased fragmentation of cement.[1,24,26] This has resulted in the production of a durable construct[23,24,34] with no increase in the rate of radiographic radiolucencies.[28]

A number of studies have offered evidence of the biological advantages of bone grafting. These advantages include rapid union[5,30,36] and biological incorporation of the grafts.[24,26,27,30] Dorr et al.[24] demonstrated evidence of bone graft union and revascularization through tomogram, bone scan, and bone biopsy. In this study 24 bone graft constructs were followed for 3 to 6 years, and 22 grafts exhibited evidence of union with incorporation present by 6 months. Similarly good results have been reported with the use of allografts as well. Tsahakis et al.[37] reported 100% graft incorporation among 19 allografts after 1 year. Wilde et al.[38] demonstrated evidence of graft incorporation through use of a SPECT scan among 11 of 12 allografts with approximately 2 year follow-up. Furthermore, Mow and Wiedel[27] followed 15 allografts for an average of

4 years, and found no evidence of graft failure. Additional biological advantages are preservation of a greater area of native subchondral bone,[1,24,26] and the restoration of additional bone stock.[7,21–23,28,29,32] Most authors agree that bone stock preservation is a critical consideration, especially among younger and higher demand patients who may require additional procedures in the future.[4,27,30,34–36]

Concerns about the rate of infection are not unfounded. Reported infection rates of 10%[4] and 12%[39] are appreciable risks. However, it should be pointed out that these occurred in studies in which massive allografts were used. The enormous size of the defects being addressed most likely prohibited the use of prosthetic wedge augmentation. To compare these infection rates to those incurred with prosthetic wedge augmentation would be inaccurate and misleading.

## Summary

Bone grafting provides the surgeon with a biological approach to the management of bone deficiency in either primary or revision TKA. Many techniques for dealing with bone deficiency are available to the surgeon who is performing a TKA. The size, shape, and location of these defects range widely, especially in revision TKA, and each bone deficiency will possess a unique set of characteristics. The bone stock for each TKA possesses its own "personality." For this reason no single method for addressing bone defects will be the ideal treatment alternative in every case. However, whenever possible, preservation of the underlying bone is vital to the long-term success of the replacement. In primary knee replacement with autogenous bone readily available, grafting should be used. Modular wedge augments are costly, may not fit, and have problematic attachments to the baseplate which may increase debris formation. In revision total knee replacement, both allograft and autograft, in conjunction with modular revision total knee systems in the more difficult cases, seem to be the best solution at this time. Modular systems provide the flexibility needed to augment bone deficiency and also transfer load away from deficient areas to more distal sites. The long-term results with these systems, however, await the passage of time.

# References

1   Windsor RE, Insall JN, Sculco TP: Bone grafting of tibial defects in primary and revision total knee arthroplasty. *Clinical Orthopaedics and Related Research* **205**:132–137, 1986.

2   Dorr LD: Bone grafts for bone loss with total knee replacement. *Orthopaedic Clinics of North America* **20**:179–187, 1989

3   Rand JA: Bone deficiency in total knee arthroplasty: The use of metal wedge augmentation. *Clinical Orthopaedics and Related Research* **271**:63–71, 1991.

4   Ghazavi MT, Stockley I, Yee G *et al.*: Reconstruction of massive bone defects with allograft in revision total knee arthroplasty. *Journal of Bone and Joint Surgery* [Am] **79**:17–25, 1997.

5   Engh GA, Ammeen DJ: Classification and preoperative radiographic evaluation: Knee. *Orthopaedic Clinics of North America* **29**:205–217, 1998.

6   Sculco TP: Bone grafting in total knee arthroplasty. In *Revision total knee replacement*, ed. WN Scott, pp. 1333–1344. Mosby, St. Louis, 1994.

7   Sculco TP, Choi JC: Management of severe bone loss: The role and results of bone grafting in revision total knee replacement. In *Revision total knee arthroplasty*, ed. PA Lotke, JP Garino, pp. 197–206. Lippincott-Raven, Philadelphia, 1999.

8   Laskin RS, Saddler SC: Bone defects in total knee arthroplasty. In *Knee surgery*, eds. FH Fu, CD Harner, KG Vince, pp. 1399–1405. Williams and Wilkins, Baltimore, 1994.

9   Mason JB, Scott RD: Management of severe bone loss: Prosthetic modularity and custom implants. In *Revision total knee arthroplasty*, ed. PA Lotke, JP Garino, pp. 207–216. Lippincott-Raven, Philadelphia, 1999.

10  Laskin RS: Tricon-M uncemented total knee arthroplasty. *Journal of Arthroplasty* **3**:27–38, 1988.

11  Lotke PA, Wong R, Ecker M: The management of large tibial defects in primary total knee replacement. *Orthopaedic Transactions* **9**:425, 1985.

12  Scott RD: Bone loss: prosthetic and augmentation methods. *Orthopedics* **18**:923–926, 1995.

13  Hvid I: Trabecular bone strength at the knee. *Clinical Orthopaedics and Related Research* **227**:210–221, 1988.

14  Sneppen D, Christensen P, Larsen H, Vang PS: Mechanical testing of trabecular bone in total knee replacement. Development of an osteopenetrometer. *International Orthopaedics (SICOT)* **5**:251–256, 1981.

15  Dorr LD, Conaty JP, Schreiber R *et al.*: 1985 Technical factors that influence mechanical loosening of total knee arthroplasty. In *The Knee*, ed. LD Dorr, pp. 121–135. University Park Press, Baltimore.

16  Ritter M: Screw and cement fixation of large tibial defects in total knee arthroplasty. *Journal of Arthroplasty* **1**:125–129, 1986.

17  Ritter M, Keating M, Faris P: Screw and cement fixation of large tibial defects in total knee arthroplasty: A sequel. *Journal of Arthroplasty* **8**:63–65, 1993.

18  Brooks PJ, Walker PS, Scott RD: Tibial component fixation in deficient tibial bone stock. *Clinical Orthopaedics and Related Research* **184**:302–308, 1984.

19  Freeman MAR, Bradley GW, Revell PA: Observations upon the interface between bone and polymethylmethacrylate cement. *Journal of Bone and Joint Surgery* [Br] **64**:489–493, 1982.

20  Ginther JR, Ritter MA: The management of severe bone loss: Methylmethacrylate cement as fill. In *Revision total knee arthroplasty*, ed. PA Lotke, JP Garino, pp. 217–225. Lippincott-Raven, Philadelphia, 1999.

21  Rand JA: Modular augments in revision total knee arthroplasty. *Orthopedic Clinics of North America* **29**:347–353, 1998.

22  Dennis DA: Repairing minor bone defects: Augmentation and autograft. *Orthopedics* **21**:1036–1038, 1998.

23  Brand MG, Daley RJ, Ewald FC, Scott RC: Tibial tray augmentation with modular metal wedges for tibial bone stock deficiency. *Clinical Orthopaedics and Related Research* **248**:74–79, 1989.

24  Dorr LD Ranawat CS, Sculco TP *et al.* 1995 Bone graft for defects in total knee arthroplasty. *Clinical Orthopedics and Related Research* **205**:153–165.

25  Scott RD: Revision total knee arthroplasty. *Clinical Orthopaedics and Related Research* **226**:65–77, 1988.

26  Scuderi GR, Insall JN, Haas SB *et al.*: Inlay autogeneic bone grafting of tibial defects in primary total knee arthroplasty. *Clinical Orthopaedics and Related Research* **248**:93–97, 1989.

27  Mow CS, Wiedel JD: Structural allografting in revision total knee arthroplasty. *Journal of Arthroplasty* **11**:235–241, 1996.

28  Altchek D, Sculco TP, Rawlins B: Autogenous bone grafting for severe angular deformity in total knee arthroplasty. *Journal of Arthroplasty* **4**:151–155, 1989.

29  Rorabeck CH, Smith PN: 1998 Results of revision total knee arthroplasty in the face of significant bone deficiency. *Orthopedic Clinics of North America* **29**:361–371.

30  Engh GA, Parks NL: The management of bone defects in revision total knee arthroplasty. *Instructional Course Lectures* **46**:227–236, 1997.

31  Rand JA: Augmentation of a total knee arthroplasty with a modular metal wedge: a case report. *Journal of Bone and Joint Surgery* [Am] **77**:266–268, 1995.

32  Laskin RS: Total knee replacement in the presence of large bony defects of the tibia and marked knee instability. *Clinical Orthopaedics and Related Research* **248**:66–70, 1989.

33  Rosenberg AG: The use of bone graft for managing bone defects in complex total knee arthroplasty. *American Journal of Knee Surgery* **10**:42–48, 1997.

34  Whiteside LA, Bichallo PS: Radiologic and histologic analysis of morselized allograft in revision total knee arthroplasty. *Clinical Orthopaedics and Related Research* **357**:149–156, 1998.

35  Aligetti P, Buzzi R, Scrobe F: Autologous bone grafting for medial tibial defects in total knee arthroplasty. *Journal of Arthroplasty* **6**:287–294, 1991.

36  Ries MD: Impacted cancellous autograft for contained bone defects in total knee arthroplasty. *American Journal of Knee Surgery* **9**:51–54, 1996.

37  Tsahakis PJ, Beaver WG, Brick GW: Technique and results of allograft reconstruction in revision total knee replacement. *Clinical Orthopaedics and Related Research* **303**:86–92, 1994.

38  Wilde AH, Schickendantz MS, Stulberg BN, Go RT: The incorporation of tibial allograft in total knee arthroplasty. *Journal of Bone and Joint Surgery* [Am] **72**:815–823, 1990.

39  Lord CF, Gebhardt MC, Tomford WW, Mankin HJ: Infection in bone grafts: incidence, nature, and treatment. *Journal of Bone and Joint Surgery* [Am] **70**:369–378, 1988.

## Questions and answers

*Moderator:* Dr. Sculco, do you have any age limit on using bone grafts for defects in primary knees? Should older patients have augments?

*Dr. Sculco:* In primary total knee replacement with severe bone loss, patient age has not been a factor in selection of autogenous bone grafting to deal with these defects. However, bone quality is a consideration. Osteopenic bone is uncommon, and indeed the bed of the defect tends to be somewhat sclerotic even after resection and shaping. If however very inferior bone is present, then I prefer prosthetic augmentation. In evaluation of results in over 50 patients with autogenous grafts for tibial defects, chronological age *per se* was not a factor in graft incorporation.

*Moderator:* Dr. Rand, although you have stated that although you do use modular augments, you will at times also use bone graft. Could you lay out for us your algorithm that helps you make your decision. Is age a consideration for you?

*Dr. Rand:* The appropriate use of a bone graft in revision surgery is dependent on the age of the patient, as well as the extent of the bone deficiency. In the patient of physiological younger age, bone graft is preferred to the use of a large customized implant or large bone augment, as the potential exists for the replacement of bone stock. Unfortunately, retrieval studies of bone graft have shown limited incorporation and revasculaization of the bone graft at 5–7 years. The larger the bone graft, the less potential exists for revascularization, unless it is a morselized graft. Modular metal augments are preferred for type 2 bone deficiencies. The results of histological analysis of 9 structural bone grafts in 4 patients at 62 months were reported by Parks and Engh in 1997. Of the 4 knees, 2 were revision and 2 primary arthroplasties. Two core biopsies of grafts were taken during revision surgery. Although the graft showed no signs of trabecular collapse or resorption, the bone was acellular and had not been revascularized. At the host bone graft junction, there was evidence of new bone deposition on the dead graft. Only the autograft showed viable bone trabecula within the graft. The results of structural bone grafts in revision TKA have been variable. In a META analysis of 136 structural bone grafts in 131 knees with follow-up of 2–4.5 years, union occurred in 92%. Graft collapse occurred in 16 (12%). The failure of union or collapse of the graft is a concern when using large structural bone grafts. Modular bone augments do not require healing and do not collapse. However, type 3 bone defects are not well suited to modular bone augments, as the bone–cement interdigitation in the remaining sclerotic bone provides poor fixation. In contrast to the results of structural graft, morselized bone graft displays a different process of healing. Whiteside and Bicallo in 1998 obtained biopsies in 14 patients at reoperation, 3 weeks to 37 months following particulate bone grafting for revision arthroplasty. There was evidence of enchondral ossification within the grafts with woven bone and lamellar bone present at 18 months. Dead trabecular bone became encased in new bone by 37 months.

*Moderator:* Dr. Sculco, are you using any types of bone augmentation materials with your bone graft such as Grafton? What are your thoughts regarding this materials to supplement your graft?

*Dr. Sculco:* In the primary knee, bone defects are easily handled with autogenous bone that is available from bone resected as part of the procedure. It is important that intimate coaptation be achieved between the base of the defdect and the bone graft. The bed of the tibial defect must also be primarily autogenous with the sclerotic surface resected. Therefore in the primary knee, graft supplements are not necessary. In the revision knee, since there is less autogenous bone available (although some will be present as part of the recutting of the surfaces), bone supplements may be used to augment grafts. There are a number of suitable bone augmentation supplements materials available, including Collograft, Grafton, and Opteform.

*Moderator:* Now that you brought up the topic of availability of bone in revision surgery, do you use iliac crest bone graft? If so, do you really believe that an iliac crest bone graft is a lesser procedure than a metallic augmentation in these cases? Can you really accept the reported 20% incidence of iliac crest donor site pain reported in the literature?

*Dr. Sculco:* I rarely use iliac crest bone as autogenous supplement to bone deficiency in the revision total knee replacement patient. The ideal situation would be in the younger patients with bone loss where reconstitution of bone is crucial should further revision procedures be necessary at a later date. When iliac crest is used, usually small segments are used or just the intercortical cancellous bone alone, and therefore complications related to the donor site tend to be less that when large full-thickness grafts are used.

*Moderator:* Dr. Rand, do you have an algorithm for which type of augment you use, a block or a wedge. By the way, we should all consider calling these devices augments, since the term a "block wedge" is an oxymoron.

*Dr. Rand:* I feel that a wedge augment is appropriate for defects that are angled less than 10–15°. For wider-angled peripheral defects on the tibia, a block augment is utilized as this provides less shear forces across the augment-bone interface.

*Moderator:* When you have to revise a femoral component, we have often found soft osteopenic bone in the trochlear area that often is removed hen the femoral component is removed. What do you use for this area, augments or bone graft?

*Dr. Rand:* The bone that is found in the trochlear area during revision is often osteopenic. This area had been stress protected by the trochlear design of the femoral component, accounting for its osteopenia. Bone loss in this area is best treated by cement filling and there is rarely a need to consider bone graft or augments to treat this. A long stemmed implant is utilized to stress relief past this area of the bone.

*Moderator:* I would like to get back to Dr. Sculco again to discuss the exact type of bone graft that he uses. Is the bone you take for these cases freeze dried or frozen? Have you had problems with patients accepting the potential risks of allograft bone?

*Dr. Sculco:* When larger allografts segments are needed for significant bone deficiency in the revision setting, either freeze dried or frozen bone can be used. I prefer to use frozen bone as the handling proprieties are often superior, particularly for strut grating. The danger with disease transmission is always present when cadaveric bone is used, even though most commercial bone banks are extremely thorough in donor screening and bone preparation. The risks must be discussed with the patient and most are amenable to the use of bone when its advantages are explained. Biologic reconstitution of deficient bone is advantageous particularly in younger patients undergoing revision knee replacement, and most patients are willing to accept the minimal risks related to disease transmission when weighed against the benefits of allografting large areas of bone loss.

*Moderator:* Dr. Sculco has said that all augments require the surgeon to sacrifice bone, while bone grafting adds bone. How do you respond to this?

*Dr. Rand:* Modular bone augments are used to treat bone that is already deficient. In a primary knee, if a block augment is used on the tibia, some minimal additional bone is resected to accommodate the augment. With a wedge augment, very little bone is removed as the wedge often corresponds to the shape of the bone deficiency. In revision surgery, there is deficient bone on the femur and tibia that is considerably greater than that encountered in primary arthroplasty. Modular bone augments replace the deficient bone and generally do not sacrifice any appreciable amount of additional remaining bone with their use. Although structural bone grafts can be utilized to compensate for the bone deficiency, they probably act more as prosthesis than living bone, and their long-term ability to replace the deficient bone remains unknown.

*Moderator:* Augments cost money but autologous bone does not. Do the results using the augments justify the added cost?

*Dr. Rand:* Although autologous bone is present at primary arthroplasty, it is generally not available locally at the time of revision arthroplasty. In these situations, autologous bone requires harvesting of a remote source such as the iliac crest with the associated morbidity and cost of operating time. Iliac crest bone grafts do not fit well into bone deficiencies encountered at the time of revision arthroplasty. Structural allografts used in revision surgery are expensive, and are more costly than modular metal augments. Contouring the structural grafts to fit the bone defects is complex, and the increased operating time and its associated cost probably outweigh any potential cost saving, compared to the use of a simple modular metallic augment.

*Moderator:* Have you ever had to go back in on a knee that was bone grafted to ascertain the viability of your large grafts? Have you done any biopsies of the grafted knee? Has anyone? If not, how can you be sure that you just don't have a large piece of inanimate material there (much like you would with a prosthetic augment)?

*Dr. Sculco:* Viability of autogenous grafting has been evaluated *in vivo* both by myself and by Dr. Dorr at the time of revision surgery. Histological examination has demonstrated viable bone at the interface with dead (although structurally sound) bone at the peripheral areas and particularly in areas with significant cortical bone. When revision surgery has been performed after autogenous grafting, structural support is maintained at the graft site for implantation and stability of the revision components. There has been some peripheral resorption of the autogenous bone grafts in about 15% of patients but this has not led to loss of implant position. When larger allografts are used, most of the graft is not viable but structurally sound. Incorporation of the graft to the underlying host bone is present, however, and this interface *is* viable. The advantage, even though this bone is largely not viable, is that there is bone that is attached to the host and should revision surgery be necessary, this gives a larger area to accept the revision prosthesis. There is a real advantage to this biological setting, rather than using costly and often poorly fitting prosthetic filler devices that may gain poor fixation and have large level arms that may accelerate prosthetic failure.

## 4

*In the normal knee, the posterior cruciate ligament is an important restraint to posterior directed forces on the tibia. Its insertion on to the tibia is below the joint line, enabling its retention when the tibia plateau is resected. We can save it, but should we?*

# The posterior cruciate ligament should routinely be salvaged during total knee replacement

## Pro: Sandeep Munjal and Kenneth A. Krackow

In total knee arthroplasty (TKA), two different approaches are taken with regard to the posterior cruciate ligament (PCL):

- maintaining the ligament (PCL-retaining, PCR prostheses)
- substituting for the ligament (PCL-substituting or posterior stabilized [PS] prostheses).

The PCL provides 95% of the total restraining force to posterior tibial displacement and is therefore the primary restraint to posterior tibial translation. All other ligamentous and soft tissue structures provide the remaining 5% of the secondary restraint.[1] In addition, the PCL is believed to facilitate the "screw-home" mechanism as the knee is brought to full extension.[2]

In the normal knee, a large range of motion is achieved through a combination of bone geometry and ligament constraint. As the knee flexes, the insertion point of the PCL on the lateral aspect of the medial femoral condyle begins to displace anteriorly, increasing tension in the PCL. As flexion continues the insertion point would continue to proceed anteriorly, but the PCL checks this motion causing a posterior displacement or rollback of the femur on the tibia with increasing flexion. This posterior translation assures that the femoral shaft will not impinge on the posterior tibial plateau, permitting flexion approaching 140°. Without this mechanism, impingement of the soft tissues of the knee, and also the bony margins of the posterior rim of the tibia and the posterior aspect of the femur, would limit flexion to between 90 and 105°.

This femoral rollback during knee flexion is also thought to be beneficial in providing an effective increase in the extensor mechanism lever arm. As the femoral tibial contact location moves posteriorly away from the patellar tendon[3,4] there is resultant anteriorization of the tibial tubercle relative to the axis of knee flexion.

The PCL is also seen to be a secondary stabilizer to varus and valgus laxity (2–10°).[3] The axes of tibial rotation with respect to the femur during varus–valgus "testing," i.e., while varus or valgus moments are placed on an extended or partially flexed knee, must lie within or even outside the respective lateral and medial compartments of the knee. That is, they could not be coincident with the center of the knee unless somehow the tibia were "swinging" on the PCL. When one is trying to effect lateral opening with a varus stress, if and when that opening occurs, it is obvious that the rotation must be occurring at some point of contact of the femur and tibia in the medial compartment. Or if the medial compartment is also distractible, then this rotation must be occurring even beyond the medial edge of the knee. With the PCLs being situated approximately in the center of the knee and therefore tending to prevent tibiofemoral distraction in this region, one can understand the mechanism of this secondary stabilization.

The issue of prosthetic selection in TKA, in terms of PCL retention versus sacrifice, is not clear to many; even the most experienced knee surgeons debate this issue. We believe that the PCL should be routinely preserved in TKA, and we base our practice on many of the points described below.

## Bone loss

It is important to spare bone in TKA, an operation which is, in truth, joint resurfacing. For most routine TKAs the bone cuts are made as conservatively as possible (measured resection) to give a well-balanced knee. Posterior cruciate substitution requires removal of significant amount of bone (5–8 cm$^3$) from the intercondylar notch to provide room for the post and cam mechanism. The femoral component must fit tightly "comfortably" into this area. Inadequate bone resection and subsequent hammering of the component can even result in intercondylar fracture.[5] The bone removed, particularly the cortical-like intercondylar bone from each of the medial and lateral femoral condyles, as well as the firm bone which is the roof of the intercondylar notch, seem to represent strong supporting material whose removal surely must be suboptimal. Particularly in rheumatoid and other patients with mild to significant amounts of osteopenia, this wholesale, or at least routine, removal is unattractive.

In the event of revision, although most cruciate-sparing TKAs can be revised to cruciate-substituting total knees, the latter may seem more likely to require revision to a higher constraint, i.e., a total stabilized or CCK type of TKA. It is particularly cautioned that the apparent success of PS primary total knee replacement cannot casually be extrapolated to infer comparable long-term success for these more conformed intercondylar mechanisms.[6]

## Kinematics

It is the major goal for many surgeons and inherent in the design of many prostheses to reproduce normal or as near normal kinematics of the knee as possible. Preservation of the PCL in TKA has been recognized by many authors to reproduce more normal knee kinematics, preserve anatomic femoral rollback, and increase the range of motion [2–4,7–10]. In the normal knee, femoral rollback can also increase the quadriceps efficiency.

Sorger et al.[10] studied the knee kinematics of intact knees, of PCL-retaining, TKAs, and of PCL-substituting TKAs. Their results showed that the PCL was able to prevent posterior translation and maintain femoral rollback when it was preserved during TKA. To optimize rollback and range of motion after total knee replacement with cruciate retention, it may be important to match the tibial slope and recess the PCL if tight.

In addition, retention of the PCL can also preserve anterior tibiofemoral contact during extension, which may be important during the heel strike phase of gait.[8]

## Proprioception

The cruciate ligaments accommodate morphologically different sensory nerve endings (Ruffini endings, Pacinian corpuscles, Golgi tendon organ-like endings, and free nerve endings), with different capabilities of providing the central nervous system with information not only about noxious and chemical events, but also about characteristics of movements and position-related stretches of these ligaments. The sensory system of the cruciate ligaments is able to contribute significantly to the functional stability of the knee joint.[11]

The current literature does not support a marked advantage for either cruciate-retaining or cruciate-substituting designs.[12–16] Recent sensitive immunohistochemical analysis[17] revealed plentiful and varied types of encapsulated mechanoreceptors found in even the arthritic PCL, suggesting a rich proprioceptive role. These findings tend to support those clinical reports of improved proprioception after PCL-retaining versus PCL-substituting TKAs. The presence of many and varied types of mechanoreceptors may account for the improved stair-climbing reported, and may contribute to a more normal feeling in patients with PCL-retained knees.

## Gait analysis

Gait usually undergoes excellent improvement after TKA. Nevertheless, some abnormalities persist even after a long period of time. The abnormal knee patterns have been attributed to several possible causes, such as implant geometry, surgical technique, PCL retention/substitution, pre-operative stiff knee pattern due to pain and altered biomechanics, weakness of extensor muscles, pre-operative arthritic pattern, and multi-joint degenerative involvement. Even for patients with an excellent functional score, the duration of implant survival may be compromised by an altered control of the knee.

In the three-dimensional knee motion, study of the PCL retaining and substituting knee by Ishii et al.,[18] although motion during the swing phase of gait was similar for both knee groups, abduction, adduction and proximal and distal translation were larger for the patients with PS implants, suggesting that the substituted surface may not reliably provide as much stability in these directions as does retention of the PCL.

Andriacchi has shown that by maintaining the increased quadriceps lever arm with a stabilized posterior tibiofemoral axis, patients with PCL retained arthroplasties have better function in stairclimbing. Also, the retained PCL as a secondary stabilizer to varus–valgus stress helps prevent lateral lift-off and stress loading of the medial compartment as the knee assumes a more adducted position in the stance phase of walking.[3,19]

## Deformity

Posterior cruciate sacrifice and substitution for major fixed varus and valgus deformities has been proposed.[7,8,20] We agree that PCL release or substitution may facilitate these corrections for severe cases. Furthermore, if *these* varus–valgus deformities are present in combination with flexion contracture, PCL release *may* be appropriate. However, this is not the same thing as agreeing that performing PCL resection *primarily for flexion contracture management* is appropriate. This is an important point because it commonly is stated that flexion contracture release requires sacrifice of the PCL.[5] If we consider a few simple arguments, we can see that the statement *must* be wrong.

To say that PCL release is necessary for flexion contracture management suggests that the flexion contracture is somehow caused or sustained by the PCL, and, if that sustentation is caused by the PCL, and one feels or "finds" that *release* improves the situation, the implication must be that the PCL is somehow tight, or contracted. A tight PCL however, would only serve to displace the tibia anteriorly. One even sees very clearly at surgery that the tight PCL obviously does "pull" the tibia anteriorly. Moving the tibia anterior with the knee in any degree of flexion does not cause or contribute to a flexion contracture. A tight anterior cruciate ligament, pulling the tibia posteriorly, could cause or participation the development and sustentation of flexion contracture, not a tight PCL. Again, a tight PCL draws the tibia anteriorly. How can this possibly create a flexion contracture?

Furthermore, laboratory work of the senior author[21] shows that the PCL release actually leads principally to a relative increase in the size of the flexion space and should, in itself, be *antagonistic* to improving many flexion contractures. This conclusion is also stated informally by both L. Whiteside (St Louis, MO, USA) and L. Dorr (Los Angeles, CA, USA). As a result, release of the PCL to deal with "pure" flexion contracture, i.e., flexion deformity without significant varus or valgus malalignment, will instead tend to thwart one's attempts to manage the flexion contracture. This result is seen because the increased thickness of tibial spacer required to provide stability of the knee at 90° of flexion, due to the relatively larger flexion space, will prohibit full extension and may require additional distal femoral resection to achieve full flexion.

The data from this study suggest that PCL sacrifice would lead either to a worsening of the flexion contracture, or to some measure of flexion instability with no improvement in the extension point.

In cases in which major flexion contractures exist in conjunction with severe varus or valgus deformities, we recognize that PCL release/sacrifice may be necessary as part of the management of *varus–valgus deformity*, but not as a part of flexion contracture management.

Also, in very extreme, typically rheumatoid situations, with major 70–90° flexion contractures, one may see true PCL and collateral ligament contractures of a great degree. In these very rare cases, PCL excision will be necessary. It is done not so much to "manage" the flexion contracture, bur rather to provide tibiofemoral separation necessary for simply getting the components into position.

## Stability

The PCL is present in 99% of the knees undergoing TKA. It is the view of many, including ourselves, that the retained PCL can share many tibiofemoral translational forces and some varus–valgus ones, thereby unloading the implant interface, unlike more conforming PCL-sacrificed knees. Those must rely not only on careful balancing of the flexion and extension spaces to achieve stability, but also on the higher conformity of the tibiofemoral articulation which must transfer much of the "ligament" load to the bone cement interface surrounding each implant.[12]

PCL substitution designs do provide a passive restraint against posterior instability, although without appropriate balance of the flexion and extension gaps, dislocation of the PS knee is possible.[20] A number of case reports in the literature have highlighted the concerns about dislocation with the PS TKA. In several large series of PS TKAS, posterior dislocation was reported in 2–2.6%, and further revision surgery was carried out in 0.6–0.8% of cases.[22,23]

## Summary

The longevity of TKA is well established.[24–28] The survivorship of both the PCL-substituting and PCL-retaining procedures is over 95% at 10 years.

Our preference for using a PCL-retaining TKA is based upon its being relatively bone sparing and having excellent kinematics. Also, recent identification of plentiful and varied mechanoreceptors found in arthritic PCLs, better three-dimensional understanding of gait pattern, and stability issues of PCL sacrifice are favorable considerations for retaining the PCL.

However, we do propose the selection of PCL-sacrificing prostheses (PS implants) in the following situations, which is only a very small fraction of the total number of TKAs in our practice:

- when the flexion space is too tight
- with *major* varus–valgus deformity
- in the chronically subluxed knee
- for residual A/P translation instability.

# References

1   Noyes FR, Stowers SF, Grood ES: Posterior subluxations of the medial and lateral tibiofemoral compartments. an in vitro ligament sectioning study in cadaveric knees. *American Journal of Sports Medicine* **21**:407–414, 1993.

2   Detenbeck LC: Function of the cruciate ligaments in knee stability. *American Journal of Sports Medicine* **2**:217–221, 1974.

3   Andriacchi TP, Galante JO: Retention of the posterior cruciate in total knee arthroplasty. *Journal of Arthroplasty* **3**(suppl): 513, 1988.

4   Draganich LF, Andriacchi TP, Anderson GBJ: Interaction between intrinsic knee mechanics and the knee extensor mechanism. *Journal of Orthopaedic Research* **5**:539, 1987.

5   Garino JP, Lotke P: Sacrificing the posterior cruciate ligament with and without substitution in total knee arthroplasty. In *Knee surgery*, ed. FH Fu, CD Harner, KG Vince, Vol. 2, pp. 1321–29. William and Wilkins, Baltimore, 1994.

6   Krackow KA: Surgical Principles in total knee arthroplasty: alignment, deformity, approaches and bone cuts: In *Orthopaedic knowledge update: hip and knee reconstruction*, pp. 269–76. American Academy of Orthopaedic Surgeons, Rosedale, IL, 1995.

7   Rand JA: Posterior cruciate retaining total knee arthroplasty. In *Reconstructive Surgery of the Joints*, 2nd edn, ed. BF Morrey, Vol. 2, pp. 1401–1408. Churchill Livingstone, New York, 1996.

8   Barnes CL, Sledge CB: Total Knee replacement with posterior cruciate ligament retention designs. In *Surgery of the Kneè*, 2nd edn, ed. JN Insall, RE Windsor, WN Scott *et al.*, Vol. 2, pp. 815–827. Churchill Livingstone, New York, 1993.

9   Scott RD, Thornhill TS: Posterior cruciate supplementing total knee replacement using conforming inserts and cruciate recession: effect on range of motion and radiolucent lines. *Clinical Orthopaedics and Related Research* **309**:146–149, 1994.

10  Sorger JI, Federle D, Kirk PG *et al.*: The posterior cruciate ligament in total knee arthroplasty. *Journal of Arthroplasty* **8**:869–879, 1997.

11  Johansson H, Sjolander P, Sojka P: A sensory role for the cruciate ligaments. *Clinical Orthopedics* **268**: 161–178, 1991.

12  Pagnano MW, Cushner FD, Scott WN: Role of the posterior cruciate ligament in total knee arthroplasty. *Journal of the American Academy of Orthopaedic Surgeons* **6**(3):176–187, 1998

13  Warren PJ, Olanlokum TK, Cobb AG, Bentley G: Proprioception after knee arthroplasty: the influence of prosthetic design. *Clinical Orthopedics* **297**:182–187, 1993.

14  Simmons S, Lephart S, Rubash H *et al.*: Proprioception after unicondylar knee arthroplasty versus total knee arthroplasty. *Clinical Orthopedics* **331**:179–184, 1996.

15  Becker MW, Insall JN, Faris PM: Bilateral total knee arthroplasty: one cruciate retaining and one cruciate substituting. *Clinical Orthopedics* **271**:122–124. 1991;

16  Cash RM, Gonzalez MH, Garst J *et al.*: Proprioception after arthroplasty: role of the posterior cruciate ligament. *Clinical Orthopedics* **331**:172–178, 1996.

17  DelValle ME, Harvin SF, Maestro A *et al.* Immunohistochemical analysis of mechanoreceptors in the human posterior cruciate ligament: a demonstration of its proprioceptive role and clinical relevance. *Journal of Arthroplasty* **13**(8):916–922, 1998.

18  Ishii Y, Terajima K, Koga Y *et al.*: Gait analysis after total knee arthroplasty. comparison of posterior cruciate retention and substitution. *Journal of Orthopedic Science* **3**(6):310–317, 1998.

19  Andriacchi T: Gait analysis and total knee replacement. In *Current concepts in primary and revision total knee arthroplasty*, eds J Insall, W Scott, GR Scuderi. Lippincott-Raven, Philadelphia, 1996.

20  Stern, SH, Insall JN: Total knee arthroplasty with posterior cruciate ligament substitution designs. In *Surgery of the knee*, 2nd edn, ed. JN Insall, RE Windsor, WN Scott *et al.*, Vol. 2, pp. 829–867. Churchill Livingstone, New York, 1994.

21  Mihalko WM, Krackow KA. Posterior cruciate ligament effects on the flexion space in total knee arthroplasty. *Clinical Orthopaedics and Related Research* **360**:243–250, 1999.

22  Ranawat CS, Luessenhop CP, Rodriguez JA: The press-fit condylar modular total knee system: four-to-six year results with a posterior cruciate substitution design. *Journal of Bone and Joint Surgery* [Am] **79**:342–348, 1997.

23  Colizza WA, Insall JN, Scuderi GR: The Posterior stabilized total knee prosthesis: assessment of polyethylene damage and osteolysis after a ten year minimum follow up. *Journal of Bone and Joint Surgery* [Am] **77**:1713–1720, 1995.

24  Scott RD, Volatile TB: Twelve years experience with posterior cruciate retaining total knee arthroplasty. *Clinical Orthopedics* **205**:100–107, 1986.

25  Ritter MA, Campbell E, Faris PM, Keating EM. Long term survival analysis of the posterior cruciate condylar total knee arthroplasty: a 10 year evaluation. *Journal of Arthroplasty* **4**:293–296, 1989.

26  Ranawat CS, Boachie-Adjel O. Survivorship analysis and results of total condylar knee arthroplasty, eight to eleven year follow up period. *Clinical Orthopedics* **226**:6–13, 1988.

27  Vince KG, Insall JN, Kelly M. The Total condylar prosthesis, ten to twelve year results of a cemented knee replacement. *Journal of Bone and Joint Surgery* [Am] **70**:1163–1173, 1988.

28  Scuderi GR, Insall JN. The posterior stabilized knee prosthesis. *Orthopedic Clinics of North America* **20**:71–78, 1989.

# Con: Steven B. Haas and Khalin J. Saleh

TKA has proven to be a highly successful procedure, with over 250 000 performed annually in the USA.[1] Controversies do, however, still persist. One such controversy involves the surgical approach to the PCL. A recent survey of the Knee Society revealed that 49.6% of the surgeons prefer to routinely save or recess the PCL during TKA, whereas 50.4% routinely sacrifice the PCL and use knee implants which substitute for PCL function.[2]

The origins of PCL sacrifice and substitution philosophy date back to the early 1970s, with the design and introduction of the Total Condylar knee implant in 1974.[3] The Total Condylar knee, designed by J. Insall, C. Ranawat, and P. Walker required excision of the PCL. Flexion stability was provided by a precise balancing of the flexion and extension spaces and by highly conforming articulating surfaces. The Total Condylar implant was found in numerous studies to provide good improvement in pain and function and has also been shown to have good long-term survival.[4-8] In addition, the implant was not found to have significant polyethylene wear problems. Vince and Insall[8] reported on results of Total Condylar knees with a minimum of 10 year follow-up. They found that 87% of patients had a good or excellent result. Ranawat[6] also reported on the 8–11 year survivorship of his first 112 primary Total Condylar knees and found clinical and radiographic survival of 95% and 89% respectively (1988). Scuderi and Insall[7] reported the 15 year survivorship of 224 Total Condylar prostheses; the cumulative survival was 91%. There were, however, several limitations of the Total Condylar design. Occasional posterior instability was noted and proper implantation required precise balance of the flexion and extension spaces. The posterior instability was most often seen in the patients with severe rheumatoid arthritis. Patients who received the Total Condylar knee also had less than optimal range of motion with an average flexion angle of 95°. Clinicians also noted limitations in stair-climbing ability in patients who received the Total Condylar implant. John Insall and Albert Burstein[9] felt that the limitations of the Total Condylar knee were primarily due to the lack of posterior stabilization and controlled femoral rollback. Insall and Burstein did not feel that consistent and adequate posterior stabilization and tibiofemoral kinematics could be achieved with retention of the PCL, and felt that substitution of the PCL should be incorporated into the implant design. This led to the introduction of the Insall–Burstein (IB) PS knee in 1978.[9] The IB design incorporated a femoral cam and tibial peg that controlled rollback of the femoral component on the tibial component and simultaneously improved flexion.

The IB PS knee gave better results than the Total Condylar knee. Stern and Insall[10] reported 9–12 year follow-ups of 289 original IB knees and found that 87% of the patients have a good or an excellent result with an average range of motion of 110°. The authors reported an overall 12 year survivorship of 94%. The incidence of femoral subluxation was also significantly decreased, even in patients with rheumatoid arthritis. Survivorship also appeared to be even better than that of the Total Condylar knee with a 16 year survivorship of 94% as reported by Font-Rodriguez and Insall.[4] Newer PS designs, which employ modifications of the original IB design, are currently available.

The fundamental concept of PS design incorporates a femoral cam and a tibial spine[9] (Fig. 4.1). The cam and post are designed to contact at approximately 60-70° of flexion. The engagement of the femoral cam and tibial spine causes the tibiofemoral contact point to move posteriorly with further knee flexion. This leads to a controlled rollback and increased flexion of the knee. The femoral cam and tibial spines prevent anterior sliding as well as posterior subluxation

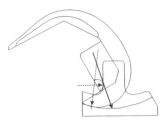

**Fig. 4.1**

The cam and spine mechanism leads to controlled femoral rollback and the resulting force vector passes distally through the tibial stem.

of the knee. Additionally, tibiofemoral articular conformity has been greater in PS knee designs because the femoral rollback can be induced without increasing tension in the PCL, potentially limiting flexion.

Opponents of the PS design criticized the transverse forces created by the contact of the tibial spine and femoral cam. The original design engineers however, pointed out that the magnitude of the transverse forces created by the cam and post were much smaller than that of the tibiofemoral contact force. The net resultant force was directed centrally down the tibial shaft.[9] Therefore, the total forces created in this design led to a compressive force on the tibial component rather than a shear type force. These conclusions were ultimately confirmed by long-term survivorship studies and by the low rate of tibial loosening.

## Why use a PS design?

Both PCL-retaining and PS knee designs have shown good clinical results; however, there are several indications that PS designs have

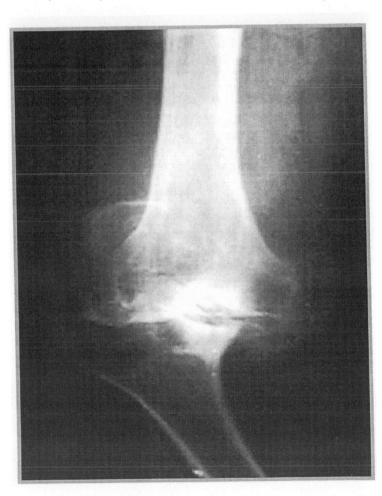

**Fig. 4.2**

Arthritic knee with greater than 20° of varus alignment.

shown superior clinical outcome. Laskin, in 1996,[11] compared PCL-retaining and PS knee arthroplasty in severely deformed knees at 10 years. Patients who received PCL-retaining prostheses were found to have more pain, decreased flexion arc, higher rate of bone cement radiolucenies, and decreased survivorship. Laskin, therefore, felt that PS knees should be used in patients with more than 15° of tibiofemoral varus or valgus and in patients with combined varus and flexion contractures greater than 15° (Fig. 4.2). Laskin also compared the results of PCL retention or substitution in patients with rheumatoid arthritis.[12] He found that patients with rheumatoid arthritis who received a PCL-retaining knee arthroplasty have lower knee scores. Additionally, many of those patients developed late posterior subluxation and instability. The inferior results obtained with PCL-retaining implants were felt to be due to the involvement of the PCL in the inflammatory disease and late stretching of the ligament. Kleinbart[13] histologically studied 24 PCLs harvested at the time of TKA for osteoarthritis and compared the results to 36 age-matched specimens harvested from above-knee amputation procedures, cadavers, and bone bank donors. Only 17% of the specimens in the TKA group demonstrated normal PCLs, compared to 45% in the control group. In the TKA group 63% of the ligaments had marked degenerative changes, compared to zero in the control group. These results further corroborate Laskin's conclusions.

The basic premise of PCL retention is that appropriate balance of the PCL can be obtained. Lotke[14] has shown that appropriate balance of the PCL is not commonly achieved. He examined 10 TKAs with PCL-retaining implants. He used strain gauge analysis of the PCL to determine if it was appropriately tensioned. He found the PCL was excessively loose in 6, too tight in 3, and balanced to appropriate

**Fig. 4.3**

*In vivo* anterioposterior contact point with knee flexion. (a) normal; (b) ACL deficient; (c) PCL substitution; (d) PCL sparing.

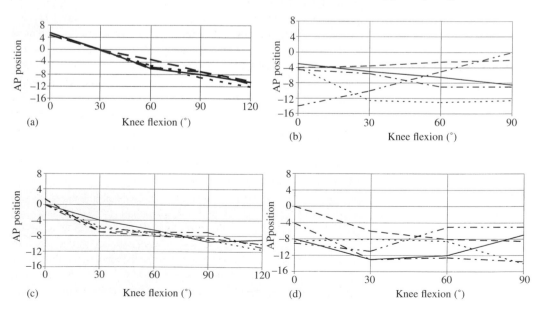

(a)  Knee flexion (°)

(b)  Knee flexion (°)

(c)  Knee flexion (°)

(d)  Knee flexion (°)

tension in only 1. An unbalanced PCL is unlikely to provide the appropriate and predicted kinematics in knee arthroplasty and may lead to limited flexion or posterior subluxation.

Stiehl *et al.* have elaborately studied the *in vivo* kinematics of PCL-retaining and PS arthroplasty. They employed two-dimensional fluoroscopy and did three-dimensional computer matching with templates of the implanted components. The bone was subsequently digitally subtracted and tibiofemoral contact points were mapped.

Dennis *et al.*[15] compared contact points for four groups: normal knees, anterior crucial ligament (ACL) deficient knees, PCL-sparing TKA and PCL-substituting TKA. The results for five individual patients in each of these groups are shown in Fig. 4.3. The kinematics in the normal knees of the five test subjects were consistent throughout flexion. The contact points were anterior in full extension and moved posterior throughout the 120° flexion arc. The PCL-substituting knee arthroplasty patients also had consistent kinematics. The contact points in these patients were generally more centralized in full extension. Femoral rollback with flexion was consistent and similar for all patients. When Dennis examined the ACL-deficient knee he found erratic and inconsistent kinematics among the test subjects. The contact points in full extension were slightly posterior in some patients and even more posterior in others. Some patients subluxed forward with flexion, whereas in others the contact point moved posteriorly. The PCL-sparing TKAs behaved very similarly to the ACL-deficient knees. Kinematics were erratic and inconsistent amongst the test subjects. Contact points in full extension were variable, with flexion contact points moved anteriorly in some patients and posteriorly in others.

The findings of these studies indicate that consistent and predicted kinematics are not reproduced in the PCL-retaining knee designs and in fact act more similar to an ACL-deficient knee. This erratic nature of tibiofemoral contact can be detrimental to the polyethylene. These conclusions are fortified by earlier work. Stiehl[16] demonstrated the tibiofemoral contact point was posterior in extension and translated anteriorly with knee flexion in PCL-retaining designs. The authors were concerned about accelerated polyethylene wear as a result of this paradoxical anterior femoral translation with knee flexion in PCL-retaining designs. In contrast, the PCL-substituting knees behaved in a more consistent and predictable fashion. This has the potential advantage of decreasing polyethylene wear and producing a more consistent clinical outcome.

Results of gait analysis have shown inconsistent findings when PCL retention and substitution have been compared. Andriacchi, in 1982,[17] reported better stair-climbing with PCL retaining implants. Many of the implants used in this study were older designs that are not currently in use. Wilson *et al.*[18] also compared stair-climbing in PCL-retaining and PCL-substituting knee arthroplasties. He found no significant or consistent difference in gate and stair-climbing ability.

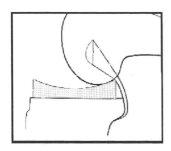

**Fig. 4.4**

Kinematic conflict occurs as PCL forces the contact tibiofemoral point posterior while the dished articulation increases the tension in the PCL.

Since the 1980s many arguments have been put forward for saving the PCL, but most of them have subsequently been proved incorrect. An original design requirement for PCL retention was that the polyethylene should be flat. It was felt that conformity in the polyethylene would lead to increased stress at the implant–bone interface. It was also felt that a curved polyethylene surface could lead to a kinematic conflict (Fig. 4.4). Curving of the posterior tibial articulation would cause the PCL to tighten further as the femur rolled back onto the tibia, essentially causing the femur to roll up a hill, and thus causing excessive tightness of the PCL.

Most current PCL-retaining implants have eliminated flat polyethylene tibial inserts as a result of the increased shear forces created, decreased contact area, and accelerated polyethylene wear (Fig. 4.5). Increasing polyethylene conformity may eliminate some of the excessive wear problems found in the first generation of PCL-retaining designs.

Most of the long-term data on PCL-retaining designs to date are with implants that utilized low-conforming polyethylene tibial inserts. The use of more conforming or "dished" polyethylene tibial inserts may lead to a kinematic conflict by producing a tight PCL and thus reducing flexion. There are few long-term studies that report on the results of highly conforming posterior PCL-retaining implants.

Another argument for PCL retention was that these designs could lead to increased knee flexion. This again has proven incorrect. Lotke reported on 242 consecutive TKAs composed of three surgical groups (Fig. 4.6). In group 1 the PCL was completely released, in group 2 the PCL was saved, and in group 3 a PCL-substituting design

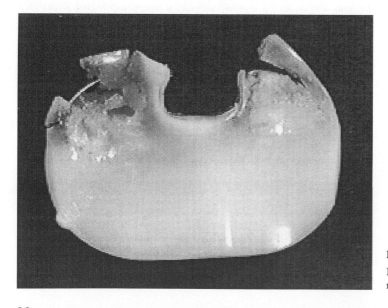

**Fig. 4.5**

Flat tibial articulation with massive polyethylene wear.

**Fig. 4.6**

Knee flexion using three designs: PCL sacrificing (white bar, average flexion 103°); PCL retention (grey bar, average flexion 104°); PCL substitution (black bar, average flexion 112°). $N = 242$; $p < 0.001$.

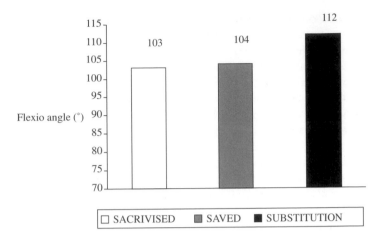

was used. Groups 1 and 2 had similar ranges of motion (103° and 104° respectively)whereas group 3, the PCL-substituting design, had significantly greater motion (112°). Numerous other studies have shown no difference in range of motion between these implant designs. There are, however, reports of patients with excessively restricted motion due to a tight PCL.

Critics of PS designs argue that the increased stress caused by the tibial peg/femoral cam mechanism along with the increased conformity may lead to early loosening and inferior survivorship compared to PCL-retaining designs. This argument has been disproved.[4] Long-term survivorship of PCL-substituting designs has been excellent, with 16 years survivorship for all-polyethylene tibial components exceeding 94%. The 14 year survivorship of metal-backed IB I implants are reported at 98%.[4] These results are at least as good as for PCL-retaining designs.

The primary arguments for PCL-retaining designs which appear to have the most merit include increased intercondylar bone resection and the occasional patella "clunk" syndrome.[19] Newer designs, which are modifications of the original IB PS knee, allow for decreased intercondylar bone resection, improved patella–femoral articulations, and the elimination of patellar clunks.

In contrast to the changing philosophy of PCL-sparing arthroplasty, the fundamental concepts and principles of PCL substitution have remained the same. The advantages of PCL substitution are that:

- it provides easier surgical exposure
- it offers an effective means of correcting knee deformity
- it provides consistent and reproducible kinematics to the knee
- it avoids the complexity of "balancing" the PCL
- it circumvents the possible risk of late attenuation or rupture as seen in rheumatoid patients.

89

PCL substitution eliminates the risk of an excessively tight PCL with the use of a less conforming tibial insert, which can restrict motion. We believe that the concern for a tight PCL may become more prevalent with the current generation of more conforming PCL-retaining designs. Finally, we believe that PCL-substituting designs may provide for better durability of the polyethylene. Polyethylene wear continues to be the greatest risk to the long-term survival of a knee arthroplasty. Erratic kinematics with anterior sliding can lead to polyethylene damage and wear problems. Additionally, PCL-substituting designs are still generally more conforming with lower contact stresses than PCL-retaining implants. Additionally, resection of the PCL may allow for placement of a slightly thicker polyethylene insert.

In summary, TKA with PCL-substituting implants has been shown to be a simple and reproducible technique with excellent results and survivorship. Although it is not universal, there is a growing consensus that PS knees are advantageous in the severely deformed, inflammatory, and revision arthroplasty situations. Additionally, we feel that routine use of the PCL-substituting knees has several advantages, most importantly the potential for decreased polyethylene wear.

Finally, as with any surgical technique, the surgeons should make a decision as to what is best for each individual patient.

# References

1 National Center for Health Statistics: *American Academy and American Association Orthopaedic Surgeons Bulletin* **47**(3):14, 1999.
2 Saleh KJ, MacAulay A, Gross A *et al.*: The Knee Society Index of Severity (KSIS) for failed total knee arthroplasty. Presented before the combined AAHICS and Knee Society Specialty Day, AAOS Orlando, March 2000.
3 Insall J: *Surgery of the knee*. Churchill Livingstone, New York, 1993.
4 Font-Rodriguez DF, Scuderi GR, Insall JN: Survivorship of total knee arthroplasty. Presented before the Knee Society, Atlanta, February 1996.
5 Insall J, Scott WN, Ranawat C: The total condylar knee prosthesis: a report of two hundred and twenty cases. *Journal of Bone and Joint Surgery* [Am], **61**:173–180, 1979.
6 Ranawat C, Boachie-Adjei O: Survivorship analysis and results of total condylar knee arthroplasty. *Clinical Orthopedics* **226**:6–13, 1988.
7 Scuderi G, Insall J, Windsor R *et al.*: Survivorship of cemented knee replacements. *Journal of Bone and Joint Surgery* [Br] **71**:798:1989.
8 Vince KG, Insall JN, Kelly MA: The total condylar prosthesis: 10 to 12 year results of a cemented knee replacement. *Journal of Bone and Joint Surgery* [Br] **71**:793–797, 1989.
9 Insall JN, Lachiewicz PF, Burstein AH: The posterior stabilized condylar prosthesis: A modification of the total condylar design—two to four year clinical experience. *Journal of Bone and Joint Surgery* [Am] **64**:1317–23, 1982.
10 Stern SH, Insall JN: Posterior stabilized prosthesis: Results after follow-up of nine to twelve years. *Journal of Bone and Joint Surgery* [Am] **74**:980–6, 1992.

11 Laskin RS: Total knee replacement with posterior cruciate ligament retention in patients with a fixed varus deformity. *Clinical Orthopedics* **331**:329–334, 1996.

12 Laskin RS: Total condylar knee replacement in patients who have rheumatoid arthritis. A ten-year follow-up study. *Journal of Bone and Joint Surgery* [Am] **72**:529–35, 1990.

13 Kleinbart FA, Bryk E, Evangelista J *et al.*: Histologic comparison of posterior cruciate ligaments from arthritic and age-matched knee specimens. *Journal of Arthroplasty* **11**:726–31, 1996.

14 Lotke P, Corces A, Williams JL, Hirsch H: Strain characteristics of the posterior cruciate ligament after total knee arthroplasty. *American Journal of Knee Surgery* **6**:104–107, 1993.

15 Dennis DA, Komistek RD, Hoff WA, Gabriel SM: In vivo knee kinematics derived using an inverse perspective technique. *Clinical Orthopedics* **331**:107–117, 1996.

16 Stiehl JB, Komistek RD, Dennis DA, *et al*: Fluoroscopic analysis of kinematics after posterior and auclate retaining total knee arthroplasty. *Journal of Bone and Joint Surgery* **118**:884–889, 1995.

17 Andriacchi TP, Galante JO, Fermier RW: Influence of total knee replacement design on walking and stair climbing. *Journal of Bone and Joint Surgery* [Am], 1328–1335, 1982.

18 Wilson SA, McCann PD, Gotlin RS *et al.*: Comprehensive gait analysis in posterior-stabilized knee arthroplasty. *Journal of Arthroplasty* **11**:359–367, 1996.

19 Hozack W, Rothman R, Booth R *et al.*: The patellar clunk syndrome. A complication of posterior stabilized total knee arthroplasty. *Clinical Orthopedics* **241**:203–208, 1989.

## Questions and answers

*Moderator:* Dr. Krackow, you propose that PS prosthesis can be used with a *major* varus deformity. For you, how major is major?

*Dr. Krackow:* 15° and above. The complete answer to this is rather difficult. It also depends upon one's taste with regard to avoiding the kinematics of a "two ligament" knee in combination with use of a plastic that is designed for rollback. It is clear that in moderate to severe varus and valgus deformities correct "collateral" balance is facilitated by releasing the PCL. Otherwise the PCL tethers or blocks the effective opening one seeks with the collateral release. It is frequently possible to get symmetric enough flexion and extension spaces and to get equal enough spaces so that the roller in trough aspects of a "two ligament" knee, i.e., the old total condylar situation, do provide adequate stability. However, one could argue that in the absence of highly conforming tibial geometry, generally not present in a tibial component designed for rollback, that the tibiofemoral kinematics and the implications for polyethylene wear are not as good and predictable if one avoids the PS type of prosthesis. Having said all of that, there are many of us PCR users who still only use the PS when there is an apparent or suspected subluxation situation against which one needs to protect. And, otherwise, when things seem stable enough, the nonPS prosthesis, i.e., PCR, is used.

*Moderator:* Obviously all PS knees are not alike. Admittedly some PS designs remove less femoral bone stock than others, but all remove some bone. Don't you find this problematic, Dr. Haas?

*Dr. Haas:* The major drawback of intercondylar bone resection for PS designs is the increased risk for intercondylar fracture. The fracture rate at most centers that routinely perform PS knee arthroplasty is quite low. Additionally, several current PS designs have significantly reduced the amount of bone resection in the intercondylar notch. The bone resection is less problematic at revision, since most revisions require a PS design anyway, and the notch bone will need to be resected in almost all cases.

*Moderator:* A similar type of question for you, Dr. Krackow. All PCL-retaining prostheses are not alike. At this stage in your career with over 20 years of experience, what do you feel that the optimal configuration of the articulated surface of a PCL retaining implant should be?

*Dr. Krackow:* Quite conforming, permitting only a few millimeters of roll-back; having a moderate anterior, uphill dish; and also having as large as possible intercondylar hump, to block against translational instability.

*Moderator:* Dr. Haas, most comparisons of PS vs. PCL-retaining knees that are used by PS devotees use first-generation tibial components, which were flat and thin. This is an unfair comparison since the present designs are more conforming and thicker. How do PS designs fare against these implants?

*Dr. Haas:* It is true that most comparisons of PS and PCL-retaining knees have discussed first-generation tibial components, with less conforming tibial articulations. Despite these flat articulations, the range of motion in many series has been the same or less than in PS designs. Additionally, these less conforming articulations were more prone to polyethylene wear. The current generation of PCL-retaining designs employ more conforming polyethylene inserts. The PCL may be more difficult to balance with the more conforming polyethylene insert, and range of motion may be even worse. Although the fundamental principles of PCL substitution have remained the same and have been well studied in long-term follow-up the results of PCL-retaining designs with more conforming polyethylene inserts is less well studied.

*Moderator:* Dr. Krackow, what is your response to the PS surgeons who state that the PCL is not normal histologically in an arthritic knee and that you may be preserving a macroscopic, scarred, poorly functioning ligament?

*Dr. Krackow:* Who cares? It still functions as a ligament. You will never convince me otherwise!

*Moderator:* If you resect the PCL during a total knee (either purposely or inadvertently), Dr. Haas, do you think that you then need to insert a PS implant? If so, why? If not, why not?

*Dr. Haas:* I believe that if the PCL is found to be incompetent or cut at the time of knee arthroplasty, that a standard PCL-retaining design is not optimal. I believe that acceptable alternatives would be a PS component with a femoral cam and tibial spine or alternatively a more congruent articulation or "deep dish" design as they are often called. Providing a PS or "deep dish" design will minimize the risk of a posterior subluxation and improve the kinematics of the knee.

*Moderator:* Let me vary this question for you Dr. Krackow. Although you save the PCL do you at times have to perform a PCL resection? If so, when do you do it? How do you do it?

*Dr. Krackow:* Our greatest use of PCL resection likely occurs during performance of the routine tibial cut. We do not think that "balancing" of the PCL has a *major* influence on opening the flexion space to avoid excessive roll-back and/or excessive flexion space tightening. Division of the PCL in the cadaver knee has been found and published by us only to open the flexion space on average by 4 mm. Therefore, we do not see partial release as having a *major* effect. Nonetheless, if we wind up with a totally intact PCL and excessive rollback or flexion space tightness are present, we will start by release of the anterior PCL fibers from the femur. If this action is not enough, we will release the entire PCL and then decide if it is necessary to change to PS components.

*Moderator:* To follow up on this question, Dr. Haas, there have been real concerns that in patients who obtain large amounts of flexion after surgery in their activities of daily living (i.e., patients in the Orient), this hyperflexion can lead to a jumping of the PS post. Should we therefore not be using a PS knee in this group of patients?

*Dr. Haas:* I would argue that patients requiring a large degree of flexion might be better served with a PS design. I believe that a high degree of flexion can be more consistently reproduced with a PS design since the femoral rollback and kinematics of the knee are more controlled. Jumping of the PS post is a rare problem and was most commonly associated with knees that had a large valgus deformity and underwent extensive lateral ligament releases. In a well-balanced knee arthroplasty, jumping of the PS post should be rare, regardless of the range of motion.

*Moderator:* What percentage of the people in the USA do you believe routinely save the PCL, Dr. Krackow?

*Dr. Krackow:* Sixty per cent.

*Moderator:* As a follow up question, it has been alluded that it is more difficult to perform a PCL-retaining TKR than a PS TKR since you have one extra ligament to balance. Realizing that most TKRs in the US are performed by general orthopaedic surgeons at a rate of less than 20 per year, would they not be better served using PS prosthesis?

*Dr. Krackow:* It is probably easier to manipulate the tibia, i.e., to get better exposure with removal of the PCL. However, performance of the box cut and preparation of the femur are not easier. The ligament balancing is only "easier" for the more severe deformities in which the PCL will be totally released or removed anyway. We say therefore, that this has to be decided by the individual surgeon; perfect balance may not be easy in difficult cases, but it should also be remembered that retention of the ligament may provide more posterior stability in these difficult cases.

*Moderator:* Despite your statement, Dr. Haas, that almost half of the members of the Knee Society use a PCL-sacrificing design of some sort, you must realize that worldwide over 70% of the total knees that are sold are of the posterior PCL-retaining design. Why do you think that you are in the minority and how could change the majority opinion?

*Dr. Haas:* I believe that the reason that the majority of surgeons in the world retain the PCL during a TKA is that that was the way they were trained to do knee replacement. Since most of these surgeons obtain satisfactory results with this design, they have not changed to a PS design. There is, however, a trend towards PS arthroplasty since many surgeons have begun to realize the potential benefits of posterior stabilization. Some have switched because they had had trouble consistently achieving good range of motion especially with more conforming articulations in some PCL-sparing implants.

# 5

*The normal knee exhibits a phenomenom known as rollback in which one (or both?) femoral condyles displace posteriorly as the joint flexes. Most would agree that this rollback is beneficial in the normal knee. Is it, hower, beneficial in the prosthetic knee? Furthermore, even if it is beneficial, can we obtain rollback using the types of prostheses presently available? This chapter contains three points of view, the Pro, the Con, and the "not sure."*

# Femoral rollback is obtainable and beneficial in the total knee patient

## Pro: Thomas P. Andriacchi, Chris O. Dyrby, and Eugene J. Alexander

The anterior–posterior (AP) motion of the knee associated with femoral rollback is needed to maintain normal function. Femoral rollback occurs in the normal knee and should be maintained in the knee following total knee replacement. The ability to restore the kinematic features of the knee that have the greatest influence on patient function is the critical issue for total knee replacement.

Historically, femoral rollback in the normal knee and in the knee after total knee replacement has been reported to influence passive range of motion as well as function during activities of daily living such as stair-climbing.[1] Improved ability to climb stairs has been related to femoral rollback.[2,3] Rollback of the femur increases the lever arm of the quadriceps muscles at a critical phase of the stair-climbing cycle and provides increased mechanical advantage for the quadriceps muscle to extend the knee.

One of the key features of the functional abnormality in total knee replacement patients while ascending stairs was a reduction in the moment sustained by the net quadriceps contraction.[1] Patients with posterior cruciate ligament (PCL)-sacrificing knee replacements had a tendency to reduce the moment sustained by the quadriceps by leaning forward during the portion of the support phase of ascending stairs when the quadriceps moment would normally reach a peak value. This finding was also consistent with a study in which electromyelographic (EMG) activity was measured during stair-climbing.[4] In that study, maximum quadriceps activity was reported for patients with PCL-retaining and PCL-sacrificing designs. However, patients with PCL-sacrificing designs required increased use of the soleus muscle while stair-climbing. The increased soleus activity suggested a forward lean was occurring in the PCL-sacrificing designs similar to that described in other studies.[4]

In a more recent study by Wilson *et al.*,[5] patients with PCL-sacrificing designs were compared to normal subjects while walking and stair-climbing. Although the study did not report a statistical difference, there was a 25% reduction in the peak flexion moment during stair-climbing between normal subjects and patients following total knee replacement. The lack of a statistically significant difference in that study may have been associated with the sample size of the test population.

The finding of reduced quadriceps moment in patients with PCL-sacrificing designs has been explained by the dynamic interaction between the PCL, tibiofemoral rollback with flexion, and the changing lever arm of the quadriceps.[2] The functional adaptations seen in patients with PCL-sacrificing designs were likely associated with the need to compensate for the lack of normal femoral rollback. The interpretation of these results was based on inferring rollback from passive measurements of rollback based on cadaver studies,[6] since direct measurements of *in vivo* rollback were not obtained. Although increasing the muscle lever arm during flexion is beneficial for stair-climbing, the mechanism for changing muscle lever arms during dynamic activities with large muscle forces is not well understood.

Recent advances in the methods to capture *in vivo* motion during activities of daily living have made it possible to measure *in vivo* the six-degree-of-freedom movement of the knee.[7] Using these methods it is possible to gain new insights into the relationships between *in vivo* knee kinematic and patient function.

Thus, the question of obtaining femoral rollback in the total replacement patient should be addressed in the context of *in vivo* function. The purpose of this paper is to examine femoral rollback in the context of the interplay between the geometry of the articular surfaces, constraints imposed by passive soft tissue, and forces generated by muscle contraction.

## Passive characteristics of the knee

Under passive loading, the contact location of the femur has been described as rolling posteriorly in early flexion (0–20°).[6] The rolling motion was greater on the lateral plateau than the medial plateau. Beyond approximately 20°, the contact location remains relatively fixed indicating sliding motion. Sliding at the surface can occur when the knee translates without flexion or the knee flexes without translation (Fig. 5.1).

The mechanics of rolling and sliding provide a basis for examining the relationship between the passive motion of the knee joint, the geometry of the articular surfaces, and restraints provided by the passive soft tissue surrounding the joint.[8] For example, consider the motion of the tibiofemoral joint. The distal radius of the lateral and medial femoral condyles is substantially different (Fig. 5.2). The radius of a

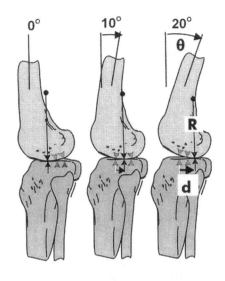

(a)

(b)

(c)

**Fig. 5.1**

(a) The contact between the tibia and femur moves posteriorly with flexion under conditions of pure rolling. Rolling will produce a one-to-one correspondence between the angle of knee flexion and the location of tibiofemoral contact. Typically rolling without sliding occurs during flexion between 0 and 20°. (b) Sliding with flexion occurs when the knee flexes and the contact remains in the same position. Typically sliding with flexion occurs beyond 20° of flexion. (c) Sliding with fixed flexion can occur when the knee displaces without flexion. An anterior drawer test is an example of sliding at a fixed flexion angle.

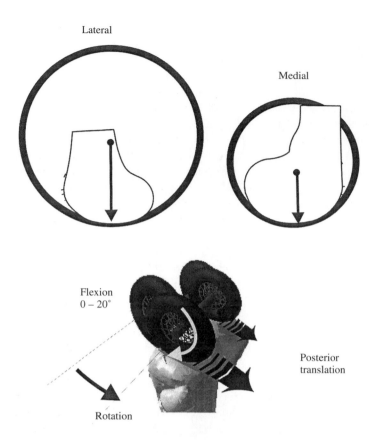

Lateral

Medial

Flexion
0 – 20°

Posterior
translation

Rotation

**Fig. 5.2**

The distal femoral radius with a lateral condyle is substantially larger than the medial femoral condyle. Thus, during pure rolling (typically between 0 and 20°), the lateral femoral condyle will displace a posteriorly greater distance than the medial femoral condyle. Thus, rotation of the femur will be coupled with flexion under conditions of pure rolling between 0 and 20°.

circle placed through the distal portion of the medial femoral condyle is approximately half that of the lateral femoral condyle. Under conditions of pure rolling from full extension, the lateral condyle will translate further than the medial condyle during flexion, since the lateral condyle has a larger distal radius. Thus, rollback with flexion must be coupled to external rotation of the femur relative to the tibia. This coupling of motion between flexion and rotation of the knee has been observed during passive motion and described as screw-home movement.[9] It should be noted that this movement takes place because passively the femoral condyle rolls over the surface of the tibia between 0 and 20° of flexion. Beyond 20° of flexion, and during activities where the movement of the femur with respect to the tibia is influenced by external forces such as active muscle contraction, the femur can slip relative to the tibia. Passively, beyond 20° of flexion the relative femoral tibial movement is dominated by slip at the interface between the femur and the tibia. If rolling continued with flexion, the femur would roll off the back of the tibia.

The anatomy and structure of the soft tissue surrounding the knee is also compatible with the coupling between rollback flexion and rotation.[9] Consider the menisci: both menisci are fixed to the tibia at their anterior and posterior horns but the rest of the structure is

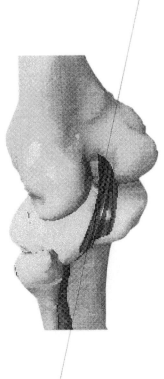

**Fig. 5.3**

The oblique orientation of the PCL. The orientation of this ligament is compatible with the asymmetry in the curvature of the distal femoral condyles in the coupling of rotation during early flexion.

freely mobile. The medial meniscus is more securely attached to the surface of the tibia and has less mobility than the lateral meniscus. The relatively greater mobility of the lateral meniscus is consistent with the difference in the motion of the lateral and medial femoral condyles during flexion from full extension (Fig. 5.2). Similarly, the oblique orientation of the PCL is compatible with the asymmetry in the geometry of the distal femoral condyles (Fig. 5.3). The lateral femoral condyle will move posteriorly a greater distance than the medial femoral condyle during rolling with flexion. As a result, the femur will rotate externally with flexion relative to the tibia. This axis of rotation is compatible with the oblique orientation of the PCL and permits maintenance of normal tension in this ligament during the early ranges of flexion. This geometric interaction between the anatomy of the PCL and the geometry of the distal femoral condyles is likely an important consideration in the design of knee replacements where retention of the PCL is considered. Clearly, the interaction of the femoral condyles and the orientation of the cruciate ligament play a fundamental role in the function of the knee joint.

The passive anatomy of the knee joint will guide the knee to a position where the passive soft tissue is in balance at any angle of knee flexion. This position of balance has been described as the neutral position of the passive knee joint.[10] In the neutral position, the passive knee joint will move within a certain range with minimal resistance to applied loads. When the knee is in the neutral position its resistance to movement over a certain range of displacements (envelope of movement) is extremely low. Beyond this envelope, the resistance to movement increases substantially, as indicated by the increased slope of the force displacement curve (Fig. 5.4). This envelope of movement has been shown to be a function of the angle of the flexion.

At full extension the envelope of motion is quite small and the knee remains quite stable. As the knee flexes portions of the ligaments relax and the envelope of movement from the neutral position increases. The envelope of passive movement can be described for motion in AP, abduction–adduction, and internal–external rotation directions. For the purposes of this paper only the AP motion of the femur will be discussed.

The changing envelope of stability at the knee is important from a functional viewpoint.[11] At full extension, the knee is passively stable allowing for standing posture with a minimal amount of muscular demand. During dynamic activities, such as walking, (where the knee typically flexes to approximately 20° during mid-stance) the ligaments are relatively relaxed and large muscle forces generated by muscle contraction provide the dynamic stability. Thus, at any position of flexion passive soft tissue and articular surfaces can guide the knee to a neutral position. However, external forces due to muscle contraction or external forces acting at the knee can displace the knee easily within the envelope of passive motion as illustrated in Fig. 5.5.

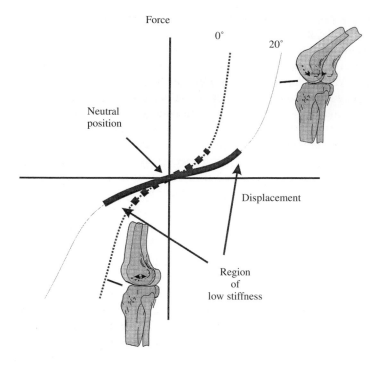

**Fig. 5.4**

The relationship between the force displacement characteristics of the knee joint at 0 and 20° of flexion. The heavy line about the neutral position represents a region where displacement can occur with relatively small force applied. As the knee flexes, the region of low stiffness (high mobility) of the knee increases. Thus, the knee has an envelope of possible AP positions that can occur depending on the magnitude of the applied force. It should be noted that as the knee displacement increases, the slope of the force–displacement curve increases substantially indicating resistance to further displacement.

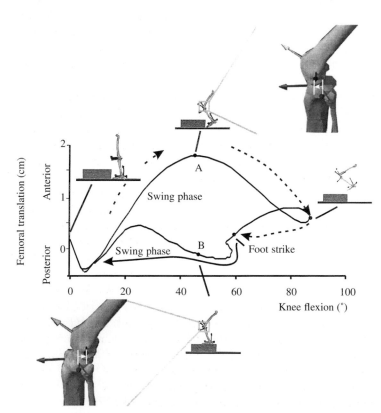

**Fig. 5.5**

The relationship between the AP movement of the femur and the angle of knee flexion during the swing and stance phase of the stair-climbing cycle. At full extension, the knee begins in the neutral position and the femur moves anteriorly with flexion during the swing phase of the stair climbing cycle. At point A (approximately 45° of knee flexion) the knee begins to move posteriorly with flexion until a point of maximum flexion. The AP movement of the femur during swing phase determines its location at foot strike where it is approximately maintained through the remainder of stance phase. It is important to note that there is a maximum offset between the anterior and posterior position of the knee during swing phase and stance phase with the knee flexed at approximately 45°. This hysteresis is likely driven by the generation of muscle forces during the stair-climbing cycle.

Beyond this envelope the passive resistance will increase substantially (due to passive soft tissue strain) and limit the AP displacement of the femur. In addition, the stretch of passive soft tissue can generate sensory feedback causing muscle-firing patterns to be adjusted to provide additional stability to the joint. The phenomenon of interaction between passive structures and muscle firing patterns is best evaluated during *in vivo* testing of natural activities of daily living.

## *In vivo* testing

As previously noted, stair-climbing provides important information on *in vivo* function of the knee joint with regard to femoral rollback. Abnormal rollback during stair-climbing is one explanation for the reduced quadriceps moment following total knee replacement.[2] However, there has not been a direct measure of femoral rollback during natural stair-climbing conditions. Previously reported fluoroscopic studies do not include the entire stair-climbing cycle.[12]

A recently described motion acquisition method permits measurement of the six-degree-of-freedom movement of the femur and tibia using a cluster of points distributed on the thigh and shank segments.[7] The cluster consists of a set of retro-reflective markers located in three dimensions using a four-camera optoelectronic system.

This technology has recently been used to study the AP movement of the femur during natural stair-climbing.[13] This study has provided new insight into the kinematics of the knee during *in vivo* conditions. It has been shown that the AP motion of the knee joint is highly dependent on the phase of the stair-climbing cycle and can be associated directly with patterns of muscle contraction. The study tracked the AP position of a reference point located at the midpoint of the transepicondylar axis relative to a reference point fixed in the tibia.

The results of that study demonstrated that the AP movement of the femur does not follow a pathway that is dependent on the angle of knee flexion. Thus, there is not a direct correspondence between the angle of the flexion and the AP position of the femur during *in vivo* activities. As illustrated in Fig. 5.5, there was an offset between the swing phase position of the femur and stance phase position for identical angles of knee flexion. For normal subjects the average offset was approximately 19 mm. The results would suggest to the casual observer that the knee "paradoxically" rolls forward during flexion during the early swing phase of the stair-climbing cycle. When examining these results in the context of the patterns of muscle contraction, this result is not paradoxical. The knee is moving within a passive envelope of AP displacement that is driven by the hamstring muscle contracting to flex the knee during the swing phase. As the hamstrings generate force with the knee flexed, the tibia is pulled posteriorly producing a net forward motion of the femur. The forward motion of the femur is likely constrained by both the passive envelope of motion and inhibitory muscle response associated with stretch of the passive soft tissue surrounding the knee.

The hysteresis illustrated in Fig. 5.5 appears to be generated primarily by the force of muscle contraction, with the largest offset from the swing phase due to the quadriceps contracting during stance phase. The maximum offset typically occurs at approximately 60° of knee flexion. These results suggest that the AP movement of the femur during stair-climbing is likely driven by the patterns of muscle firing. If this is the case, the ligaments act primarily as cables providing end-point restraints to this AP motion, as they become taut.

The observation that the muscles are driving the AP movement of the femur on the tibia is consistent with the patterns of femoral AP movement measured in patients following total knee replacement.[13] The maximum AP translation for the normal population had an average value of 1.9 cm ± 0.6 cm. This value was significantly less than either group of patients following total knee replacement. The cruciate retaining group was 2.9 cm ± 0.6 cm and the posterior stabilized group was 3.3 cm ± 0.8 cm. There was also a difference in the characteristics of the AP movement-knee flexion curves for each of the three groups (Fig. 5.6). The posterior stabilized group reahed the greatest anterior position at approximately 65° of knee flexion, the PCL-retaining group at approximately 55°, and the normal group at approximately 45°(Fig. 5.5).

## Role of neuromuscular system

Adaptive changes during locomotion can have a profound influence on the loading and motion of the knee joint. Often these changes are a response to a deficit such as instability or weakness and manifest as a reprogramming of the locomotor process. Forces generated from muscle contraction can have a substantial influence on the kinetic and kinematics of the knee joint (Fig. 5.7). Muscle forces can control the position of the contact between the femur and the tibia in the absence of passive constraints. The ability of the neuromuscular system to maintain normal kinematics in the absence of passive constraint has been illustrated in functional studies of patients with ante-

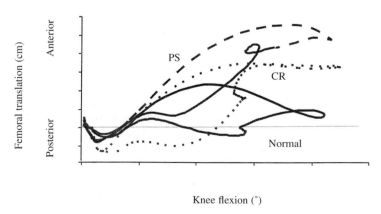

Knee flexion (°)

**Fig. 5.6**

The patterns of AP displacement vs. flexion angle during stair climbing were similar or close to normal, cruciate retaining (CR) and posterior substituting (PS) groups. However, the magnitude of the displacement was different for each group. The PS group had the largest anterior translation of the femur during swing phase. The CR group, although closer to normal, also had increased anterior displacement during swing phase relative to the normal group.

**Fig. 5.7**

An illustration of the ability of the extensor and flexor muscle groups at the knee to generate AP translation of the joint. The muscles can also act to tense an otherwise slack PCL. Therefore, the PCL can be thought to behave as a cable resisting external forces within an envelope of functional performance.

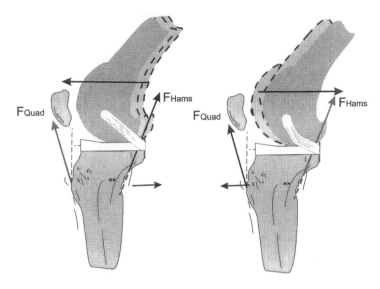

**Fig. 5.8**

An illustration of the regions of wear found in retrieved Miller–Galante components with unconstrained articular surfaces. It is important to note that the typical pattern of retrieval in a well functioning knee demonstrates central contact. This dominance of central contact is likely governed by patterns of muscle contraction adapted by patients following total knee replacement

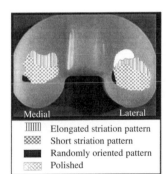

rior cruciate ligament (ACL) deficiencies. Some patients with ACL-deficient knees adapt a gait pattern that reduces or avoids the moment tending to flex the knee during stance phase.[14,15] It has been shown that the development of adaptive gait changes occurs over a period of several years after the index injury.[16] The nature of these adaptations suggests a reprogramming of the locomotor process to alter the pattern of muscle contraction prior to destabilizing events, since the latency time for muscle contraction would be too slow to respond instantaneously to a rapid stimulus.

Similar types of anticipatory adaptations have been reported in studies of patients following total knee replacement. Several studies have suggested that PCL-retaining patients demonstrate a more normal quadriceps function ascending stairs than patients with PCL-sacrificing knee designs.[1,5] Patients with PCL-sacrificing knee replacements have a tendency to reduce the moment sustained by the quadriceps by leaning forward during the portion of the support phase of ascending stairs when the quadriceps moment normally would reach a peak value.

Another example of the potential of the neuromuscular system to maintain normal functional kinematics in the absence of passive constraints can be found in retrieval studies. The centrally located (Fig. 5.8) wear patterns in retrieved components with flat unconstrained tibial geometry is likely maintained by the neuromuscular system through adaptive changes in the pattern of muscle contraction.[17] Clearly patients can dynamically stabilize the knee in the absence of passive constraints. These observations imply that constraint forces can be distributed to soft tissue structures rather than polyethylene surfaces. Future improvements in implant design could benefit from integrating the characteristics of these adaptations.

## Conclusion

Femoral rollback can and should be obtained in patients following total knee replacement. The intrinsic anatomy of the knee joint is designed to permit passive rollback during flexion. These characteristics are important for the restoration of normal function, since, among other factors, AP motion of the knee permits the muscles to function normally. The normal function of the joint is compatible with passively guiding the knee to a neutral position of maximum mobility at any angle of flexion. At any angle of flexion there is a passive envelope where the knee can displace with minimal force. Beyond this envelope, the resistance to passive force increases substantially. Studies of *in vivo* motion clearly demonstrate that the knee can displace in an AP direction within this envelope. The forces generated during a particular activity determine the amount of displacement.

The results (Figs 5.5 and 5.6) from a recent kinematic study of knee function during stair-climbing provide new insights into the relationship between femoral rollback and *in vivo* function. In particular, the AP movement of the knee joint during stair-climbing follows a consistent and characteristic pattern of movement, which is substantially different during swing phase than during stance phase. This difference is best illustrated by the hysteresis or offset between the loaded position of the femur versus the unloaded position of the femur (Figs 5.5 and 5.6). During the swing phase, between 20° and 50° of knee flexion, the femoral position moves anterior with flexion. At first, this observation appears to contradict the normal concepts of femoral rollback. However, the pattern of AP movement of the femur on the tibia can be related to patterns of muscle firing at the knee. These results suggest that the AP movement of the femur during stair-climbing is likely driven by the patterns of muscle firing. If this is the case, the ligaments act as cables providing end-point restraints to this AP motion, as they become taut. Further, as the knee approaches the extremes of the passive envelope stretch receptors in the surrounding capsule and ligaments will control the position of the knee through altering muscle firing patterns based on sensory feedback. Even in the absence of ligamentous constraint, receptors in tendon and capsule can produce sensory signals that can control the positional stability of the knee joint. The recent finding of centrally located wear patterns in unconstrained retrieved tibial components supports the interpretation that the neuromuscular system can adapt a pattern of muscle firing that dynamically maintains knee stability during locomotion.

Posterior rollback and patient function are still important considerations in total knee replacement. However, there is new information on the dynamic interactions that can take place during natural function. These interactions will likely play an important role in future considerations in the design of total knee replacement. These observations suggest that much of the constraint stresses needed to maintain AP stability can be sustained by passive soft tissue as well as through appropriate control of the neuromuscular system. Implants that constrain motion will not permit the normal sensory signals generated through soft tissue receptors to be generated. Therefore, AP stability must come from stress generated at the tibiofemoral articulation. This stress will cause increased damage to the articular surface and limit the longevity of the implant. Future improvements in implant design could benefit from integrating the role of the neuromuscular system to permit the knee to achieve normal kinematics.

# References

1   Andriacchi TP, Galante JO *et al.*: The influence of total knee-replacement design on walking and stair-climbing. *Journal of Bone and Joint Surgery* [Am] **64**(9):1328–1335, 1982.

2   Andriacchi TP, Stanwyck TS *et al.*: Knee biomechanics and total knee replacement. *Arthroplasty* **1**(3):211–219, 1986.

3   Kelman GJ, Biden EN *et al.*: Gait laboratory analysis of a posterior cruciate-sparing total knee arthroplasty in stair ascent and descent. *Clinical Orthopaedics and Related Research* **248**:21–26, 1989.

4   Dorr LD, Ochsner JL *et al.*: Functional comparison of posterior cruciate-retained versus cruciate-sacrificed total knee arthroplasty. *Clinical Orthopaedics and Related Research* **236**:36–43, 1988.

5   Wilson SA, McCann PD *et al.*: Comprehensive gait analysis in posterior-stabilized knee arthroplasty. *Journal of Arthroplasty* **11**(4):359–367, 1996.

6   Draganich LF, Andriacchi TP *et al.*: Interaction between intrinsic knee mechanics and the knee extensor mechanism. *Journal of Orthopaedic Research* **5**(4):539–547, 1987.

7   Andriacchi TP, Alexander EJ *et al.*: A point cluster method for *in vivo* motion analysis: applied to a study of knee kinematics. *Journal of Biomechanics Engineering* **120**(6):743–749, 1998.

8   Wimmer MA, Andriacchi TP: Tractive forces during rolling motion of the knee: implications for wear in total knee replacement. *Journal of Biomechanics* **30**(2):131–137, 1997.

9   Kapandji IA: *The physiology of the joints: annotated diagrams of the mechanics of the human joints: lower limb.* Churchill Livingstone, New York, 1988.

10  Markolf KL, Bargar WL *et al.*: The role of joint load in knee stability. *Journal of Bone and Joint Surgery* [Am] **63**(4):570–585, 1981.

11  Dye SF: The knee as a biologic transmission with an envelope of function: a theory. *Clinical Orthopaedics and Related Research* **325**:10–18, 1996.

12  Banks SA, Hodge WA: Accurate measurement of 3-dimensional knee replacement kinematics using single-plane fluoroscopy. *IEEE Transactions on Biomedical Engineering* **43**(6):638–649, 1996.

13  Andriacchi TP, Tarnowski LE *et al.*: 1999 New insights into femoral rollback during stair climbing and posterior cruciate ligament. *Transactions of the 45th Annual Meeting of the ORS* **24**:20.

14  Berchuck M, Andriacchi TP *et al.*: Gait adaptations by patients who have a deficient anterior cruciate ligament. *Journal of Bone and Joint Surgery* [Am] **72**(6):871–877, 1990.

15 Andriacchi TP, Birac D: Functional testing in the anterior cruciate ligament-deficient knee. *Clinical Orthopaedics and Related Research*
**288**:40–47, 1993.

16 Wexler G, Hurwitz DE *et al.*: Functional gait adaptations in patients
with anterior cruciate ligament deficiency over time. *Clinical
Orthopaedics and Related Research* **348**:166–175, 1998.

17 Wimmer MA, Andriacchi TP *et al.*: 1998 A Striated pattern of wear in
ultrahigh-molecular-weight polyethylene components of
Miller–Galante total knee arthroplasty. *Journal of Arthroplasty*
**13**(1):8–16.

# Con: Hiro Iwaki, Vera Pinskerova, and Michael Freeman

In this chapter femoral rollback will be defined as a posterior displacement of both femoral condyles with flexion. The important
emphasis in this definition is on the word "both." It will be argued
that the lateral femoral condyle tends to move backwards with flexion
in the normal knee. On the contrary, the medial femoral condyle
does not move backwards. It is obvious that a combination of an AP
motionless medial femoral condyle and backward displacement of
the lateral femoral condyle is simply a way of describing femoral
external rotation (or tibial internal rotation) with flexion. To say that
the tibia rotates on the femur as the knee flexes is one thing. To say
that the whole femur moves backwards across the tibia is another.
Only the latter will be regarded as rollback.

Strictly the "motion" to be argued in this contribution is that such
rollback is "unobtainable and undesirable." This position cannot in
fact be sustained. It is clear that a prosthesis can be designed (for
example the Insall–Burstein knee) in which a cam mechanism forces
the femur to move backwards with flexion. Thus rollback is certainly
obtainable. Whether or not rollback is desirable can be debated but
first the question must be addressed "Is it *necessary* and, in particular, is it *normal*?" If it were to be shown that the normal knee did
not rollback (in the sense defined) with flexion, the onus of proof
would lie with those who would wish to produce a prosthetic knee
that moved in a fashion quite different from that of the natural
knee.

So far as the present authors are aware, three lines of argument
have been adduced to support the view that rollback is desirable.
These are:

• that in the normal knee PCL tension causes "rollback" and that
this should be replicated after TKR
• that backward movement of the trochlea and patella occurs as a
consequence of rollback and is desirable because it lengthens the
extension lever arm in the flexed knee
• that rollback is necessary in order to obtain full flexion.

## Is the PCL tense throughout flexion and does "rollback" occur in the natural knee?

The concept of rollback was introduced in 1904 by Zuppinger,[1] who was the first to study the cadaveric knee using X-rays and wrote in German. He asserted that the cruciate ligaments represented the crossed-bars in a four-bar kinematic chain. He recognized that for this chain to function in such a way as to produce backward displacement of the femur, all four bars and specifically the two cruciate ligaments, would have to be rigid (i.e., tense) at all times. Zuppinger produced no evidence in support of the belief that the cruciate ligaments were tense at all times and his radiographs (which are shown only as traces in his original paper) do not clearly distinguish between rollback (i.e., backward displacement of both femoral condyles) as against rotation (i.e., backward displacement of only one femoral condyle).

In 1917, Strasser,[2] also writing in German, addressed the issue of the "rigidity" of the four-bar kinematic chain. He reported observations in support of his belief that no such chain existed because the cruciate ligaments were not tense at all times. Specifically, Strasser made the point that (save in extreme extension) the PCL was not tense in early flexion. Unfortunately for the subject of knee kinematics, Strasser published a drawing based on the work of Zuppinger showing the cruciate ligaments as lines of the same length throughout flexion to illustrate the concept of the four-bar chain that he was refuting. It would appear that subsequent authors may not have read Strasser's text and instead may have concluded from his illustrations that Strasser in fact was the originator and indeed a supporter of the concept. Since Strasser's argument was exactly the opposite, it is ironic that this conclusion should have been drawn.

The subject appears to have excited little interest from then until the 1950s when a number of authors revisited the topic. Huson,[3] who wrote both in German and English, analysed the motion of the knee on the basis of a rigid four-bar chain, but in his introduction specifically stated that the whole concept rested on the assumption (which he proposed to make) that both cruciate ligaments were indeed tense at all times. Menschik,[4] writing in German, published a complex analysis of the kinematics of the knee based on a rigid four-bar chain and leading to a description of the sagittal section of the femur as being helical in shape. Menschik published a figure (Figure 1 in his text) showing the appearance of the cruciate ligaments coated in radio-opaque material and then radiographed in the cadaveric knee in various degrees of flexion. This figure does indeed appear to show both cruciate ligaments as being tense throughout the range of flexion, with each ligament constant in length throughout the range. However, scrutiny of this figure shows that the tibial attachment of the PCL has in some way "displaced" itself forwards in the flexed knee. It is in fact only by "producing" this displacement that a ligament of constant length can be illustrated as being always tense. Kapandji,[5] in his widely read text-book dealing with the physiology of joints, produced line drawings illustrating the action of a rigid four-bar chain. Kapandji (personal communication) states that he obtained this idea from the work of Strasser. Müller[6] similarly illustrated the action of a four-bar chain by publishing photographs of a model in which the cruciate ligaments were replaced by rigid bars. Finally (and perhaps best known in the English literature) the work of O'Connor[7] again reproduced the rigid four-bar link mechanism. It is not entirely clear to the present authors what anatomical observations these workers made, particularly with respect to the PCL, to support the concept of its constant tension, but such tension (in both cruciate ligaments) is an important feature of the computer models upon which their subsequent work rests.

More recently other workers have suggested that the knee essentially rotates around an unmoving axis[8,9] and yet others have failed to identify rollback in cadaveric studies.[10]

The questions therefore arise:

- are the cruciate ligaments tense throughout the range of flexion: specifically, is the PCL tense throughout the range of flexion?
- do both femoral condyles move backwards as the knee flexes, i.e., does rollback occur?

The present authors have carried out a study of the unloaded normal cadaveric human knee using both dissection and magnetic resonance imaging (MRI). The method and the details of the results are published elsewhere and will not be repeated here.[11,12] The essential technique was to obtain fresh cadaveric knees and to attach them to a wooden board using wooden pegs passed through the tibia and femur into the board. Without opening the capsule, MRIs were obtained in various degrees of flexion and internal or external rotation. The knee was then dissected, again attached to the board to replicate the various positions of flexion for which MR images had been obtained. In this way the MRIs could be validated by anatomical photographs.

Figure 5.9 shows the appearance of the PCL at "–5°" and 90° of flexion. Similar MRIs in a living knee are shown in Fig. 5.10. It can be seen that the ligament appears straighter, and by measurement it can be seen that the distance between its tibial and femoral attachments is greater, at 90° than it is earlier in flexion. Figure 5.11 shows a dissection of the knee in which the lateral femoral condyle has been removed to enable the PCL to be photographed from its lateral aspect in corresponding positions of flexion. Once again the PCL can be seen to be somewhat slack (and thus deflectable with a piece of tape in Fig. 5.11) as compared with its situation at 90° of flexion when it is more vertical and tight. As the knee extends from about 5° of flexion to hyperextension, a small, inconstant band (called the posterior

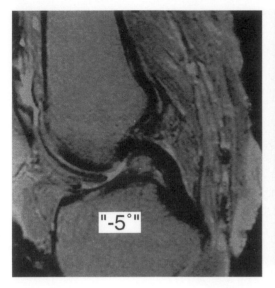
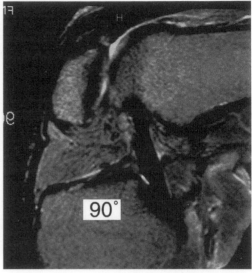

a                                                    b

**Fig. 5.9**

The PCL in the cadaver on MRI. Left (labelled "–5°") full extension. Right 90°. In full extension the PCL appears relaxed in comparison with its appearance at 90°.

oblique component of the PCL by Fuss[13]) located at the back of the ligament, again becomes tense. The change in length of the PCL as measured by two independent observers in six knees on MRI, between –5° and 120° is shown in Fig 5.12. It will be seen that the ligament elongates by about 22% with knee flexion, i.e., by more than the elongation which would be permitted by strain in the ligament.

Thus, it would appear that the PCL (as Strasser argued) is not tense throughout the range of flexion and therefore that there is no *rigid* four-bar kinematic chain in the knee. The PCL appears to tighten from 45° to 90° and to remain tight from 90° to 120°. The significance of this is discussed below.

To answer the question "Do both the femoral condyles move posteriorly with flexion?" it is necessary to study the shapes of the femoral condyles and to locate the centres of any circular articular surfaces that may be present in the sagittal plane.[11,12] Our own cadaveric studies[11,12] confirm the observations of Meyer[14] and of Albrecht.[15] The femoral condyles are composed, where they articulate with the tibia, of arcs of two circles as shown in Fig. 5.13. From an indeterminate zone between 10° and 30°, the medial femoral condyle rotates around the centre of the posterior arc (the "flexion facet") to full flexion. Between 10° and full extension, the condyle rotates around the anterior arc, the "extension facet," but its position can still be located by reference to the centre of the posterior arc if suitable allowance is made for the displacement of the centre of the flexion facet as it rotates around the centre of the extension facet.[11,12] On the lateral side the flexion facet contacts the tibia from 10° to full flexion. In some knees this contact is maintained to full extension but in

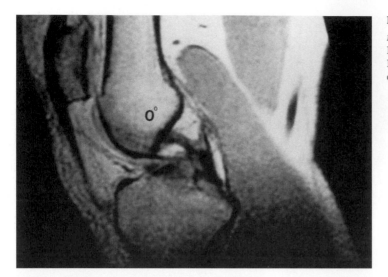

a

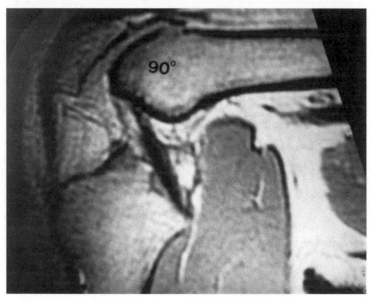

b

**Fig. 5.10**

MRIS corresponding to those in Fig. 5.8 in living volunteers. Full extension is now labelled 0°.

some knees there is a second anterior arc which subtends a smaller angle than on the medial side.

The position of both the flexion facet centres (adjusted towards extension to account for rotation around the extension facet centre) is shown for various positions in the flexion/extension cycle in Fig. 5.14. It will be seen that as the knee flexes the lateral condyle moves backwards but the medial does not. At about 30/45° flexion a line connecting the medial and lateral flexion facet centres (i.e., the

**Fig. 5.11**

Dissections corresponding to the MRIs in Fig. 5.8. A tape has been passed round the PCL in full extension to show that the ligament can be deflected by light tension exerted through the fingers.

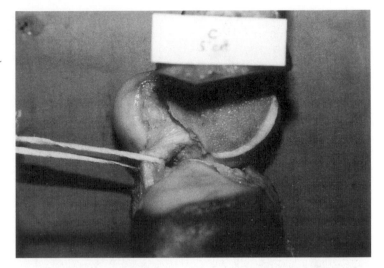

a

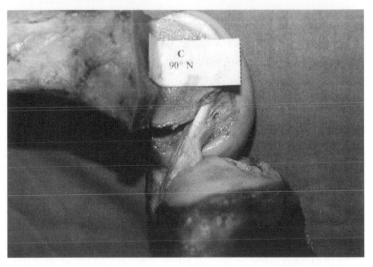

b

posterior femoral condyles) in the male knee (all the cadavers studied were male) is perpendicular to the long axis of the foot.[22] As the knee flexes from full extension, there are about 6° of tibial internal rotation until 20° is reached. From 20° to 45° rotation is negligible. From 45° to full flexion the tibia internally rotates a further 14°.

The observation that the tibia tends to rotate internally as the knee flexes has been in the literature for more than 100 years.[16] Brantigan and Voshell,[17] among many other authors, reported, as part of a general anatomical study of the knee, that the medial femoral condyle moved very little with flexion whereas the lateral condyle was much more mobile. Lafortune et al.[18] have demonstrated that the total arc of longitudinal rotation occurring during gait in the normal

111

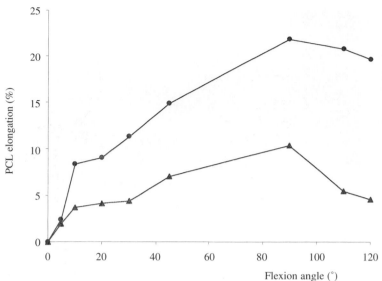

**Fig. 5.12**

PCL elongation expressed as a percentage increase of its length at full extension ($0°$). Observations by two independent observers (VP and HI). Measurements were made from a central position on the tibial and femoral attachments (central band, black circles) and posterolaterally (posterolateral band, black triangles). The separation between all parts of the ligament increases with flexion but to a lesser extent posteriorly.

knee is about 10°. This combination (i.e., of 10° internal rotation and 60° of flexion during the whole gait cycle) corresponds with our cadaver observations (Table 5.1). During the stance phase of gait (i.e., up to about 35° flexion), there are only about 8° rotation in the cadaveric knee, as in the knees studied by Lafortune et al.[18] Thus although the femur rotates externally (tibia internally) as the knee flexes, the knee is not far from being a uniaxial hinge during the stance phase of gait.

If the femur is forcibly rotated internally in the cadaveric knee flexed at 90°, the rotation occurring between 30° and 90° as the knee flexes can be abolished. Thus it would seem that the natural knee, were it to be flexed in combination with femoral internal rotation, would move without rollback or rotation from 0° to 90°.

We conclude that "normal" gait involves no AP displacement on the medial side but does involve posterior displacement on the lateral side. This equates to tibial internal rotation (or femoral external) rotation. There is no evidence of rollback. (In saying that rollback does not occur we concede that if the femur is internally rotated while the knee flexes, the condyles remain parallel between 30° and 90° but move backwards about 2 mm: this backward displacement of the condyles could be viewed as rollback.)

In summary of the arguments so far:

- We conclude that there is no rigid four-bar kinematic chain in the knee, because the PCL (and probably the ACL, not discussed here) is not tense at all times.
- This fits with the observation in the cadaveric and living knee that as the knee flexes the medial femoral condyle does not move backwards but that the lateral femoral condyle does, i.e., the

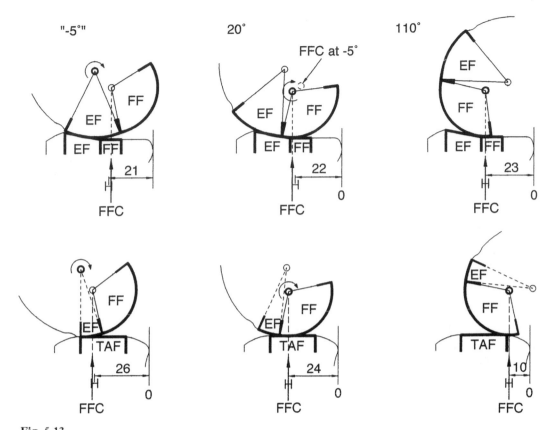

**Fig. 5.13**

Appearance of the femur and tibia in sagittal MRIs taken through the centre of the medial femoral condyle (top line) and the lateral femoral condyle (bottom line).

Medially the femoral condyle is composed of the arcs of two circles with separate geometric centres. Initially the femoral condyle slides on the tibia rotating round the anterior centre. At about 20° the posterior arc contacts the tibia and thereafter the femur moves with almost pure sliding relative to the tibia rotating around the centre of the posterior circle (FFC in the diagram; EF, extension facet; FF, flexion facet; TAF, tibial articular facet).

Laterally the motion is about 40% rolling, 60% sliding, so that the lateral femoral condyle tends to move backwards with flexion. A combination of no AP motion medially and backward motion of the femur laterally equates to femoral ER (tibial IR) with flexion (Reproduced from *Surgery of the Knee*, 3rd edition, ed. Insall J. N., Scott W. N., by kind permission of W. B. Saunders Co., Philadelphia).

femur externally rotates. This backward lateral displacement can be suppressed by flexing the knee whilst applying femoral internal rotation.

- Thus, rollback (as here defined) is not a feature of the natural knee and therefore there would seem to be no reason to produce it in the replaced knee.

Although it is not central to our argument, we suggest that the PCL is (in part) responsible for femoral external rotation with flexion. As the ligament tightens from 45° onwards it may (as suggested by the

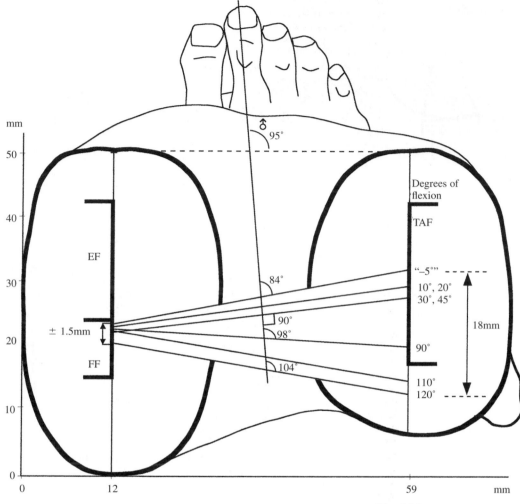

**Fig. 5.14**

The proximal tibia showing the tibial facets identified in Fig. 5.12 (EF, FF and TAF). The lines connect the position of the femoral flexion facet centres as shown in Fig. 5.12 at various degrees of flexion to demonstrate the femoral external rotation that occurs as the knee flexes. The midline of the knee moves backwards, with its transverse axis remaining roughly perpendicular to the long axis of the foot (Reproduced from *Surgery of the Knee*, 3rd edn, ed. Insall J. N., Scott W. N., by kind permission of W. B. Saunders Co., Philadelphia).

**Table 5.1** Femoral external rotation during the stance phase of gait

| Percentage of stance phase of gait | Flexion (°) corresponding to % gait cycle[18] | Femoral external rotation (°) corresponding to % gait cycle[18] | Degrees of flexion[11,12] |
|---|---|---|---|
| 0 (= heel strike) | 0 | 0 | 0 (at "–5°") |
| 20 | 20 | 4 | 6 |
| 40 | 20 | 4 | 6 |
| 60 | 5 | 4 | 4 |
| 80 | 5 | 3 | 4 |
| 100 (= toe-off) | 35 | 8 | 6 |
| Total arc | 35 | 8 | 6 |

"four-bar chain" concept) draw the midline of the femur backwards. At the same time the posterior horn of the medial meniscus, being firmly fixed to the tibia by the coronary ligaments,[17] may prevent backward movement of the medial femoral condyle. No such restraint exists laterally. In the presence of a "fixed" medial femoral condyle and a mobile lateral femoral condyle, backward movement of the femoral midline (due to PCL tension) would produce femoral external rotation, not femoral rollback.

## Is rollback necessary for backward displacement of the patella with flexion?

The outline of the trochlea in mid-sagittal MRIs in a cadaver knee is shown in Fig. 5.9. It can be seen that the trochlea (and therefore in life the patella) has moved back relative to the tibia by about 60 mm from −5° to 120°. In this knee femoral external rotation with flexion moved the midline of the femur back about 8 mm relative to the tibia. This represents about 13% of the total backward displacement

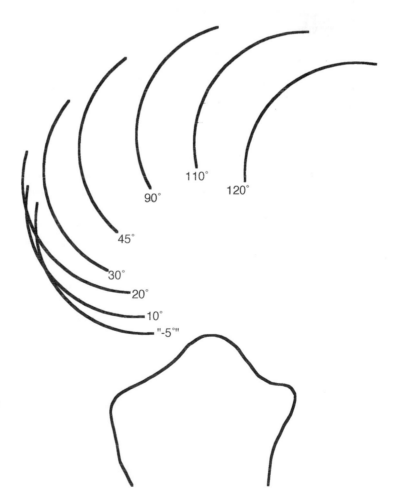

**Fig. 5.15**

Outlines of the trochlea taken from mid-sagittal MRIs at various degrees of flexion as shown in the diagram. Note that the trochlea moves upwards and then backwards relative to the tibia. The explanation for this movement is in the text (Reproduced from *Surgery of the Knee*, 3rd edition, ed. Insall J. N., Scott W. N., by kind permission of W. B. Saunders Co., Philadelphia).

of the trochlea shown in Fig. 5.15. The remainder is due to the relative positions within the femur of the flexion axis and the trochlea itself.

Space prevents a detailed description of the position of the flexion axis in the knee: it has been described elsewhere.[12] In summary the axis in the extended knee lies posterior to the trochlea. As the knee flexes therefore, the trochlea is moved first upwards and then backwards simply as a consequence of the rotation of the femur around the flexion axis (as it were from 10 o'clock to 3 o'clock). It is this displacement which is responsible for 87% of the posterior trochlea displacement with flexion.

In summary: posterior displacement of the trochlea (and thus of the patella) as the natural knee flexes is due mainly to the position of the trochlea relative to the flexion axis. To some extent it is also due to the femoral external rotation which usually accompanies flexion. It is not due to femoral rollback. Even in a knee prosthesis which does not permit rotation, the relative positions of the trochlea and the flexion axis can be arranged so as to replicate the normal and thus produce posterior displacement of the trochlea (and thus of the patella) with flexion.

## Is rollback necessary for full flexion?

Walker *et al.*[19] demonstrated in 1972 that full flexion could be obtained in a cadaveric knee that had been implanted with a variable-axis hinge, a prosthesis that did not permit rollback. For many years it has been known that patients implanted with fixed-axis hinges could obtain full flexion provided the axis was placed posteriorly. In the natural knee, full flexion occurs without significant backward displacement of the medial femoral condyle. These observations demonstrate that it is not necessary to provide rollback in order to obtain full flexion.

Having said that rollback is not a prerequisite of full flexion, it should be noted that the design of the posterior lip of the tibial component may well affect the flexion range if the femur does not move backwards across the tibia: if the posterior lip is curved strongly upwards, it may impinge upon the posterior femur before full flexion is obtained.

## Conclusion

It seems to the authors that the concept of "rollback" in the context of total condylar knee replacement was introduced in the 1970s as part of a kinematic view used to justify the retention of the PCL (after resection of the anterior cruciate ligament) in total knee replacement. We have argued in this chapter that there is no rigid four-bar kinematic chain in the natural knee and therefore that there is no physiological basis for rollback (defining rollback as a bodily backward displacement of the whole of the femur as distinct from backward displacement of the lateral femoral condyle in isolation). The femur does tend to rotate externally with flexion to 90°. Whether rotation around a medial axis (such as occurs in the unloaded natural knee) is really desirable in the replaced knee is not clear. The arguments for providing no rollback whatsoever centre around the fact that the medial and lateral femoral condyles can then be designed with a single radius matching a corresponding radius on the tibia. This increases the contact area and may thus reduce wear.[20] The same conforming geometry can, however, be provided in the medial femoral compartment alone and combined with rotation by designing the medial side as a ball-in-a-socket, allowing the lateral femoral condyle to track back by providing nonconforming surfaces between it and the lateral tibial condyle.

We would thus accept that rollback is obtainable in the replaced knee but we argue that this does not replicate normality. We believe that it is possible to design a knee which approaches normal kinematics by providing a medial ball-and-socket geometry. This would allow, as in the normal knee, posterior femoral displacement on the lateral side as the knee flexes, equating to longitudinal rotation not to rollback. Whether such an arrangement would have demonstrable clinical advantages, compared with conformity on both sides and thus neither rotation nor rollback, is not clear.

There appears to be no argument based on the extension lever arm nor on the range of movement for providing bodily backward displacement of the whole of the femur, i.e., rollback, in the replaced knee.

# References

1    Zuppinger H: *Die aktive Flexion im unbelasteten Kniegelenk*, p. 703. Züricher Habilitationschrift, Bergmann, Wiesbaden, 1904.

2    Strasser H: *Lehrbuch der Muskel - und Gelenkmechanik. III Band. Die untere Extemität.* J Springer, Berlin, 1917.

3    Huson A: The knee joint: Recent advances in basic research and clinical aspects. Congenital and postural deformities: The functional anatomy of the knee joint: the closed kinematic chain as a model of the knee joint. *Excerpta Medica International Congress Series* **324**:163–8, 1974.

4    Menschik A: Mechanik des Kniegelenks. *Zeitschrift für Orthopädie* **112**:481, 1974.

5    Kapandji IA: The mechanical role of the cruciate ligaments. *In The Physiology of the Joints* 2 ed., p. 120. Churchill Livingstone, Edinburgh.

6    Müller W: *Das Knie.* Springer-Verlag, Berlin, 1982.

7    O'Connor J, Shercliff T, FitzPatrick D *et al.*: Geometry of the knee. In *Knee ligaments: structure, function, injury and repair,* ed. D Daniel *et al.*, p. 163. Raven Press, New York, 1990.

8    Churchill DL, Incavo SJ, Johnson CC *et al.*: A comparison of the transepicondylar line with the optimal flexion/extension axis of the knee. *Transactions of the ORS 44th Annual Meeting,* 169, 1998.

9    Hollister AM, Jatana S, Singh AK *et al.*: The axes of rotation of the knee. *Clinical Orthopedics* **290**:259, 1993.

10 Blankevoort L: Passive motion characteristics of the human knee joint. PhDThesis, University of Nijmegen, 1991.

11 Iwaki H, Pinskerova V, Freeman MAR. Journal of Bone and Joint Surgery [Br] 2000 In press.

12 Pinskerova V, Iwaki H, Freeman MAR. The shapes and relative movements of the femur and tibia in the unloaded cadaveric knee: A study using MRI as an anatomical tool. In *Surgery of the knee*, 3rd edn, ed. JN Insall, WN Scott. WB Saunders, Philadelphia, In press 2000.

14 Fuss FK: Anatomy of the cruciate ligaments and their function in extension and flexion of the human knee. *Journal of Anatomy* **184**:165, 1989.

14 Meyer H: Die Mechanik des Kniegelenks. *Arkiv für Anatomie und Physiologie* p. 497, 1853.

15 Albrecht H: Zur Anatomie des Kniegelenkes. *Diss. Deutsche Zeits. u Chirurgie* **III**:433, 1876.

16 Bugnion E: *Le mécanisme du genou.* Ch Viret-Genton, Lausanne, 1892.

17 Brantigan OC, Voshell AF: The mechanics of the ligaments and menisci of the knee joint. *Journal of Bone and Joint Surgery* [Br] **22**:44, 1941.

18 Lafortune MA, Cavanagh PR, Sommer HJ et al.: Three-dimensional kinematics of the human knee during walking. *Journal of Biomechanics* **4**:347, 1992.

19 Walker PS, Shoji H, Erkman MJ: The rotational axis of the knee and its significance to prosthesis design. *Clinical Orthopedics* **89**:160, 1972.

20 Plante-Bordeneuve P, Freeman MAR: Tibial high density polyethylene wear in conforming tibiofemoral prostheses. *Journal of Bone and Joint Surgery* [Br] **75**:630–636, 1993.

# Not sure

## James B. Stiehl

The question of whether or not the knee rolls back in total knee arthroplasty (TKA) is a critical point of discussion, as it is presupposes that the technique of TKA has the ability to capture normal knee kinematics. The second issue is how rollback or the lack of it influences ambulatory function after TKA. I will begin by reviewing current knowledge of normal knee function.

According to Kapandji et al.,[1] flexion of the knee is a result of a combination of rolling gliding and rotation of the femoral condyles over the tibial plateau. The contact on the lateral side moves a greater distance than does that on the medial side. Draganich has suggested that rollback occurs with a change of tibiofemoral contact of approximately 10 mm from full extension to flexion.[2] Kurosawa et al.,[3] studying cadavers and normal subjects found that the center of the medial condyle seemed to move forward 4.4 mm to midrange of flexion and then backward 4.0 mm as the knee flexed further. The center of the lateral condyle moved steadily backward for a total of 15 mm and the rate of excursion decreased with flexion. There was a resultant tibial internal rotation of 17° at 120° of flexion.

LaFortune et al.[4] placed Steinman pins in 5 healthy subjects and then studied them using high-speed cine cameras. He found that stance phase tibial internal rotation was 9.4°. Tibiofemoral contact was 1.3 mm anterior to the midpoint of the proximal tibia and translated up to 14.3 mm posteriorly during swing phase of gait. Ishii *et al.*[5] used an intracortical pin placement with an instrumented spatial linkage system in 5 healthy volunteers finding 5.2° of posterior femoral rollback and 10.6° of tibial internal rotation. Neither of these studies could specifically differentiate medial from lateral tibiofemoral contact.

Freeman has argued the presence of a more complex kinematic motion, which has been confirmed by recent MRI studies. There is little if any rollback or motion of the medial femoral condyle (3–4 mm) through a functional range. This shift in part could be explained by liftoff of the anterior portion of the relatively flat cam-shaped medial femoral condyle. The lateral condyle has a greater potential for rolling and sliding motion and can actually translate posteriorly 15–18 mm. With a fixed medial pivot point and a mobile posteriorly translating lateral condyle, the rollback noted is really more a case of tibial internal rotation relative to the tibia.[6,7] This then defines what we now understand as the normal knee kinematics. There appears to be a complex interaction of motion deriving from a relatively stationary position of the medial condyle and posterior translation of the lateral condyle to describe resultant tibial internal rotation.

## Anterior cruciate deficient kinematics

Draganich *et al.*[8] defined a total of 13.5 mm of posterior displacement of tibiofemoral contact from 0° to 90° in normal knees. With anterior cruciate resection, all of the tibiofemoral contact points shifted posteriorly with resultant anterior displacement of the tibia. Posterior rollback persisted with the greatest displacement of 3–4 mm during the first 20° of flexion. With both cruciates incised, after 20° there was anterior displacement of the tibia laterally and after 40° of flexion, medially. A subsequent study revealed that the PCL does not resist anterior translation of tibiofemoral contact, only posterior.[9] With *in vivo* weightbearing studies, Andriacchi found that ACL-deficient knees had exaggerated contraction of hamstring muscles with a relative quadriceps avoidance from 0° to 40° flexion. This would negate the effect of the patellar tendon pull to displace tibiofemoral contact anteriorly. At greater degrees of flexion (beyond 40°), this effect tended to disappear.[10]

Karrholm,[11,12] using photogrammetry (RSA) to assess tibiofemoral relationships of the ACL-deficient knee, found a relative external tibial rotation of the knee. It was suggested that varus position was exaggerated and that internal rotation normally seen with flexion was reduced in the ACL-deficient knee. Dejour[13] analyzed tibiofemoral translation in ACL-deficient knees, finding excessive AP translation in the medial compartment compared to the lateral. In summary, absence of the ACL causes a relative posterior displacement of tibiofemoral contact, especially on the lateral tibial plateau. Furthermore, normal internal rotation seen with the swing phase of gait can be reduced with this position, and the normal medial condyle pivot may be lost due the ACL deficiency.

## Nonfluoroscopic kinematic analysis of TKA

For reasons that will become obvious in the subsequent discussion, determination of three-dimensional tibiofemoral kinematics has dramatically improved with the introduction of *in vivo* weightbearing fluoroscopic studies. It is now believed that these techniques are highly accurate and reproducible as compared to earlier non fluoroscopic methods. From literature review, those techniques included *in vitro* cadaver studies, invivo nonweightbearing radiographic studies, gait analysis, goniometric studies, and photogrammetry (RSA). *In vitro* cadaver studies basically measured the effects of the primary and secondary ligament constraints and were unable to add the physiologic muscle forces or the dynamic loading of actual human weightbearing. The disadvantage of gait studies and goniometric fixtures was the significant error introduced by nonstationary soft tissues. Roentgenographic stereophotogrammetry (RSA) is highly precise with accuracy of 0.03 mm but the method only evaluates a nonweightbearing situation as subjects are not able to walk, stair-climb, or deep knee bend for the test.

Without exception, all published *in vitro* cadaveric studies have suggested that PCL-retaining TKA specimens allow posterior tibiofemoral rollback as described by the normal knee. Schlepckow *et al.*[14] measured the ligamentous versus prosthetic constraint of three different implant designs: unconstrained (LCS), semiconstrained (TriconM), and constrained (MARK II). Though posterior rollback and rotation of the total knees was stated, a concern about implant stability was noted with increasing flexion. This was to imply that the normal roll–slide movement of the implants as well as rotational movements became irregular and unpredictable. Menchetti and Walker[15] utilized the radiographic cadaver technique described by Kurosawa to analyze a mobile-bearing TKA (MBK). Posterior rollback from −14 to −7.0 mm (net 4.6 mm) was seen from 0° to 120° flexion. Lateral condyle translation accounted for tibial internal rotation.

Garg and Walker[16] used a computer generated model based on 23 anatomical specimens to assess flexion and rollback. Then concluded that rollback was possible if the PCL was maintained and the posterior slope of the tibia matched that of the normal knee. Using similar methods, Soudry *et al.*[17] concluded that rollback was present in PCL-retaining designs and was not influenced by weightbearing loads. Their study did not, however, examine weightbearing loads.

El Nahass *et al.*[18] used a electrogoniometric fixture to assess AP translation and internal–external rotation of the tibia in weightbearing gait and stair-climbing. For total knees, there was 5–10° of internal rotation and 9–14 mm of posterior femoral rollback from 0° to

90°.[19] Andriacchi, *et al.* reported recently that total knees had AP translation of 2.9 cm with normal knees moving 1.9 cm. The method used was a point cluster system that possibly suffers error due to soft tissue translation.

Nilsson *et al.*[20] used RSA to evaluate total knee kinematics. He placed tantulum markers in the bone about implants and obtained perpendicular radiographs of the knees. Spatial calculations of the markers were used to determine tibiofemoral movements. This method was done nonweightbearing in the prone position with simple loads applied. Nilsson studied a fixed (MG I) and mobile-bearing (LCS) PCL-retaining design and a PCL-sacrificing design. He found an increased posterior position in extension though there appeared to be significant posterior translation or rollback with increasing flexion. Prosthetic knees showed 3–4° of internal rotation with flexion and normal knees averaged 6.5° of internal rotation.[21] Lateral radiographs of these subjects confirmed the relatively posterior tibiofemoral contact position. Kim *et al.*[22] performed a similar nonweightbearing study utilizing lateral radiographs at 0° and 90° flexion, finding essentially no change in AP position, and concluded that there was no rollback.

## *In vivo* weightbearing fluoroscopic studies

The idea of studying a subject by fluoroscopy following TKA began with Banks and Hodge in 1993.[23] They studied four LCS meniscal-bearing implants and found a paradoxical anterior translation of tibiofemoral contact with flexion. We modified this technique slightly using a two-dimensional computer vector analysis to study AP translation of the lateral condyle. The lateral condyle was chosen from the belief that the greatest motion would be seen on the lateral side. We found that the lateral condyle started about 10 mm posterior to the midsagital plane of the tibia in extension and translated anteriorly 15 mm to a point 5 mm anterior to the midsagital tibia. It was noted that the pattern of motion in total knees was highly variable and was irreproducible, showing jerky discontinuous motion.[24]

It was postulated that in the normal knee the ACL was maximally loaded in extension whereas the PCL was minimally loaded. The PCL without the restraint of the ACL tended to pull the femur posteriorly during full extension, hence the posterior tibiofemoral contact position. On weightbearing, the normally posteriorly directed shear force on the proximal tibia caused the prosthetic femur to translate anteriorly. An interesting feature of the early study was that five different posterior cruciate retaining "flat on flat" condylar total knee designs were evaluated from nine community surgeons. Despite the diversity of results, the patterns of motion were uniform. This study suffered early criticism as it was felt that the surgeons were not skilled in correctly balancing the PCL. Also, the analysis was done only with a deep knee bend position, not felt to be a realisitic measure of normal gait. We were drawn, however to the clearcut results, and the implication of not having reproducible posterior femoral rollback with these "flat on flat" condylar implants.

Dennis et al.[25] refined the computer vector analysis to use three-dimensional computer-assisted design models of the tibial and femoral components. A large library of three-dimensional images (861) for each prosthesis then described spatial orientation through six degrees of freedom. The computer technician then matched the appropriately oriented image to the two-dimensional image, and then subtracted that image allowing computer analysis. Dennis et al. evaluated in vivo passive versus weightbearing range of motion in these patients, finding that all knees, including normal, PCL-retaining TKA, and PCL-substituting TKA had significantly less active weight-bearing versus passive range of motion ($p < 0.02$). This could result from the increased constraint of combining ligament restraints with articular surface geometry, muscle contraction, and tibiofemoral kinematics. On in vivo weightbearing, PCL-retaining TKA had significantly less motion that PCL-substituting TKA ($p < 0.05$) with a maximum flexion of 103° versus 130° in PS knees. From the authors' perspective, rollback or posterior translation seemed to be preserved in the PS TKA although paradoxical anterior tibiofemoral translation of PCR TKA may limit the amount of flexion possible.[26]

ACL-deficient knees were evaluated using the fluoroscopic method finding a posterior tibiofemoral contact in extension followed by varying and erratic° of anterior translation from 30° to 90° of flexion. On average, this amounted to 0.5 mm but one case translated as far as 13.7 mm through flexion. According to Dennis, posterior cruciate retaining TKA started with an average position 5.1 mm posterior to the midsagital tibia in extension with anterior translation from 30° to 90°. One knee moved anteriorly 7 mm. PS total knees started at the midline and translated posteriorly on average 7.71 mm.

Appropriate conclusions from Dennis's study were that PCL-retaining total knees suffered from ACL-deficient kinematics and that weightbearing kinematics in TKAs were substantially effected by both implant geometry and ligamentous constraints as determined by surgical technique. Thusly, tight PCL tensioning caused the implant to remain posterior through range of motion whereas laxity caused the tibiofemoral contact to translate anteriorly, occasionally in exaggerated fashion.

More recently, Komistek et al.[27] have developed a sophisticated computer method of interactive model fitting that allows true three-dimensional spatial determination. This fourth-generation method allows calculation of all six degrees of freedom: sagittal plane AP motion, internal/external (screw-home) rotation, and abduction/adduction (condylar liftoff). For purposes of this discussion, the most obvious enlightenment was simultaneous calculation of medial and lateral condyle tibiofemoral contact—earlier studies had evaluated only lateral condyle position.

We investigated medial and lateral tibiofemoral contact in a variety of total knees to assess *in vivo* kinematics. The "flat on flat" condylar Whiteside prosthesis demonstrated posterior contact of both condyles in extension, exaggerated medial condylar sliding, and relative lateral condyle pivot on deep knee bend. Though not as prominent with gait, anterior medial sliding was still greater than lateral motion and no rollback was demonstrated. Rotation was unpredictable, showing up to 9° of internal rotation and 1.5° of external rotation. Our greatest concern was the detrimental medial condyle sliding of considerable distance of 6–14 mm which could result in significant in significant pattern wear.[28] Blunn *et al.*[29] have implicated a sliding, ploughing motion as the most likely cause of polyethylene implant delamination and catastrophic wear. Retrieval studies of other "flat on flat" condylar designs have shown similar pattern wear. Gabriel *et al.*[30] suggested an additional problem with exaggeration of tibial fixation interface stresses resulting from posterior tibiofemoral contact.

A mobile-bearing TKA was investigated with posterior cruciate retention, sacrifice, or substitution. The implant was the LCS which has very high conformity from 0° to 40° of flexion and diminished line contact with further flexion. The implant has a femoral condylar shape with decreasing radii of curvature into deep flexion. The only implant difference in this study was the surgical technique with reference to the PCL. The PCL-retaining LCS meniscal-bearing implant demonstrated consistent tibiofemoral contact posterior to the midsagital tibial reference point. There was early posterior rollback up to 30° but anterior translation was noted at 60° and 90° of flexion. The PCL-sacrificing LCS rotating platform design remained virtually midline on the proximal tibia throughout the range of motion. There was, however, a minor trend for early rollback with anterior translation in deep flexion.[31] The posterior stabilized LCS-PS, a recent design development, showed a similar midline position but with consistent posterior rollback throughout flexion. For the LCS prosthetic design, the interpretation is that PCL retention results in ACL-deficient kinematics. PCL sacrifice allows tibiofemoral contact to reflect implant geometry and congruency. With PCL substitution, the greatest constraint of tibiofemoral contact is exerted on the implant as the cam/post mechanism forces posterior femoral rollback. Our clinical experience with the LCS-PS would suggest that posterior femoral rollback will result in greater range of motion, similar to the results of Dennis *et al.*[25]

A separate study evaluated the results of a bicruciate or ACL-retaining TKA, the Cloutier prosthesis. This implant had spherical line contact but would be considered an unconstrained implant, similar to the Whiteside prosthesis. This implant overall resulted in posterior femoral rollback on early flexion with some anterior translation in deep flexion. However, all implant positions were posterior to the midsagital tibial line. Our conclusion was that although about 50% of cases had an improvement over PCL-retaining implants, the remainder probably had a nonfunctioning ACL. A number of cases had a flexion contracture of 10–15°, which could represent a minor imbalance or tightness of the ACL.[32]

Dennis et al.[33] recently compared the PFC TKA with options of a flat, dished, or posterior stabilized tibial polyethylene insert utilizing gait and stair-climbing modes. The dished and PCL-substituting implants had similar kinematics with treadmill gait whereas the flat condylar tibial insert demonstrated significantly greater sliding translation and variability.

## Discussion

The summary of known kinematic information regarding the knee can be stated as follows. The normal knee has a complex pattern of motion with tibial internal rotation on flexion related to posterior translation or rollback of the lateral condyle about a relatively fixed medial pivot point. PCL-retaining TKAs have abnormal kinematics that most likely relate to surgical technique, specific implant geometry, and absence of the ACL. There is posterior tibiofemoral contact in extension followed by varying degrees of anterior translation with flexion and virtually no predictable rollback. "Flat on flat" condylar designs were popularized to allow retention of the PCL and a simplified surgical technique. Tibial insert design was flat to minimize constraint suggested to be the most likely cause of failure, i.e., mechanical loosening of the tibial tray. Virtually no attention was given to the impact this approach may have to implant wear.

We have been able to demonstrate abnormal medial condylar sliding or rollforward seen with some "flat on flat" condylar designs. In the case of a young, high demand patient, this mechanism can explain the wear problems of osteolysis and catastrophic implant failure seen with these designs. An additional feature of abnormal kinematics is loss of normal "screw-home" rotation or internal rotation in certain cases. Although internal rotation of up to 10° has been confirmed in TKA, external rotation of over 6° is also seen. With abnormal tibial component placement, this irregularity can cause potential component wear in certain fixed-bearing designs.

Those implant designs with high conformity, such as the mobile-bearing LCS, or PS designs that have a cam/post mechanism for articulated AP motion have obligatory posterior femoral rollback as a function of implant geometry. Stated simply, the design engineer can enforce a degree of posterior rollback by creating a unique design. Ultimately, knee function relates to a complex interaction of weight-bearing forces, muscle contractions, and kinematic features which are likely to be abnormal or nonphysiologic in total knee patients. In vivo weightbearing fluoroscopic studies have revolutionized our understanding of these complex relationships of surgical technique and implant design.

# References

1 Kapandji IA: *The physiology of the joints*, pp. 114–123. Churchill Livingstone, New York, 1970.

2 Andriacchi TP, Galante JO: Retention of the posterior cruciate in total knee arthroplasty. *Journal of Arthroplasty* **1**,Suppl:13–19, 1988.

3 Kurosaw H, Walker PS, Abe S *et al.*: Geometry and motion of the knee for implant and orthotic design. *Journal of Biomechanics* **18**:487–499, 1985.

4 LaFortune, MA, Cavanagh PR, Sommer HJ, Kalenak A: Three-dimensional kinematics of the human knee during walking. *Journal of Biomechanics* **25**:347–357, 1992.

5 Ishii Y, Terashima K, Terashima S, Koga Y: Three-dimensional kinematics of the human knee with intracortical pin fixation. *Clinical Orthopaedics and Related Research* **343**:144–150, 1997.

6 Freeman MAR, Railton GT: Should the posterior cruciate ligament be retained or resected in condylar nonmeniscal knee arthroplasty? *Journal of Arthroplasty* **1**, Suppl:3–12, 1988.

7 Pinskerova V, Iwaki, H, Freeman MAR: 1999 The movements of the knee: A cadaveric magnetic resonance imaging and dissection study. *Transactions of the Annual Meeting of the American Academy of Orthopaedic Surgeons*, 5–8 February 1999, Anaheim, CA, p. 82.

8 Draganich LF, Andriacchi TP, Andersson GBJ: Interaction between intrinsic knee mechanics and the knee extensor mechanism. *Journal of Orthopaedic Research* **5**:539–547, 1987.

9 Vahey JW, Draganich LF: Tensions in the anterior and posterior cruciate ligaments of the knee during passive loading: predicting ligament loads from insitu measurements. *Journal of Orthopaedic Research* **9**:529–538, 1991.

10 Andriacchi TP, Birac D: Functional testing in the anterior cruciate ligament-deficient knee. *Clinical Orthopaedics and Related Research* **288**:40–47, 1993.

11 Kärrholm J, Selvik, G, Elmqvist LG, Hansson LI: Active knee motion after curciate ligament rupture. *Acta Orthopaedica Scandanavia* **59**:158–164, 1988.

12 Jonsson H, Kärrholm, J: Three-dimensional knee joint movements during a step-up: Evaluation after anterior cruciate ligament rupture. *Journal of Orthopaedic Research* **12**:769–779, 1994.

13 Dejour H, Bonnin M: Tibial translation after anterior cruciate ligament rupture. *Journal of Bone and Joint Surgery* [Br] **76**:745–749, 1994.

14 Schlepckow P: Three-dimensional kinematics of total knee replacment systems. *Archives of Orthopaedic and Trauma Surgery* **111**:204–209, 1992.

15 Menchetti PP, Walker PS: Mechanical evaluation of mobile bearing knees. *American Journal of Knee Surgery* **10**:73–81, 1997.

16 Garg A, Walker PS: Prediction of total knee motion using a three-dimensional computer-graphics model. *Journal of Biomechanics* **23**:45–58, 1990.

17 Soudry M, Walker PS, Reilly DT *et al.*: 1986 Effects of total knee replacement design on femoral-tibial contact conditions. *Journal of Arthroplasty* **1**:35–45.

18 El Nahass B, Madson NM, Walker PS: Motion of the knee after concylar resurfacing—an invivo study. *Journal of Biomechanics* **24**:1107–1117, 1991.

19 Andriacchi TP, Tanrowski LE, Berger RA, Galante JO: New insights into femoral rollback during stair climbing and posterior cruciate

ligament function. *Transactions of the 45th Annual Meeting of the Orthopaedic Research Society*, February 1999, Anaheim, Ca., p. 20, 1999.

20  Nilsson KG, Kärrholm, J, Ekelund L: Knee motion in total knee arthroplasty. A roentgen stereophotogrammetric analysis of kinematics of the Tricon-M knee prosthesis. *Clinical Orthopaedics and Related Research* **256**:147–161, 1990.

21  Nilsson KG, Kärrholm J, Gadegaard P: Abnormal kinematics of the artificial knee. Roentgen stereophotogrammetric analysis of 10 Miller–Galante and five New Jersey LCS Knee. *Acta Orthopaedica Scandanavia* **62**:440–446, 1991.

22  Kim, H, Pelker RR, Gibson DH *et al.*: Rollback in posterior cruciate ligamanent-retaining total knee arthroplasty. *Journal of Arthroplasty* **12**:553–561, 1997.

23  Banks SC, Hodge WA: Direct measurement of 3D knee prosthesis kinematics using single plane fluoroscopy. *Proceedings of the Orthopaedic Research Society* **18**:428, 1993.

24  Stiehl JB, Komistek RD, Dennis DA, Paxson RD: Fluoroscopic analysis of kinematics after posterior cruciate-retaining knee arthroplasty. *Journal of Bone and Joint Surgery* [Br] **77**, 884–889, 1995.

25  Dennis DA, Komistek RD, Hoff WA, Gabriel SM: *In vivo* kinematics derived using an inverse perspective technique. *Clinical Orthopaedics and Related Research* **331**:107–117, 1996.

26  Dennis DA, Komistek RD, Stiehl JB *et al.*: Range of motion after total knee arthroplasty. *Journal of Arthroplasty* **13**:748–752, 1998.

27  Hoff WA, Komistek RD, Dennis DA *et al*: A three dimensional determination of femorotibial contact positions under in vivo conditions using fluoroscopy. *Journal of Clinical Biomechanics* **13**:455–470, 1988.

28  Stiehl JB, Dennis DA, Komistek RD: Detrimental kinematics of a 'flat on flat' total condylar knee arthroplasty. *Clinical Orthopaedics* **365**: 139–148, 1999.

29  Blunn GW, Walker PS, Joshi, A, Hardinge, K: The dominance of cyclic sliding in producing wear in total knee replacements. *Clinical Orthopaedics and Related Research* **273**:253–260, 1991.

30  Gabriel SM, Dennis DA, Koomistek RD *et al.*: *In vivo* TKA kinematics with consequences for system stresses and strains. *Proceedings of the 42nd Annual Meeting of the Orthopaedic Research Society*, p. 201, Atlanta, Georgia, 18–22 February, 1996.

31  Stiehl JB, Dennis DA, Komistek RD, Keblish PA: In vivo kinematic comparison of posterior-cruciate-retaining and sacrificing mobile bearing total knee arthroplasty. *American Journal of Knee Surgery*, 2000.

32  Stiehl JB, Dennis DA, Komistek RD: The cruciate ligaments in total knee arthropalsty: a kinematic analysis. *Journal of Arthroplasty* **15**:545–500, 2000.

33  Dennis DA, Running D, Komistek RD, Anderson DT: *In vivo* kinematic analysis of posterior cruciate retaining and posterior stabilized knee implants during normal gait. *21st Annual Meeting of SICOT Abstract Book*, p. 438. Sydney, Australia, 18–23 April, 1999.

## Questions and answers

*Moderator:* The entire topic of femoral rollback is intertwined with many aspects of total knee replacement. Two that immediately come to mind are the debate over whether or not to save the PCL, and the debated as to whether it is beneficial to have a tibial bearing that moves. If I therefore ask you some questions of which others have previously spoken, I would like to get your personal opinions. I am sure it will not be repetitive. Let's start.

*Moderator:* Dr. Andriacchi, when we perform a knee replacement we routinely remove the ACL. Do you really think that an ACL-deficient knee can function like a normal knee? If not, how does this affect the results that you have seen in your testing?

*Dr. Andriacchi:* The way the knee dynamically functions is dependent on the activity. During walking on level ground, we have found that following total knee replacement patients tend to walk in a manner similar to patients following ACL injury. That is, they tend to walk with a reduction or an avoidance of the use of the quadriceps when the knee is near full extension. This is a reasonable response to ACL deficiency since when the knee is near full extension a force generated by the quadriceps will tend to pull the tibia anteriorly in the absence of the ACL. It appears that a number of patients reprogram their pattern of muscle firing during locomotion and adept a slight variation in gait during walking on level ground. The testing methodology to detect this type of gait change is an important consideration since the gait abnormality can only be detected under normal or near normal walking conditions. Care must be taken in conducting these tests to avoid causing another stimulus that may influence a change in muscle firing patterns resulting in an adaptation to the test environment that is not reflective of the normal function of the patient. During activities such as stair-climbing, there is an interaction between the PCL and patterns of muscle firing. Thus, the absence of the ACL during a stair climbing activity does not appear to have a major influence on knee function. Again, it is important to replicate the conditions of the normal activity to test these effects.

*Moderator:* As a follow-up question, Jim Stiehl and Doug Dennis have shown erratic motion in PCL-retained knee replacements performed by talented surgeons who knew how to balance the ligaments. How do you respond to their findings, Dr. Andriacchi?

*Dr. Andriacchi:* My opinion of the fluoroscopic measurements described by Jim Stiehl and Doug Dennis are that they do not truly reflect normal *in vivo* function. The measurements were taken during an awkward single leg squat in front of a fluoroscope. Their results describe conditions of liftoff that clearly do not occur with any frequency during normal function since we do not see failures of polyethylene components related to that type of motion. Regarding issues of balance of the ligaments, our results indicate that the ligaments behave as cables that become lax or taut based on the forces generated during a specific activity. The AP motion during normal function arises primarily from forces generated during muscle contraction that are guided by a neutral position dictated by ligament tension. Clearly retrievals of unconstrained total knees show a well-contained band of contact. These retrieval studies suggest that control of AP motion is possible in knees that do not depend on polyethylene to provide the constraint forces to maintain stability.

*Moderator:* On the basis of your studies, Dr. Stiehl, it would appear that a medial ball-in-socket lateral sliding surface knee would be indicated. Do you use such a knee?

*Dr. Stiehl:* From my knowledge of the subject, there currently is a fixed-bearing design that attempts to capture the concept of a fixed medial joint with a mobile sliding unconstrained lateral joint (Advance Knee, Wright Medical Technology, Memphis, TN). I believe that the concept of trying to recreate normal knee kinematics with a reconstructed arthroplasty is rarely accomplished and there are always essential elements that are absent for normal function. As we have shown, the fundamental problem with PCL-retaining total knees is the loss of the ACL. This creates medial compartment laxity and explains the exaggerated anterior tibiofemoral motion seen both in sports injuries and in weightbearing total knees. I have been able to show this problem with the Whiteside total knee that had "flat on flat" articulating surfaces with posterior cruciate retention. Anecdotally, several retrievals of this knee revealed wear patterns consistent with abnormal medial compartment laxity. Blunn, *et al.*, with a large number of retrievals, demonstrated predominant wear on the medial joint surfaces after total knee replacement. My concern with any knee that attempts to artificially make a constrained medial pivot joint is that the innate laxity of reconstructed total knee may cause exaggerated loosening and wear in some cases. This was the typical fate of the old Geomedic prosthesis that was constrained in the medial compartment and used PCL retention. Kinematic data do not support the concept that ACL-deficient knees retain the medial pivot, and if anything, the pivot may be more laterally placed. For these reasons, I would not favor the medial pivot concept.

*Moderator:* Mr. Freeman, do you think that one can obtain proper posterior stability in a medially conforming knee (such as the Medial Pivot Knee) without limiting flexion by posterior impingement.

*Mr. Freeman:* I think that much of that question has already been answered in my contribution in the section headed "Is rollback necessary for full flexion." By posterior stability I am sure you mean posterior stability of the tibia on the femur. Assuming you do mean this, the relevant stability is supplied by the anterior lip of the medial compartment that can be as high as you like (in the case of my prosthesis, 11 mm) without interfering with flexion. It does raise questions about the exact shape of the anterior part of the femoral component as the knee extends, but that is a different matter.

*Moderator:* Let me ask that question in a slightly different way. To what extent to you think that we can have full flexion without rollback in both compartments?

*Mr. Freeman:* We have an MRI study of a Japanese patient fully flexing the knee. What it shows is that the Japanese fully flex by combining flexion with internal rotation. The result is that the medial femoral condyle does not go appreciably back, but rather the lateral femoral condyle goes so far back as effectively to lose contact with the tibia altogether. Obviously one could not produce this situation in a prosthesis and it is not clear to me (or to anyone else) whether or not it is possible fully to flex the normal knee in combination with tibial external rotation so as to keep the lateral femoral condyle forwards. For those readers who are interested we have submitted a paper on this topic for publication.

*Moderator:* There obviously is tremendous debate about whether the knee rolls or slides or both, Dr. Andriacchi. What are your feelings about the medial pivot knee as reproducing the "normal" rolling and sliding pattern of the knee? Do you think it works or is it more hope than truth?

*Dr. Andriacchi:* In my opinion and based on the results of our testing, the knee moves by both a rolling and sliding mechanism. Again, the nature of the knee movement is highly dependent on the activity. Even during a routine activity such as level walking, the knee will assume an internally and externally rotated position at the same angle of flexion during different periods in the walking cycle. Therefore, there is not a single axis of motion or a medial pivot. Much of the data describing motion based on a single axis have been derived from cadaver measurements and do not reflect the type of knee movement seen during activities where normal patterns of muscle firing occur.

*Moderator:* Dr. Stiehl, do you presently save the PCL in any of your knee replacements?

*Dr. Stiehl:* No, but I would like to if I could reconcile the abnormal knee kinematics with reasonable bearing mechanics. I personally used several contemporary "flat on flat" fixed-bearing PCL-retaining prosthetics over a 10 year period. The fundamental problem is abnormal tibiofemoral sagittal plane kinematics that leads to anterior translation with increasing flexion. Component liftoff is also probable. These features may predispose the articulation to increased wear and diminished weightbearing range of motion. A very clear understanding of this was shown when we compared the kinematics of the PCL-retaining meniscal-bearing LCS with the PCL-sacrificing rotating platform LCS. One had abnormal kinematics resulting from loss of the anterior cruciate ligament, whereas the other demonstrated excellent midline positioning through the range of motion but suffered from joint line elevation, and thus diminished extensor mechanics.

*Moderator:* To change tracks a bit, Dr. Stiehl, many of the problems in the past with PCL-retaining knees were in those with thin, very flat, gamma-irradiated polyethylene inserts. What are your feelings about "modern" PCL-retaining knees with thicker, more conforming, poly-ethylene inserts that are not gamma-irradiated in air?

*Dr. Stiehl:* From my perspective there were two major problems that led to many reports of osteolysis after PCL retaining TKA: "bad kine-matics," and "bad poly." Clearly the second issue will go away with recent technical advances such as thicker polyethylene, more con-forming surfaces, and nongamma-irradiated polyethylene. What this means in the real world is that designer surgeons who typically put in large numbers of joints with great expertise will no longer see early osteolysis in any of their patients. The kinematic issues will become much more difficult to recognize, except in poorly done TKAs. Average surgeons who do limited numbers of cases will still have problems with the kinematic issues and still may have wear in certain cases. We have all seen these cases where there is early failure from pain, swelling, and chronic instability.

*Moderator:* Dr. Andriacchi, you did not mention the "four-bar linkage" at all in your contribution. Do you think that this concept really is applicable to the knee, either before or after replacement? Obviously Mr. Freeman does not.

*Dr. Andriacchi:* As we look at more advanced kinematic studies of the knee joint during true *in vivo* function, it is clear that the knee does not follow the constraints of a four-bar linkage under dynamic function. It is rather a system guided by cables that are tense or slack at end-points of motion. These cables (cruciate ligaments) act to provide end-point constraints as well as feedback that allow the neu-romuscular system to program a pattern of muscle firing that main-tains dynamic stability. In my opinion, the future of enhancing knee replacement under conditions of minimally invading the joint with prosthetic material is to obtain a better understanding of the way the neuromuscular system interacts with the kinematics and utilize this understanding in evolving procedures which take advantage of these dynamic adaptations.

*Moderator:* Dr. Stiehl, do you feel that the PS post is obligatory if you remove the PCL? I already know that Mr. Freeman does not feel that it is necessary and that stability can be obtained through a cupped-type bearing.

*Dr. Stiehl:* The question can be answered by comparing the results of early total condylar total knees that sacrificed the posterior cruci-ate with the subsequent evolutionary PCL-substituting designs that added obligatory tibiofemoral rollback with a cam/post mechanism. From the studies of Ranawat, we know that PCL-sacrificing knees have performed extremely well over long periods. However, PCL-sub-stituting TKAs clearly have better range of motion and better extensor function because of the obligatory rollback. The dis-advantge, though, is increased patellofemoral problems from clunk, fracture, or subluxation which, though poorly understood, could result in part from this increased loading and the area of the patellofemoral groove that is uncovered by the cam mechanism. The choice for the PS post is a difficult tradeoff, better motion and function versus the greater chance of revision and problems from the patellofemoral joint. I personally favor the PS choice.

*Moderator:* Final question, Dr. Stiehl; you have mentioned a rotating-bearing insert with a PS post. Could this type of design not lead to dislocation of the post from the femoral component if there was any degree of laxity of the flexion and extension spaces?

*Dr. Stiehl:* Absolutely! In fact we redesigned the rotating platform LCS design to a PS implant in order to gain advantages of the cam/post mechanism and to also to prevent spinouts. However, if technique is poor and the extension and flexion spaces are not balanced well, there is little to prevent dislocation. I have used the mobile-bearing LCS for 5 years and would caution any surgeon new to this technique that errors in balancing the gaps must absolutely be avoided. I remain very enthusiastic about the mobile concept, however, because wear problems have been virtually nonexistent and clinical follow-up in many series, not just the designer's, have shown excellent long-term results.

## 6

*An infection in the knee is one of the most devastating complications that can occur after knee joint replacement. In the early days of joint arthroplasty, infection almost invariably led to marked diminution of function, limited motion, chronic pain, and severe systemic disease. Recently, however, with a better understanding of the pathogensis of this infection and by a refining of our methods of treatment, many patients who have an infected prosthesis can be treated effectively and returned to a good functional situation.*

# Two-stage exchange is the optimal treatment for an infected total knee replacement

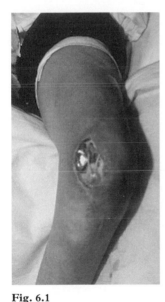

**Fig. 6.1**

Exposed, infected total knee replacement. Fortunately, exposed, infected implants are rarely encountered now. This presentation used to be common, when hinged implants were utilized in the 1960s and 1970s. Modern evaluation techniques should allow the surgeon to definitively treat the infection well before this situation occurs.

## **Pro**: Russell E. Windsor

Infection represents probably the most devastating complication of total knee replacement surgery (Fig. 6.1). Its incidence varies from 4–12% in older literature,[1–3] to 0.5–2% in more recent reports.[4] Fastidious attention to the operating room environment, laminar air flow, gown enclosures, prophylactic antibiotics, and sterile technique have decreased the rate of acute infection to an incidence of about 0.4–0.7 %. Acute and chronic infections may demand different methods of treatment. Acute infection has been defined as an infection that occurs within 3 months of primary total knee replacement implantation. Chronic infection, therefore, includes all infections that develop after 3 months. However, in a study performed by Shoifet and Morrey, success of open debridement with retention of the prosthetic components occurred in 27% of the patients that had an infection diagnosed within 3 weeks.[5] Those in whom the diagnosis was obtained after 3 weeks did not have a successful eradication of the infection. Thus, the time period of an acute infection may have to be redefined and reduced to a period of 3–4 weeks. This point is especially important if a surgeon is defining successful treatment of infection by arthrotomy and debridement versus staged re-implantation for the acute and chronic definitions.

The options for treating an infected total knee replacement include:

- antibiotic suppression alone
- surgical debridement and suppression with component retention
- single-stage exchange[6]
- two-stage exchange.[7]

Salvage options include:

- arthrodesis
- resection arthroplasty[8] (Fig. 6.2)
- amputation.

In general, antibiotic suppression alone is reserved for the medically infirm where any operation may be a threat to the patient's life.[4] Surgical debridement and suppression with retention of the components has also had limited success.[5] The procedure is reserved for the medically infirm patient who can undergo a relatively moderately invasive procedure. It is also done if the surgeon feels that infection has fallen within the acute time frame. As discussed above, the Mayo Clinic experience was not very promising. Mont has reported repeat arthrotomy and debridements with retention of components as a promising way to eradicate infection.[9] Overall, he obtained 83% retention of the prostheses out of 24 knees. All of the immediate postsurgically infected knees ($n$ = 10) were retained, but only 10 of 14 (71%) late hematogenously infected knees were retained. However, there is also the problem of subjecting a patient to many procedures. There is no guarantee that the infection is definitively eradicated and there is the likelihood of developing additional scar formation with each procedure. A single attempt at open arthrotomy

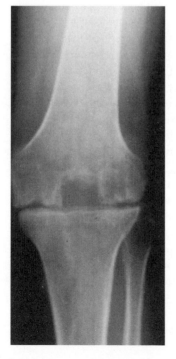 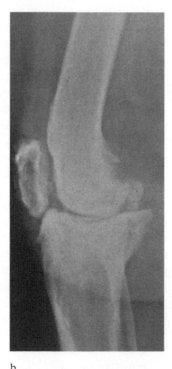

a      b

**Fig. 6.2**

(a) AP and (b) lateral radiograph of a resection arthroplasty. No acrylic cement spacer is present in the knee and the joint is immobilized for 6 months to allow the joint to stiffen.

and debridement can be done in the proper clinical setting. However, if treatment of the infection still is a failure after one arthrotomy and debridement, consideration should be given to performing a two-stage removal and reimplantation of a new knee replacement. Going directly to two-stage exchange will give a highly predictable result without having to subject the patient to multiple procedures and anesthetics.

From the above options available to the surgeon, definitive treatment of infection has been most successfully obtained by two-stage exchange of a new knee replacement. The technique involves a first-stage operation, whereby all prostheses are removed and a complete debridement of necrotic tissue with cement removal is performed.[7,10] An antibiotic-impregnated spacer block is inserted and the wound is closed. The patient undergoes a 6 week course of antibiotic treatment maintaining the serum bactericidal titer (SBT) at a minimum 1:8. The 6 week time period is counted when the SBT reaches 1 : 8. If the bacteria are particularly resistant to certain agents, it may be necessary to change the antibiotic drug or utilize synergistic effects of multiple bacteriocidal agents. Days during which the SBT falls to uncertain levels are not counted toward the 6 week interval. After 42 days of antibiotic treatment, the second operative stage is performed during which a new total knee replacement is implanted with antibiotic-impregnated cement. In the USA, the surgeon must currently mix antibiotics manually with Palacos cement. Antibiotics that are stable in powdered form in acrylic cement include tobramycin and vancomycin.

The literature is replete with studies supporting two-stage exchange. The first report by John Insall in 1983 included 11 knees that had had successful eradication of the infection with a 6 week interval between stages.[10] Rand concurrently published a series of infected total knee replacements that had had a 2 week interval of antibiotic therapy between stages.[11] However, these patients obtained dismal results and it was recommended that this time period not be used. Borden subsequently published a study showing intermediate success with a 4 week course of antibiotics between stages.[12] Currently, there have been many reports of successful treatment of an infected total knee replacement by two-stage exchange. Overall, these reports demonstrate a success rate ranging from 89% to 100% total eradication of the infectious organism.

Hanson studied 89 patients and observed an 89% success rate with the two-stage re-implantation protocol. Whiteside reported a 97% success rate in a cohort of 33 patients using this method of treatment. However, he utilized a 6 week course of antibiotic-impregnated cement beads followed by a reimplantation of a new total knee replacement by cementless means. Antibiotic-soaked allograft material was utilized and a porous, cementless implant was inserted.[13] Wasielewski reported 92% success in a group of 50 patients.[14] The fact that numerous surgeons have reproduced the successful results first obtained by John Insall[10] gives substantial support for the two-stage exchange being considered the procedure of choice for treating the infected total knee replacement. Goldman studied a cohort of 64 infected total knee replacements in 60 patients treated by two-stage exchange and found that 95% of the patients were satisfied with the decision to undergo the procedure and there was an overall 10-year predicted survivorships rate of 77.4%.[15] Backe reported 12 cases that had developed a second infected total knee replacement and underwent successful treatment by another two-stage exchange. Success was based on preserved soft tissue and a well-functioning extensor mechanism in a healthy patient.[16]

There appears to be a paucity of reports on single stage exchange for infection. Goksen and Freeman reported an 89% successful eradication of infection in a series of 18 replacements with *Staphylococcus epidermidis* and streptococcus bacteria as the infecting organisms.[6] During this procedure, the removal and debridement stage of the prosthetic components is separated from the re-implantation portion of the operation by a 30 min period of irrigation with the tourniquet deflated to allow antibiotics to reach the operative site. New instruments and draping was used during the performance of the re-implantation.

Although the two-stage technique takes an investment of 7–8 weeks to get the patient out of the hospital, the eradication of infection has been successful in 89–100% of the cases studied. Despite two stages being necessary, the success suggests that two-stage exchange will get the problem solved with less likelihood that further surgical intervention will be necessary. The appeal of single-stage exchange, despite a 70–89% eradication the infection, is a shorter period of hospitalization which decreases overall cost. The cost reduction is deceptive, however. The better ability to administer antibiotics parenterally at home by home health vendors has enabled the patient to be hospitalized for only a week after the first stage and less than a week for the second stage, thus reducing actual hospitalization time by about 4–5 weeks. Also, whereas the patient undergoing two-stage exchange receives a 6 week course of intravenous or oral antibiotic treatment between the debridement and re-implantation stages, antibiotics are completely discontinued 4 days after the second stage. On the other hand, patients who have undergone a single stage exchange will continue oral antibiotic usage for a period of 3–6 months. Depending on the concern of the infectious disease consultant and the virulence of the infecting organisms, decreasing doses of antibiotic intake may take place for up to 1 year, and some patients may receive antibiotics indefinitely.

Another issue for proponents of single-stage revision is avoidance of bone stock destruction that may occur between the debridement and re-implantation stage. If a single antibiotic spacer block is used, some bone erosion may develop during the 6 week interval between procedures. On the other hand, with the use of articulated spacers, this bone erosion is minimized. The 6 week interval allows the inflamed tissue to heal and recover from the infection. Despite scarring that occurs during the healing process, articulated spacers preserve motion while allowing the surrounding soft tissues to become better prepared for the second-stage procedure. The immune system is put in a position to heal the infection during the period of time antibiotic therapy is administered after the debridement stage. Antibiotics leach into the surrounding tissues during the 6 week period of implantation. During a single-stage revision, these inflamed tissues are still in a compromised state which may affect wound healing and overall function. The patient is frequently nutritionally depleted as a result of the immune system fighting the infection. The lymphocyte count and serum albumin may be decreased significantly and the 6 week interval of time allows the patient to get these indices back to normal physiological levels. During the 6 week period the patient's function is preserved, and the clinical results after this time interval approach those obtained after revision arthroplasty for aseptic failure.

Another issue is the preservation of knee function during the period of antibiotic treatment between stages. Proponents of single-stage exchange suggest that the rehabilitation can begin more aggressively and earlier than is possible when a spacer is implanted. It must be remembered that the inflamatory response is still ongoing and scarring may occur late after a one-stage exchange. Also, with the use of articulated spacers, acrylic prostheses (Prostalac), block spacers (Fig. 6.3) or autoclaved implants coated with antibiotic-impregnated cement, function may be preserved by a normal rehabilitative schedule that will preserve function during the time interval between the total knee replacement excision and re-implantation.

Until further literature support becomes available, two-stage exchange is the procedure of choice for treating the infected total knee replacement. It provides a successful way of treating low- and high-virulence organisms, including methicillin-resistant *Staphylococcus aureus* and gram-negative bacteria. Certainly, the proponents of single-stage exchange must provide data to support the successful eradication of infection by more virulent organisms. At present, the success rates of single-stage exchange are about 10–15% lower than those obtained with the two-stage protocol.

A controlled, randomized study of both single and two-stage exchange is needed to properly evaluate the successful eradication of the infection itself, but also to determine the functional outcomes of each procedure. A cost–benefit analysis should also be performed to compare the cost differences between one- and two-stage procedures and weigh the predictability of cure and need for subsequent procedures if infection is not successfully eradicated by the single-stage procedure.

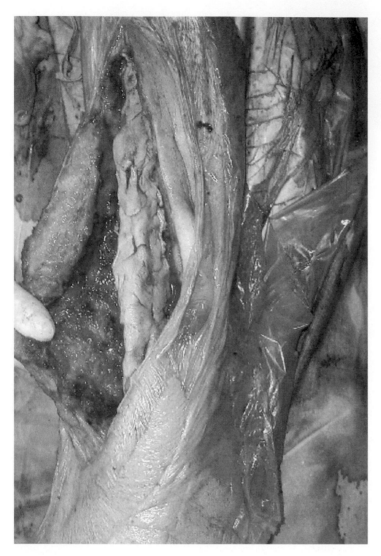

**Fig. 6.3**
A large antibiotic spacer used to maintain space after an infected, hinged prosthesis was removed for infection. The patient had the hinge implanted for limb salvage after resection of a Ewing's sarcoma in the proximal tibia.

# References

1   Deburge A, GUEPAR Group: GUEPAR hinge prosthesis: Complications and results with two years; follow-up. *Clinical Orthopedics* **120**:47–53, 1976.
2   Grogan TJ, Dorey F, Rollins J. *et al.*: Deep sepsis following total knee arthroplasty: Ten-year experience at the University of California at Los Angeles Medical Center. *Journal of Bone and Joint Surgery* [Am] **68**:226–234, 1986.
3   Rand JA, Bryan RS, Morrey BF *et al.*: Management of infected total knee arthroplasty. *Clinical Orthopedics* **205**:75–85, 1986.
4   Rand JA: Alternatives to reimplantation for salvage of the total knee arthroplasty complicated by infection. *Journal of Bone and Joint Surgery* [Am] **75**:282–289, 1993.

5   Schoifet SD, Morrey BF. Treatment of infection after total knee arthro-
    plasty be debridement with retention of the components. *Journal of
    Bone and Joint Surgery* [Am] **72**:1383–1390, 1990.

6   Goksan SB, Freeman MAR: One-stage reimplantation for infected
    total knee arthroplasty. *Journal of Bone and Joint Surgery* [Br]
    **74**:78, 1992.

7   Windsor RE, Insall JN, Urs WK *et al.*: Two-stage reimplantation for the
    salvage of total knee arthroplasty complicated by infection: Further
    follow-up and refinement of indications. *Journal of Bone and Joint
    Surgery* [Am] **72**:272–278, 1990.

8   Falahee MH, Matthews LS, Kaufer H: Resection arthroplasty as a
    salvage procedure for a knee with infection after a total knee
    arthroplasty. *Journal of Bone and Joint Surgery* [Am] **69**:1013–1021,
    1987.

9   Mont MA, Waldman B, Banerjee C *et al.*: Multiple irrigation, debride-
    ment, and retention of components in infected total knee arthro-
    plasty. *Journal of Arthroplasty* **12**:426–433, 1997.

10  Insall JN, Thompson FM, Brause BD: Two-stage reimplantation for the
    salvage of infected total knee arthroplasty. *Journal of Bone and Joint
    Surgery* [Am] **64**:1087–1098, 1983.

11  Rand JA, Bryan RS: Reimplantation for the salvage of an infected total
    knee arthroplasty. *Journal of Bone and Joint Surgery* [Am]
    **65**:1081–1986, 1983.

12  Borden LS, Gearen PF: Infected total knee arthroplasty: A protocol for
    management. *Journal of Arthroplasty* **2**:27–36, 1987.

13  Whitside LA: Treatment of infected total knee arthroplasty. *Clinical
    Orthopedics* **299**:169–172, 1994.

14  Wasielewski RC, Barden RM, Rosenberg AG: Results of different sur-
    gical procedures on total knee arthroplasty infections. *Journal of
    Arthroplasty* **11**:931–938, 1996.

15  Goldman RT, Scuderi GR, Insall JN: 2-Stage reimplantation for
    infected total knee replacement. *Clinical Orthopedics* **131**:118–124,
    1996.

16  Backe HA, Wolff DA, Windsor RE: Total knee replacement infection
    after 2-stage reimplantation.

17  Feldman DS, Lonner JH, Desai P, Zuckerman JD: The role of intraop-
    erative frozen sections in revision total joint arthroplasty. *Journal of
    Bone and Joint Surgery* **771**:1807–1813, 1995.

# Con: Klaus Steinbrink

## Acknowledgement

I would like to thank Professor H. W. Buchholz in Hamburg who
taught me the management of deep infection in the late seventies,
and Dr. Lars Frommelt, microbiologist especially for his help in
answering the moderators questions concerning germs and antibiotics.

The mean rate of infection following knee replacement surgery
(TKR) can be estimated at 1–3%. The objective of the difficult and
prolonged treatment of these infected knee implants must be to free
the patient as effectively, quickly and inexpensively as possible from
the problem.

- *Effectively* means in this context that the success of the treatment is defined by:
  - proven permanent eradication of infection in at least 80% of cases (negative C-reactive protein, sterile joint aspiration)
  - stability and functional weightbearing of the knee joint with a new implant in the majority of cases.
- *Quickly* means that the successful treatment is completed in less than 4–5 weeks.
- *Inexpensively* includes the requirement that the treatment of a septic knee prosthesis does not cost 3–4 times as much as primary arthroplasty (or twice as much as an aseptic revision of a TKR).[1]

In contrast to two- or several-stage surgical procedures, the one-stage procedure recommended by the author fulfils these criteria. This recommendation is based on the author's personal experience in the treatment of infected hip and knee prostheses during 20 years at the Endo-Klinik in Hamburg, and knowledge of the experience of the surgical team in that clinic which has performed one-stage exchange arthroplasty in more than 5000 cases of infected total hip[2–4] and 800 cases of infected total knee prostheses.[5]

After using this concept consistently for three decades to treat periprosthetic infection, the author continues to share the opinion of the surgeons at the Endo-Klinik that this therapy is the method of choice.

Without selecting patients according to local and general clinical findings, diagnosis or pathogen, the success rate for infected hips was increased with this method from 71% to 88%,[4] and for infected knees from 73% to 84%.[5] The reasons for this significant improvement in outcome lie in the disciplined operative technique, constantly increasing experience due to large numbers of patients (specialization) and consistent co-operation between surgeon and clinical microbiologist.

## Method

### Diagnosis

To treat periprosthetic infection by one-stage exchange arthroplasty it is imperative to identify the pathogen causing the infection and its antibiogram prior to operation, as antibiotics are mixed into the bone cement in order to prevent recolonization of the new implanted prosthesis.

The method of choice for obtaining a representative sample for bacteriological examination is the aspiration of joint fluid. This fluid is a good source of suitable samples because in the course of time the pathogens spread over the entire surface of the foreign body.

**Table 6.1** Accuracy of pathogen identification from preoperative joint aspiration compared with intraoperative biopsy ($n$ = 2158 cases, 1989–90)

| $n$ | Relative frequency (%) | Sample Preoperative | Intraoperative | Result (%) |
|---|---|---|---|---|
| 416 | 19.3 | Growth | Growth | Correct |
| 1589 | 73.6 | Sterile | Sterile | 92.3% |
| 93 | 4.3 | Sterile | Growth | Wrong |
| 30 | 1.4 | Growth | Sterile | 7.7% |
| 30 | 1.4 | Other/additional pathogens | | |
| 2158 | 100 | | | |

An experienced microbiologist can successfully identify the pathogen in over 90% of cases[5] (Table 6.1) provided the pre-analytical phase and the processing in the laboratory take into account the peculiarities of the pathogens and co-operation between surgeon and clinical microbiologist during the entire diagnostic procedure is maintained at all times.

If fistulae are present joint aspiration should be supplemented by bacteriological examination of a fistula specimen, obtained by curetting the fistula tract with a sharp spoon. This is important, as joint fluid and fistula specimens do not necessarily contain the same pathogen.

Specimens obtained by curetting are superior to a smear because the organisms found in the fistula wall can be more easily distinguished from colonies of surrounding skin flora, and are therefore more likely to be pathogens.

Biopsies also provide representative tissue samples if they are taken during surgical revision of the focus of infection. They are carried out in exceptional cases when identification of the pathogen is not possible preoperatively by other methods.

## Choice of antibiotics

The choice of antibiotics depends on the susceptibility of the organism on the one hand, and on the other, the effectiveness and physical properties of the antibiotic.[6]

The antibiotics in the concentration chosen by the microbiologist must have a bactericidal effect when mixed with bone cement. Concentrations which are merely bacteriostatic do not guarantee that the contaminating bacteria will be destroyed and colonization thus prevented.

The antibiotics must be eluted from the polymethylmethacrylate (PMMA) bone cement and remain stable in the presence of the tem-

**Table 6.2** Antibiotics used for PMMA bone cement/antibiotic mixtures and corresponding pathogens

| Bacteria | Antibiotics | Dose[a] |
|---|---|---|
| GRAM POSITIVE PATHOGENS | | |
| Staphylococci | | |
| Streptococci | | |
| Propionibacteria | Lincomycin | 3.0 |
| | Gentamicin | 1.0 |
| Staphylococci | | |
| Streptococci | | |
| Propionibacteria | Cefazedon | 2.0 |
| | Gentamicin | 1.0 |
| Staphylococci | Vancomycin | 2.0 |
| (highly resistant) | Ofloxacin | 1.0 |
| | Gentamicin | 0.5 |
| Enterococci | Vancomycin | 2.0 |
| | Ampicillin | 1.5 |
| | Gentamicin | 0.5 |
| GRAM NEGATIVE PATHOGENS | | |
| Enterobacteriaceae | Cefotaxime | 2.0 |
| | Gentamicin | 1.5 |
| Pseudomonas aeruginosa | Cefoperazone | 2.0 |
| | Amicacin | 2.0 |
| ACID FAST RODS | | |
| Mycobacteria | Streptomycin | 2.0 |

[a] g/40 g PMMA bone cement.

peratures which arise during polymerization of the cement. Table 6.2 shows a list of antibiotic combinations which have proved successful in local therapy.

*Operative technique*

Regardless of whether chronic periprosthetic infection is treated by a one- or two-stage procedure, there is general agreement that the removal of the infected implant is the essential element in this surgery. This means both components of the prosthesis, femoral and tibial, and also the patella replacement if present. Furthermore, if the prosthesis was fixed in position with bone cement, this must also be totally and radically removed. Any other material, such as wire or screws, can also transmit infection and must be searched for and removed.

In cases with uncemented knee prostheses, especially those with a structured surface, osteotomy and fenestration may be necessary to remove the implant. These are measures which are often complicated by intraoperative fracture of the femoral and tibial shafts.

The possibility of such fractures should, however, not induce surgeons to decide in favour of a two-stage procedure, as later re-implantation is considerably more difficult due to deformity, axial deviation, and defects even after the fracture has completely healed. Intraoperative reduction, reconstruction and stabilization with stemmed, axially linked total prostheses, even when extra-long, seems to us the better way to achieve both aims: eradication of infection and stabilization of the joint, thus preserving the function of the limb.

## Necrotomy

### SOFT TISSUES

Excision of infected and necrotic soft tissue around the knee joint in the muscle and hollow of the knee is certainly of decisive importance for the success of this therapy. It is a question of surgical experience to recognize the boundary between healthy and infected tissue and to excise into the healthy region. If present, and if possible, fistulae are integrated into the skin incision made for access to the infected joint and radically excised by following them through to the implant. We prefer the medial subvastus approach. If a fistula lies too far towards anterior or lateral in relation to this approach, then it has to be excised separately and the wound later closed primarily in several layers. Radical excision does not present a problem in the muscles close to the joint. In the vicinity of nerves and blood vessels in the hollow of the knee it does involve risks. Injuries to vessels in the hollow of the knee have, however, been extremely rare occurrences in our operations.

Perforations, fenestrated bone, and cortical defects in the femur and tibia in cases of infected stemmed prostheses always make it necessary to revise these areas separately by detaching the soft tissues, and excising and thoroughly cleaning local, sometimes demarcated abscesses. If this is not done, persistence of the infection is guaranteed. Tissue samples from all areas of revised soft tissue are sent for bacteriological examination.

### BONE

In a "normal case" of bland chronic infection, whether discovered by chance or as a result of specific diagnostic examination, there should still be cancellous bone in the region of the implant bearing which can be preserved after thorough cleaning (providing a careful implantation technique was used at primary arthroplasty). After removal of the implant the femoral and tibial bone are first subjected to a general cleaning using a sharp spoon (again samples are sent as biopsy material for bacteriological examination). Following this first general cleaning, all further tissue is removed right down to the healthy bone using elastic or ball reamers of different diameters. As with the preparation of the soft tissues, a great deal of experience is necessary in order to assess in which layer the bone is again vital, well supplied with blood, and "clean." Beyond the prosthesis tips "osteomyelitis" may have become established as an intramedullary form of the periprosthetic infection outside the implant bearing, so the medullary canals must also be thoroughly cleaned.

In severe cases of chronic infection with loss of bone stock sequestered sections of the femoral cortex or proximal tibia are found. These sections have to be sacrificed, following the principle that to eliminate the infection all sequestered tissue must be removed. Regardless of the planned re-implantation, resection of this bone must be radical when indicated. Usually this procedure is less problematic if the surgeon decides to replace these sections of long bones with metal or cement by implanting prostheses with extra-long stems. Resection of the tibia head does occasionally mean that the insertion of the patella tendon has to be sacrificed and additional plastic surgery is necessary.

After completion of the cleaning phase by preparing the bone surface with the sharp gouge, reamers and drills and resection if necessary, the site of operation is irrigated abundantly.

## Irrigation

Routinely we use a pulsating lavage to irrigate soft tissues and bone with up to 6 l of saline solution. The medullary canals can be cleaned further using special plastic brushes. This instrumentarium is not perfect and is definitely in need of improvement. The use of pressure irrigation leads to a proven reduction in the number of bacteria intraoperatively.

## Re-implantation

When the site of operation, soft tissues and bone, has been radically cleaned as described here, i.e., the maximum possible reduction of bacteria has been achieved, we see no reason why the new prosthesis should not be implanted during the same operation.

The new prosthesis is protected against possible re-infection to a large degree by the antibiotics added to the bone cement. According to the research and conclusions of A. Gristina, the infection of biomaterials, in this case the prosthesis, takes place within the first hours after implantation in a competition between bacteria and integrating cells ("race for the surface").[7,8] By analogy, re-infection of the new prosthesis also takes place within a few hours after re-implantation. Therefore, the specific antibiotic must already be on the spot when a new prosthesis is implanted following removal of an infected one. The antibiotic in the bone cement protects the prosthesis surface against recolonization by any bacteria remaining in the implant bearing. Furthermore, adjacent soft tissues are protected in the same way by the high local concentration of the antibiotic.

## The implant

Once the infected capsula synovialis and capsula fibrosa, including any affected ligaments, have been resected, it seems to us that the

**Fig. 6.4**

Rotating knee prostheses
(ENDO-Modell).

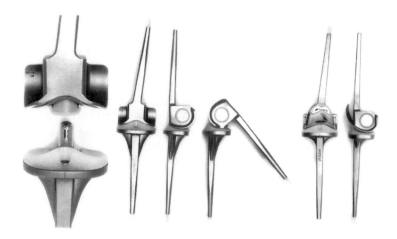

implantation of a condylar prosthesis, which needs at least the collateral ligaments to provide stability, does not offer a very good chance of success. In patients with severe infection the ligamentous apparatus is too often seriously damaged or the resection necessary to treat the infection involves the loss of the collateral ligaments (and the posterior cruciate). Therefore in every case where a condylar prosthesis has been removed we prefer to re-implant an axially linked prosthesis.

The aversion of many orthopaedic surgeons in Europe and other countries to using axially linked hinge prostheses for a primary implantation is understandable in view of the history of these prostheses and experience with antiquated designs. However, these systems have apparently become more popular in recent years with surgeons who perform large numbers of revision operations on knee prostheses. This trend is supported by the good experience we have had with intracondylar knee prostheses since 1970. Survival rates of over 90% 15 years after primary implantation give us the certainty that at least in revision cases the indication is absolutely justified.[9]

In cases where axial deviation and contracture is only slight, and where only moderate soft tissue resection is necessary, the rotating hinge model Endo, a semi-constrained, axially linked prosthesis, is adequate (Fig. 6.4). If a rotating hinge prosthesis of this kind or similar semi-constrained model has to be exchanged, or in patients with severe infection and loss of soft tissue and bone stock, a pure hinge prosthesis (Fig. 6.5) produces more reliable results. Bone defects of the tibia head, condyles, and distal femur can be adequately and securely bridged with extra-long stems, if necessary ante-curved and with a varus angle of the femoral component (Fig. 6.6).

If more than half the femur has been lost due to infection or resection, a two-stage procedure may be indicated with elimination of infection by using a so-called spacer with an extra-long femoral

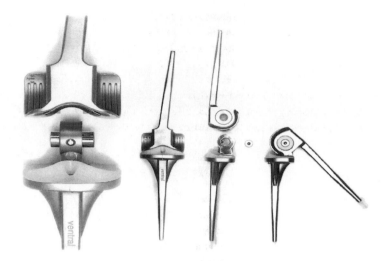

**Fig. 6.5**
Hinge knee (ENDO-Modell).

component. The aim of permanent mechanical stability can then be achieved by a total femur prosthesis which is implanted when sterile conditions have been restored after a correspondingly safe interval (Fig. 6.7).

Although the indication for a total femur prosthesis is rare (3% in the treatment of infected hip prostheses) we have achieved respectable successes with megaprostheses in some apparently hopeless cases.[10,11]

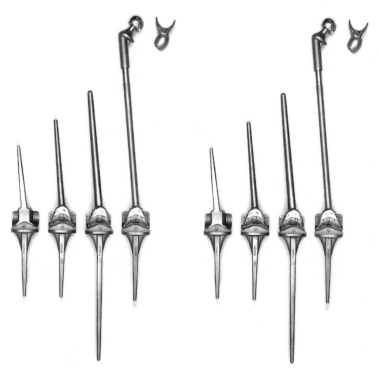

**Fig. 6.6**
Hinge knee (ENDO-Modell) with extra-long stems total femur prosthesis.

# Intracondylar prosthesis
⇩
# Intracondylar prosthesis (longer stems)
⇩
# Total femur prosthesis

a

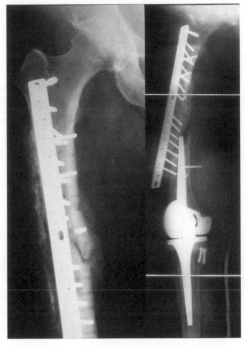

b

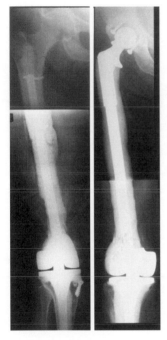

c        d

**Fig. 6.7**

Case: infected total knee replacement – spacer – total femur.

## Bone cement

The addition of antibiotics to the gentamicin PMMA bone cement is based on the recommendation of the bacteriologist and depends on the tests performed on tissue samples obtained preoperatively by joint aspiration and fistula specimen. One or two additional antibiotics specifically appropriate for each individual case are recommended for mixture with the standard cement. The total quantity of antibiotics added to cement used for fixation of implants should not be more than 4 g per 40 g of bone cement. This limit may be exceeded if the cement is used as a surface coating, e.g., for spacers, or to reshape resected condyles.

Antibiotics in crystalline form only are used for addition to bone cement, as aqueous solutions prevent the polymerization of the bone cement. Addition of antibiotics or other substances does lead to a deterioration of the mechanical properties of the cement, but this is acceptable if the 10%limit of addition is observed. The primary objective must be to eradicate the infection.

## Material (cohorts) and results

### Group 1

Between 1976 and 1985, 157 periprosthetic infections following knee arthroplasty were treated by surgery at the Endo-Klinik in

Hamburg: 118 of these underwent a one-stage exchange procedure, and 104 were analysed after a postoperative period of 5–15 years in a follow-up study.[5] In 76 patients the infection was eradicated by one one-stage operation only. In cases where the first operation failed, the procedure was repeated, raising the number of cured cases to 84. In 20 cases the one-stage method failed to eradicate periprosthetic infection. According to conventional statistical methods the rate of success in this group of patients was 73%. The second exchange operation in cases of recurrent infection raised the number of cured cases to 84 (81%). A third exchange operation performed in a few cases did not lead to a further significant increase in the success rate. In 20 cases (19%) it was not possible to bring the infection under control even by a repeat one-stage procedure. The final result was 6 arthrodeses, 5 amputations, and 9 persisting infections. The chances that the operation would be successful were much better in cases where the pathogen was staphylococcus as opposed to strepto-coccus. The outcome for cases with mixed infections, especially involving *Escherichia coli* or *Pseudomonas*, was not so good.

Survival rate analysis revealed that the majority of recurrent infec-tions occurred in the first 2 postoperative years. The probability of recurrent infection was 20% during this period. In the following 8 years only a further 13% failed, and the probability of recurrence after 10 years was approximately 33%. Aseptic failures were ex-cluded both from this analysis and from the conventional statistics (Fig. 6.8).

Five of the 84 cured patients had aseptic loosening (mostly of one component only) after 2–9 years and again underwent surgery. In 85% of cured patients the radiographs taken for follow-up examina-tions showed the prosthesis to be firmly in position; in the other 15% different degrees of radiolucency were visible and required further control.

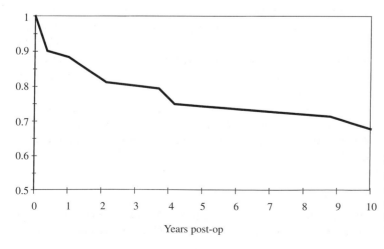

Years post-op

**Fig. 6.8**

Survival rate of all peripros-thetic infections after knee arthroplasty treated by one-stage exchange operation 1976–85 ($N$ = 118).

### Group 2

A further follow-up study was carried out on a second group of patients who were operated on in 1989. The results of this study have so far not been published. The group consisted of 46 patients, 3 of whom were not available for the study.

In group 1 the mean follow-up period was 6.3 years, in group 2 it was only 3.7 years. However, the two groups are still comparable in spite of the different follow-up periods because we know that 90% of recurrent infections occur within the first 4 postoperative years. Infection was controlled after the first one-stage exchange in 73% of the patients in group 1 and in 84% in group 2. Infection persisted after the first operation in 27% in group 1 and in 16% in group 2. A number of different measures were taken to control persistence or recurrence of infection: either a second one-stage exchange of the prosthesis, and in a few cases a third, or arthrodesis, amputation or no surgery at all.

In group 1 further surgery led to a control of infection in 7% of cases by a second one-stage exchange, in 1% by a third one-stage exchange and in 5% by arthrodesis. In group 2 the same measures led to a rise in the percentage of cured cases of 2%, 2% and 5%. Therefore, in group 1 secondary measures led to control of infection in a further 13% of cases and in group 2 in a further 9%. When these additional successes are subtracted from the failures after the first one-stage exchange there remain 14% failures in group 1 and 7% in group 2. The further course of these remaining failures was 6% persisting infections and 8% amputations in group 1, and 5% persisting infections and 2% amputations in group 2.

Table 6.3 shows the overall results and a comparison of the two groups. The results in group 2, which consisted of patients who were operated on at a later stage, were considerably better. After the first one-stage exchange, 84% had a prosthesis and infection was controlled, after a second operation the percentage rose to 86% and after a third to 88%. If the arthrodesis cases are included, 93% of infections were controlled with a follow-up period of 3.7 years.

Compared with group 1 the improvement in the results after the one-stage exchange was 11%, after the second 6%, and after the third operation 7%. If the arthrodeses are included, the improvement was 7%. The number of persisting infections fell by 1% and amputations by 6%.

The best results were achieved in cases where coagulase-negative staphylococci or *Staphylococcus aureus* were the cause of infection. The results were worst in cases of mixed infection, especially when *E. coli* or *Pseudomonas* were present.

### Summary

Periprosthetic infection of the knee can be controlled by a one-stage exchange operation in 84% of cases. This rate of success can be

**Table 6.3** Overall results and comparison of the two groups (see text for details). Figures are percentage final outcomes

|                                  | Group 1 (1976–85) | Group 2 (1989) | Improvement |
| -------------------------------- | ----------------- | -------------- | ----------- |
| Control after first one-stage    | 73                | 84             | +11         |
| Control after second one-stage   | 80                | 86             | +6          |
| Control after third one-stage    | 81                | 88             | +7          |
| Total (including arthrodesis)     | 86                | 93             | +7          |
| Persisting infection             | 6                 | 5              | −1          |
| Amputation                       | 8                 | 2              | −6          |

improved to 88% by a repeat operation and to 93% if the arthrodesis cases are included. Comparison of the two groups of patients shows that increasing experience in operative technique leads to better results. For this reason, periprosthetic infection should, as far as possible, be treated only in specialized departments. The advantage of one-stage revision in comparison with other methods is that control of infection and restoration of satisfactory function can be achieved by one single operation in the majority of cases.

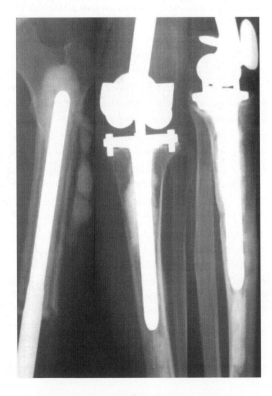

**Fig. 6.9**

Persisting deep infection (*Staphylococcus epidermis*) of a custom-made knee prosthesis in a female student from Poland after *en bloc* resection of a malignant bone tumor. Patella subluxation, femoral and tibial loosening, sinuses at the medial aspect of the knee and ventral tibia. Motion 10/0/20°.

**Fig. 6.10**

Successful one-stage revision using a custom-made hinge prosthesis with extra-long stems. The femoral component allows for transformation to a total femoral prosthesis (without exchange of the stem) in case of hip fracture or loosening of the femoral component.

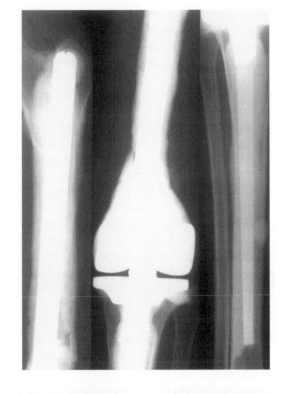

**Fig. 6.11**

Functional outcome of the patient in Figs 6.9 and 6.10, 4 years postoperatively: CRP negative, sterile aspiration, flexion of the knee 90°, patella gliding almost normally, no pain.

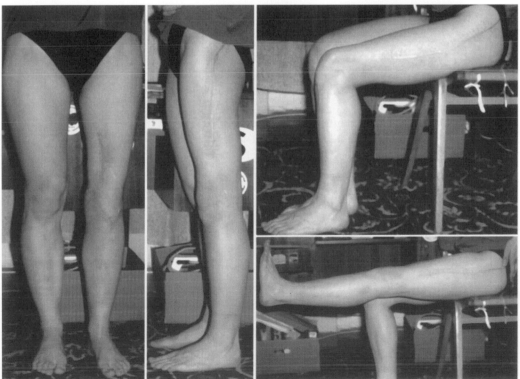

The high rate of success was achieved with exclusively topical use of antibacterials. In recent years this has been supplemented by adjuvant systemic therapy in cases with massive involvement of the soft tissues, resistant pathogens, and mixed infections. In these cases we administered systemic antibiotics for a maximum period of 1 week. As critics have remarked, it is true that this method is based exclusively on surgical and clinical empirical experience.[12]

Our conviction that this method is correct and forward-looking derives from the results of the research by A. Gristina[7,8] which virtually demand that antibiotics should be used topically. One of Gristina's recommendations is that biomaterials should be impregnated with antibiotics, because in his opinion during the primary and most vulnerable phase following implantation the antibiotic should be already on the spot, i.e., on the surface of the biomaterial, so that the competition between bacteria and integrating cells in the "race for the surface" is decided in favor of the integrating cells. Therefore antibiotics added to bone cement with proven topical effectiveness are an up-to-date therapy and not a historical one.

## Discussion

When deep periprosthetic infection of the knee occurs in the acute postoperative phase it is very improbable that long-term eradication with retention of the implanted prosthesis can be achieved. According to a report by the Mayo Clinic the success rate in such cases is only 23%.[13] Our own studies have shown that the attempt to retain the prosthesis in infected hips has a maximum success rate of 50–60%.[14]

For a number of reasons we consider two-stage procedures, permanent resection arthroplasty, or arthrodesis after implant removal to be unfavourable methods.

Removal of the infected prosthesis alone does not guarantee eradication of infection. In one of our studies we discovered that in almost 30% of resected hips the intraoperative biopsies were still positive prior to reimplantation.[15]

When a two-stage procedure is planned the patient has to undergo at least two, and often several operations before the infection is eradicated.[13] This is an important factor with regard to the physical and psychological burden on the patient, and also an economic problem in comparison with the cost of one operation and one stay in hospital, as needed for a one-stage procedure.

The method and duration of topical antibiositic treatment used in one-stage exchange arthroplasty are more favourable because the antibiotic concentration reaches a sufficiently high level locally and side-effects are not to be expected. Systemic therapy plays an adjuvant role and is always limited to a period of 7–10 days in comparison with the at least 6 week-long systemic antibiosis used in two-stage procedures with all known side-effects.

It is not the author's aim to present this method as the best in all cases and urge that it should be introduced everywhere. Certain conditions are indispensable and can only be fulfilled by specialized centres:

- A surgical team with long experience in the treatment of infected prostheses which is equipped with the appropriate instrumentarium for this operation and a range of all the revision implants which may be needed.
- Close co-operation with a competent microbiologist and a well-equipped laboratory.

We know that these conditions seldom exist, and that co-operation between surgeon and microbiologist is an exception, but this cannot mean that the concept for optimizing this treatment should be abandoned. On the contrary, special emphasis should be placed on the demand that operations of this kind and degree of difficulty should only be performed in specialized centres with the necessary personnel and equipment. The political development with regard to public health in many countries, however, is producing a situation where hospitals specializing in secondary treatment of the type described here subsidize the hospitals giving primary treatment by agreeing to perform the more expensive operation although not receiving full reimbursement of the costs. The restrictive attitude of health insurance companies and governments in this issue should not result in the suppression of optimal methods of treatment for economic reasons.

## Acknowledgement

I would like to thank Professor H. W. Buchholz in Hamburg who taught me the management of deep infection and Dr Lars Frommelt for his help with the microbiological part of the text.

## References

1 Hebert CK, Williams RE, Levy RS, Barrack RL: Cost of treating an infected total knee replacement. *Clinical Orthopaedics and Related Research* **331**:140–145, 1996.
2 Buchholz HW, Engelbrecht E, Lodenkämper H *et al.*: 1981 Management of deep infection of total hip replacement. *Journal of Bone and Joint Surgery* [Br] **63**:342.
3 Steinbrink K: The case for revision arthroplasty using antibiotic-loaded acrylic cement. *Clinical Orthopaedics and Related Research* **261**:19–22, 1990.
4 Steinbrink K, Frommelt L: Behandlung der periprothetischen Infektion der Hüfte durch einzeitige Austauschoperation. *Orthopäde* **24**:335–43, 1995.
5 Von Foerster G, Klüber D, Käbler U: Mittel- bis langfristige Ergebnisse nach Behandlung von 118 periprothetischen Infektionen

nach Kniegelenkersatz durch einzeitige Austauschoperation. *Orthopäde* **20**:244–52, 1991.

6   Lodenkämper H, Lodenkämper U, Trompa K: Über die Ausscheidung von Antibiotika aus dem Knochenzement Palacos. *Zeitschrift für Orthopädie* **120**:801, 1982.

7   Gristina AG: Biomaterial-centered infetion: Microbial adhesion versus tissue integration. *Science* **237**:1588, 1987.

8   Gristina AG, Costerton JW: Bacterial adherence to biomaterials and tissue. *Journal of Bone and Joint Surgery* [Am] **67**:264, 1985.

9   Engelbrecht E, Nieder E, Klüber D: Ten to twenty years of knee arthroplasty at the Endo-Klinik: A report on the long-term follow-up of the St. Georg Hinge and the medium-term follow-up of the Rotating Knee ENDO Model. In *Reconstruction of the knee joint*, ed. S. Niwa, S Yoshino, M Kurosaka *et al.*, pp. 86–199. Springer Verlag, Tokyo, 1997.

10  Steinbrink K: Vorgehen bei ausgedehntem oder völligem Knochensubstanzverlust des Femurs nach Schaftlockerung. *Orthopäde* **16**:277–286, 1987.

11  Steinbrink K, Engelbrecht E, Fenelon GCC: The total femoral prosthesis: A preliminary report. *Journal of Bone and Joint Surgery* [Br] **64**:305–312, 1982.

12  Scherf H: Die tiefe Infektion nach totaler Hüftendoprothese. Bakteriologie und Therapie. *Zeitschrift für antimikrobielle Chemotherapie* **6**:37, 1988.

13  Schoifet SD, Morrey BF: Treatment of infection after total knee arthroplasty by débridement with retention of the components. *Journal of Bone and Joint Surgery* [Am] **72**:1383–90, 1990.

14  Mella-Schmidt C, Steinbrink K: Stellenwert der Spül-Saugdrainage bei der Behandlung des Frühinfekts von Gelenkimplantaten. *Chirurg* **60**:791, 1989.

15  Engelbrecht E, Siegel A, Kappus M: Totale Hüftendoprothese nach Resektionsarthroplastik. *Orthopäde* **24**:344–52, 1995.

## Questions and answers

*Moderator:* Dr. Windsor, you have mentioned surgical debridement with component retention. When do you do this and in what scenario?

*Dr. Windsor:* If the patient develops acutely increased pain with erythema, and significantly worse swelling, I think of infection or a hemarthrosis as the etiology of the problem. Usually, if the patient has a substantial increase in pain after apparent improvement in symptoms after a total knee replacement, I will aspirate the knee and consider open arthrotomy and debridement. The difficulty in doing this procedure is in the proper timing of it. After a primary total knee replacement, most patients have a degree of pain for up to 2–3 months. Many have significant but normal amount of pain for 2–3 weeks after surgery. During this time it is easy to confuse normal postoperative pain with pain secondary to infection. By the time the surgeon is suspicious of infection, the patient may be beyond the 3 weeks period that Schoifet and Morrey found successful when doing debridement with retention of the components. Certainly, when confronted with the challenge of doing a two-stage exchange, both the patient and the surgeon find arthrotomy and debridement as a simple way of tackling the problem. In many cases, the patient and surgeon are willing to deal with the 23% chance of success that debridement alone will yield. My opinion is that if the patient and surgeon wish to proceed with arthrotomy and debridement, it should be done only once in the situation where the bacteria are gram-positive cocci and are sensitive to antimicrobial agents. I do not recommend the multiple debridement approach of Mond because of the potential surgical difficulties that would be encountered if the patient failed treatment and a two-stage exchange became necessary. His success rates with each debridement was only 70%. Additionally, the patient will become less confident about the definitive eradication of the infection, if multiple procedures are done. The best method is to present the success data of two-stage exchange and in many cases, the patient may opt for the most predictable results and not risk less successful outcome by a seemingly less invasive procedure.

*Moderator:* Do you think that surgical debridement and component retention should be done arthroscopically or by an open technique, and why?

*Dr. Windsor:* Surgical debridement should be done preferably by an open technique. Most prostheses make use of a modular tibial implant. With an infection, bacteria will get into the space between the polyethylene tibial insert and the metal tray. Access to this space by arthroscopic means is impossible. Thus, debridement done by arthrotomy will allow the surgeon to disassemble the tibial insert from the tray and adequately irrigate and cleanse the area. Removal of the tibial insert will also permit access to the posterior aspect of the knee, which is a notoriously difficult region to approach with the arthroscope. The only time I would consider an arthroscopic debridement is in a case of a severely medically compromised patient (e.g., associated bacterial endocarditis or florid systemic septicemia in addition to the septic knee joint). In this case, the arthroscopy would be less invasive and it would serve to allow the medical staff to control the infection during active treatment of the endocarditis. The arthroscopic debridement essentially would act as a slightly more invasive incision and drainage procedure and would not pose an extreme anesthesia risk.

*Moderator:* Not let us take the situation where you have performed a knee revision for what you felt was a nonseptic condition and several days later a positive culture appears in the chart? Do you treat it? Does it matter what the positive culture was?

*Dr. Windsor:* If the culture came back positive, it would matter if it were a positive culture in the media or broth. If there was one specimen that was positive in the broth, I would ignore the finding as a contaminant and observe the patient's symptoms. If there was a definite positive finding on media, I would check the organism's sensitivity to antibiotic treatment. A frozen section is performed during each revision to determine the possibility of infection by cell count: 5–10 WBCs per high-powered field suggest an infective process. An infectious disease specialist would be consulted and a course of parenteral antibiotics would be continued for at least 3 and in most cases 6 weeks. An oral antibiotic would be used for 1–2 years in a slowly decreasing dose. Again, as always, the clinical situation needs close attention. Thus, the patient would be treated although removal of the implants would not be done initially. If the patient showed signs of significant pain and swelling with failure of improvement, an open debridement would be performed. Also, the type of organism that was isolated would alter the course of treatment, especially if it was a gram-negative bacteria resistant to many common antibiotics or methicillin-resistant *Staphylococcus aureus*. If these organisms are encountered, an open debridement may be done first, but if the patient failed to get better, a two-stage exchange would have to be performed. For methicillin-resistant staphylococcus aureus, vancomycin would be used as the drug of choice. There have been sporadic reports of vancomycin-resistant *Staphylococcus epidermidis* and enterococcus. Fortunately, these infections are rare. During aseptic revision surgery, it is also worthwhile to consider the routine use of antibiotic-impregnated cement in cases where the patient is medically compromised or in revision surgery where the patient's wound may have had exposure to microorganisms during prior surgery.

*Moderator:* Dr. Steinbrink, you have stated that the best medium in which to obtain your culture is the joint fluid. Have you had circumstances where the joint fluid was negative but a tissue culture was positive? To continue, some people have said that culture of the fistula gives you spurious results that often represent minor skin flora. Have you found this to be the case?

*Dr. Steinbrink:* The problem is that bacteria cultured in media may be contaminants or pathogens. In our experience, the best way to obtain the pathogens is to find the same species in biopsies of tissue taken from different areas at the site of infection. In periprosthetic infection, one of the outstanding features is that bacteria colonize the surface of the indwelling medical device and spread slowly along the surface at the interface between the foreign material and bone tissue until the whole prosthesis is covered by biofilm containing the bacteria. Infectious disease starts when they leave the interface, invade the bone tissue, and provoke local osteomyelitis. In low-grade infections it takes months or even years before periprosthetic infection becomes manifest. In most cases the colonization comes into contact with the joint fluid under these circumstances, and the pathogens can be obtained easily from this specimen (Table 6.1). Only in a few cases does the invasion of bone happen very early when the colonization of the surfaces is restricted to one component of the prosthesis. In these early cases, the culture of the joint fluid remains sterile. Empirical administration of antibiotics before identification of pathogens is a common problem in patients referred to a specialist as this results in negative aspirations although deep infection is evident.

*Moderator:* I would like to second this point and stress it. We should not empirically start patients on antibiotics before obtaining proper cultures. If we do, we make a difficult problem into an extremely difficult problem.

*Moderator:* Most people use gentamicin or tobramycin in their spacer block during two-stage revision. Are other antibiotics indicated, and if so when?

*Dr. Windsor:* Other antibiotics maybe utilized during the reimplantation stage. Gentamicin and tobramycin are routinely used because the powdered form of the drug is stable during the exothermic reaction that occurs when the acrylic cement cures and hardens. Usually, 1 g of powder is mixed with 30 g of the acrylic cement powder. The liquid polymer reagent is then added to the mixture. Vancomycin powder is also heat stable in cement. This antibiotic is usually added when a methicillin-resistant *Staphylococcus aureus* infection is being treated. Ideally, it is best to place the best drug into the cement according to the antibiotic sensitivities that the microorganism displays on culture media. Even though, some bacteria may display resistance to gentamicin or tobramycin, these drugs are still used in the cement to protect the operative environment from infection by other bacteria that may be sensitive to them. On rare occasions, it may be necessary to mix both tobramycin and vancomycin together in the acrylic cement. This is usually done when there is a mixed infection with two or more infecting organisms. There is little change in the overall strength of the antibiotic-impregnated cement in comparison with cement that has no antibiotics contained within it. As discussed in a previous question, antibiotic-impregnated cement should be utilized in most, if not all, revision cases for septic and aseptic failure.

*Moderator:* Dr. Steinbrink, are all the antibiotics you list in our table truly heat stable in curing cement. I had thought that ampicillin, for example, was degraded in curing cement? As an aside, is one type of bone cement better than another for eluting antibiotics?

*Dr. Steinbrink:* The elution properties of the antibiotics mentioned in the table, both separately and in the cited combinations, have been investigated in the bacteriological department of the Endo-Klinik. The heat stability tests of the antimicrobial agents were carried out by Traub and Leonhard (*Journal of Antimicrobial Chemotherapy* (England) 1995;**35**:149), and they showed that beta-lactam antibiotics were remarkably heat-stable. The degradation of

157

beta-lactam antibiotics in the presence of humidity is another problem. The physics of the elution of antibiotics prevents these antimicrobial agents from being degraded. Within the PMMA bone cement the antibiotics are transported by very slow diffusion in an environment free of solvents (Low HT *et al.*, *Journal of Biomedical Engineering* 1986;8:149–155) and thus protected from humidity. Starting at the surface, diffusion into the tissue begins to be mediated by water that makes the substances available, but degrades them as well.

As to the bone cement itself; we have investigated exclusively the properties of Palacos-R bone cement, manufactured by the Merck Company in Darmstadt, Germany, for eluting antibiotics. Studies by Elson (1977), Bayston and Milner (1982), Wahlig and Dingeldein (1980), Kucle (1991), and Penner (1999) produced the almost universal agreement that the release of antibiotics from Palacos-R is superior to the release of antibiotics from Simplex of CMW bone cement.

*Moderator:* I would like to go into the exact details of the spacer block technique. Exactly how do you insert your spacer block? How do you size it? Do you fashion small "stem extensions" into the femur and tibia? What do you do for the patella?

*Dr. Windsor:* I wait until the cement is very doughy and can be formed into a shape. Currently I like an articulated spacer construct that permits weight bearing and some motion. I will shape the femoral piece to fill the voids left by removal of the previous prosthesis and debridement of necrotic bone. A flange is fashioned so that the patella rests on it and does not become fused to the anterior aspect of the distal femur during the 6 week course of antibiotic treatment. If the femur has a central defect, or had an implant that already had a stem attachment, I will create a "stem extension" to fit the femoral canal. This extension will improve stability of fixation. I fashion a tibial spacer in the form of a tibial implant with a central stem. The "stem extension" fits into the central defect left after removal of the stemmed tibial component. I check the size of the spacer with the implant that was removed and try to re-create its rough dimension. In the past, I would only use the tibial spacer and make it flat so that some motion can be obtained in the post-operative time period. However, I would sometimes notice significant bone erosion using this method. Because of this problem, I have more frequently used an articulating spacer construct. I do not use Prostalac spacers because they are unavailable in New York and because of the expense. Resterilization of the original, cleaned implant and coating it with antibiotic-impregnated cement is gaining more interest and enthusiasm as a spacer block option. However, the surgeon must be forewarned that a meticulous cleaning should be done followed by sterilization in an autoclave.

*Moderator:* OK, you now have placed the spacer block in and the wound has healed. You are now 6 weeks after the spacer block surgery. What exactly do you do at 6 weeks after the spacer block is inserted? Do you do another culture of the knee? What do you do if a new culture is positive?

*Dr. Windsor:* Usually, the second stage is performed with reimplantation of a new prosthesis after the 6 week period has elapsed. During this procedure, gram stain and frozen section specimens are sent for immediate analysis. If there is evidence of infection by more than 5 polymorphonuclear leukocytes per high powered field or the frozen section shows signs of persistent acute infection, the knee is debrided and closed and further antibiotic treatment is carried out. If there is no sign of persistent infection, the new prosthesis is implantated. Specimens from each bone surface are sent for routine culture and sensitivity. If the cultures come back positive for infection, the patient will continue a course of parenteral antibiotics for 2 weeks followed by a further course of oral antibiotic therapy in a decreasing dose over a period of 1–2 years. The clinical course is observed carefully. This scenario has been quite rare, but if it occurs, the surgeon must remember that the second stage also included a comprehensive debridement of the knee. If the patient's clinical course deteriorates significantly, then the surgeon will have to consider possible open debridement or another two-stage exchange. In general, antibiotics alone are usually sufficient.

*Moderator:* What has been your experience with the parenteral antibiotic access? We surely cannot use a standard peripheral venous line since it will often get thrombosed. Do you prefer one type or another of central access line and why?

*Dr. Windsor:* A PICC line is generally utilized in treatment of the infected total knee replacement. This catheter enables the patient to receive prolonged courses of intravenous antibiotics without having to consider numerous intravenous line changes during the course of treatment. The more central Broviac catheter is also utilized. This catheter is placed after the anesthesiologist gets intravenous access through the jugular vein. It must be placed in an operating room, as an incision must be made on the chest wall for placement of the access port. The Percutaneous Insertion Central Catheter (PICC line) can be placed at the bedside and is easily removed after therapy is discontinued. Thus, the PICC line is utilized more frequently.

*Moderator:* What level of parenteral antibiotics do you strive for in the treatment of infected knee prostheses, Dr. Steinbrink?

*Dr. Steinbrink:* Parenteral antibiotics should be administered intravenously at the highest recommended dosage for about 10 days postoperatively, if given in addition to one-stage revision using antibiotic-loaded cement, and if there is no other reason for their application (e.g., diffuse soft tissue infection or infection of another anatomical site)

*Moderator:* When you perform the second stage of the revision, do you use antibiotics in the cement? Do you keep the patients on antibiotics after that surgery and for how long?

*Dr. Windsor:* During the second stage of the revision, antibiotics are always used in the cement. Tobramycin powder is mixed in the cement. In cases of methicillin-resistant *Staphylococcus aureus* infections, vancomycin powder is used. Patients only receive parenteral antibiotics for another 72 h until the final intra-operative culture results are known. At this time, the antibiotic treatment is stopped with no further oral antibiotic therapy given to the patient. The operative site should be sterilized and there is no need for further treatment except for the lone exception mentioned in the above question concerning a positive culture. Routine use of oral antibiotics in two-stage exchange procedures invites the possible creation of antibiotic resistance of the patient's normal flora.

*Moderator:* Dr. Steinbrink, in the USA most surgeons are like Dr. Windsor in using an aminoglycoside as their cement antibiotic for almost all cases Since you don't appear to do this would be your response to their routine use of aminoglycosides?

*Dr. Steinbrink:* If you compare the release from PMMA bone cement of different classes of antibiotics, aminoglycoside antibiotics are most suitable. They are very heat-stable and are not degraded by other mechanisms. Unfortunately, not all bacteria are susceptible to aminoglycoside antibiotics. Furthermore, bacteria in the sessile state on the surface of foreign bodies are highly resistant because their phenotype is different to that of the planctonic brothers. Costerton reported minimal inhibitory concentration (MIC) versus tobramycin that are increased by a factor of more than 100! So we are convinced that the combination of synergistically acting antimicrobial agents is adequate for the therapy of these difficult bacteria. The aim is to obtain extremely high concentrations of effective antimicrobial agents at the site of infection without damaging the stability of the bone cement or provoking adverse effects of the antibiotics in the patient.

*Moderator:* Do you ever use longer term (or lifetime) antibiotics after a two-stage revision?

*Dr. Windsor:* Long-term antibiotics are used are in two cases. The first case scenario was discussed above where a positive postoperative culture is obtained. The second scenario is in a patient who is particularly prone to infection, immunocompromised, and on steroid therapy. These patients who are at a substantial risk of re-infection by hematogenous means are given prophylactic courses of antibiotics for a few years to life-long time periods.

*Moderator:* What is your feeling about movable spacers rather than a rigid cement block during the time of the two-stage revision?

*Dr. Windsor:* Movable spacers have become more popular than rigid cement blocks because they enable the patient to move the knee. Knee motion allows the soft tissues to remain more functionally stretchable. Since there is little scar contraction that develops during the time between procedures, the second surgical exposure is much easier. The patients also feel more functional during this difficult 6 week period. Debate centers on the best way to make movable spacers. Acrylic cement blocks can be made to coat each bone surface and allow movement. The old implants can be cleaned and resterilized and coated with antibiotic-impregnated cement. The trick in using them is to place them back on to the bone surfaces with the cement very doughy. The implants usually fit fairly well back on to the bone surface, and occasionally the patient will feel so good during the initial postoperative period, that he or she no longer wishes to consider the second stage. However, the overall construct of the implant and cement would not permit long-term survival. Prostalac spacers and prostheses, as discussed above, do provide good function, but are quite expensive because of the number of molds that must be bought and used.

*Moderator:* At the time of the second stage are there any surgical tips you can share regarding mobilizing the knee for the surgery?

*Dr. Windsor:* The major word to use during the second stage is "patience." The soft tissue should be allowed to slowly stretch and open up. I utilized the original incision whenever possible. It may be necessary to perform a quadriceps snip which is performed by extending the proximal portion of the arthrotomy cephalad and lateral across the quadriceps tendon. This incision can be repaired in a routine manner. Extraordinarily scarred knees may require a quadriceps turndown or tibial tubercle osteotomy. These are much more extensile, but carry greater morbidity. With the quadriceps turndown, there is the possibility of extension lag and devasularization of the patella. With the tibial tubercle osteotomy, stress fracture of the proximal tibia has been reported.

I usually expose the knee in a routine fashion by performing a subperiosteal dissection along the medial aspect of the tibia. The tibia is then flexed and externally rotated out from underneath the femoral condyle. This maneuver takes pressure off the patellar tendon insertion on the tibial tubercle. It is sometimes good to place a large smooth Steinman pin in the tubercle to act as a checkrein to prevent avulsion of the patellar tendon. I do not pay a lot of attention to everting the patella at an early stage. I will retract the extensor mechanism laterally and work on preparing the femur and tibia. During the time the femur and tibia are prepared and the soft tissue and scar is removed, the patella can more easily be everted. Lateral retinacular release can be performed early to facilitate eversion of the patella at a latter stage of the operation. However, the most important thing for the surgeon to remember is to take time and be patient and allow the soft tissues to stretch out. This will permit an excellent exposure without potential harm to the extensor mechanism.

*Moderator:* Dr. Steinbrink, what are your indications, if any, for a doing a two-stage exchange revision for an infected knee?

*Dr. Steinbrink:* I became familiar with the method of one-stage exchange revision to treat infected joint replacements (at whatever site) 24 years ago when I joined Professor Buchholz's team in Hamburg. Since then, as my experience and confidence with this method increased, I have (literally) never performed a two-stage revision of an infected TKR. All my operations have been one-stage procedures. The only personal indication I have for a two-stage procedure is, and will always be, the following situation: an infected TKR with an extra-long femoral component, complicated by severe loss of bone stock or fracture near the hip joint, requiring implantation of a total femur prosthesis. Treating a case like this by one-stage revision of the infected knee joint would compromise the uninfected (aseptic) hip joint in the process. So, I would treat the infection in a first operation by the insertion of a spacer. This spacer could be an extra-long femoral stem not allowing full weight bearing. In a second operation, under sterile conditions (negative CRP, sterile aspiration) and after a minimum interval of 2 months, I would then implant total femur prosthesis and allow full weight bearing (Fig. 6.7).

This is my personal standpoint. Apart for this, I can understand surgeons who do prefer two-stage revisions in the following situations:

- when the surgeon does not perform operations of this kind regularly and the causative organism is not known
- when appropriate antibiotics are not available
- where there is no suitable prosthesis available (a custom-made model is necessary)
- where the surgeon prefers a cementless procedure because when PMMA is not used the possibility of one-stage revision is excluded as there is no cement to act as a carrier for the antibiotics required
- where the reconstruction requires allografts and the implantation of a device with cementless fixation is intended.

*During the 1970s, based on the work of Sir John Charnley on hips, acrylic cement fixation of total knee prostheses became the overwhelming choice of surgeons around the world. With the pioneering work of David Hungerford, Ken Krackow, Jorge Galante, and Jo Miller, surgeons began to question whether or not fixation of implants could be obtained without having to resort to acrylic cement. The 1980s saw a surge of such uncemented implants, some of which had good results whereas others were disastrous. Surgeons then again began questioning whether to return to the acrylic cement they had used in their youth. The pendulum has still not settled on either the cemented or the uncemented side.*

# Acrylic cement is the method of choice for fixation of total knee implants

## Pro: John Insall and Giles Scuderi

Other surgeons have embraced cementless total knee replacement, but we continue to be proponents of cement fixation. Supported by the long-term clinical success and survivorship analysis, cemented total knee arthroplasty (TKA) continues to be the gold standard against which alternative means of fixation need to be compared. A well designed and properly positioned cemented total knee replacement has a greater than 90% chance of surviving more than 15 years. This success consistently surpasses the results of cementless total knee replacement. In comparison studies, the early results of cemented and cementless fixation are comparable, but cementless fixation has shown a precipitous decline in successful results with longer follow-up.

Although femoral ingowth appears to be more consistent and may be the rationale behind hybrid fixation, the tibial component is the usual site of failure because of limited bone growth. Retrieval analysis of uncemented tibial components revealed very little bone ingrowth, bringing into question the longevity of these implants.[1] In an effort to improve tibial component fixation, screws were introduced to achieve immediate tibial tray fixation. However this has introduced new problems of osteolysis and polyethylene wear from screw migration. In cementless total knee replacement, polyethylene debris may migrate through the screw holes in the tibial base plate. This particulate debris generates a biological response, both chemical and cellular, which in turn results in bone loss and osteolysis.[2-6]

163

Lewis and coworkers performed a comparative radiographic review of cementless total knee replacements specifically looking at screw osteolysis.[7] These investigators classified the appearance of the screw bone interface. When classified according to the different implant designs, cystic and cavity changes were seen in 3.8% and 2.8% of Miller Galante I knees (Zimmer, Warsaw, IN), 4.3% and 1.3% of MG II knees and 13.3% and 5.5% of Anatomic Modular Knees (DePuy, Warsaw, IN), 4 years after surgery. These radiographic findings have been the precursor to catastrophic ostelysis.[4] This problem appears to occur more frequently on the tibial side, although there are reports of osteolysis on the femoral side. The true incidence of femoral osteolyis is probably underestimated because of the limitations of radiographic imaging. Osteolysis is most likely attributable to specific articular designs, which produce greater polyethylene debris. This is particularly the case with cementless fixation, which had been coupled with posterior cruciate retaining designs. This may have unfairly hampered the early results with these designs because the surgical technique incorporated limited bone resection with a design that had a very thin flat articular surface. Designs such as the Synatomic (DePuy, Warsaw, IN) and Porous Coated Anatomic (Howmedica, Rutherford, NJ) incorporated these features. Although early outcomes were promising,[8] long-term follow-up demonstrated a precipitous decline in the successful results[9,10].

## Cement technique

Fundamental to implant longevity is meticulous technique, bone preparation, and handling of the cement. Fixation of polymethylmethacrylate (PMMA) to the cancellous bony surface is achieved by the irregular configuration of the bony surface and the penetration of the cement into the bone. Since bone penetration is critical to the intrusion of PMMA into the cancellous bone, the resected bone surfaces are cleansed with pulsatile lavage to remove blood fat and bone debris. The proper preparation allows for uninhibited penetration of the cement into the bone. Our preference is to use Simplex cement (Howmedica, Rutherford, NJ) in the doughy state. This permits easy handling and manual pressurization of the cement into the porous bone. The ideal cement penetration into the bone is 1–2 mm (Fig. 7.1). With soft rheumatoid bone, deeper cement penetration may occur. On the other hand, with hard sclerotic bone, the bone surface should be drilled or abraded to allow the cement to grasp the bone.

Our cement technique has not changed for over two decades.[11] As mentioned above, we use our cement in a doughy state so that it can be easily handled. The components are cemented in a sequential fashion using two cement mixtures. With the first batch of cement, an all-polyethylene patellar component along with the femoral component is cemented in place. While the patellar component is held in place with the patellar clamp, a small amount of cement is placed on

**Fig. 7.1**

The AP (a) and lateral
(b) radiograph demonstrate an
ideal cement mantle.

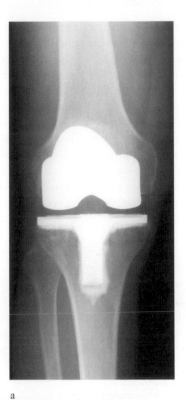

a

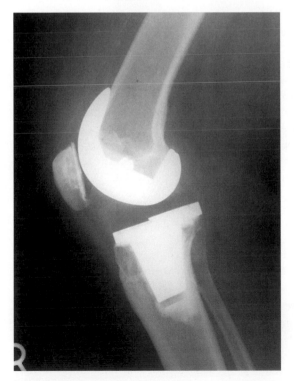

b

the posterior condyles of the femoral component. The remainder of the cement is placed in a horseshoe-shaped fashion over the anterior and distal bony surface (Figs 7.2. 7.3). The femoral component is then impacted in place and the excessive cement is removed. The precise femoral cuts allow a tight fit between the bone and prosthesis such that the resultant cement mantle is approximately 1 mm thick. The tibial component is cemented in place with the second batch of cement (Fig. 7.4). All excess cement must be removed from around the components to prevent cement particles from breaking loose (Fig. 7.5). The presence of entrapped cement between the articular surfaces leads to three-body wear and damage to the polyethylene.

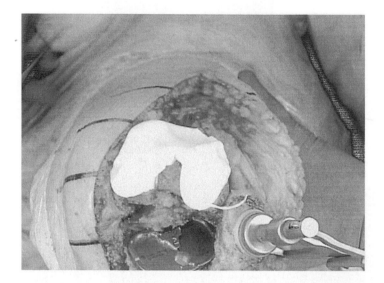

**Fig. 7.2**

The doughy cement is placed in a "horseshoe" fashion around the distal femur. See also colour plate section

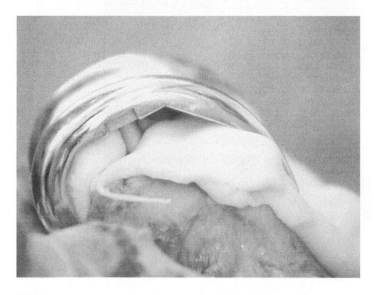

**Fig. 7.3**

Cement is placed on the posterior condyles of the femoral component prior to impaction. See also colour plate section

**Fig. 7.4**

Since the entire tibial component is cemented, cement is placed on the proximal tibial surface (a) as well as pushed into the central fixation hole (b). See also colour plate section.

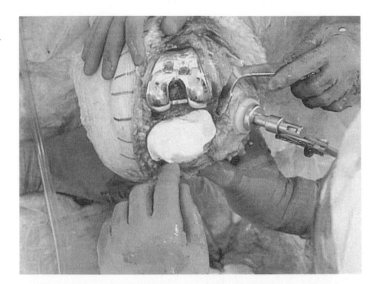

a

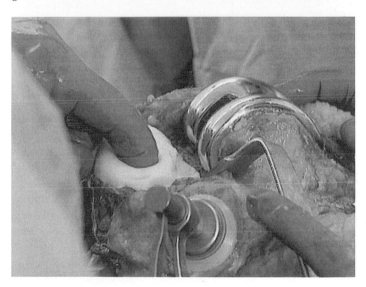

b

The importance of initial prosthetic fixation has been emphasized in the past since it has been shown that prostheses which continuously migrate will eventually loosen.[12] The most decisive time is during the operative procedure and is influenced by the surgical technique and prosthetic design. Cementing the femoral component has been standardized, but there appears to be some variation to cementing the tibial component. Some tibial tray designs have a cruciate-shape central stem, which allow "hybrid" fixation.[13] This means that the undersurface of the tray is cemented while the stem is press fit into the metaphyseal bone. Other central stem designs have an I-beam configuration and should be cemented in their

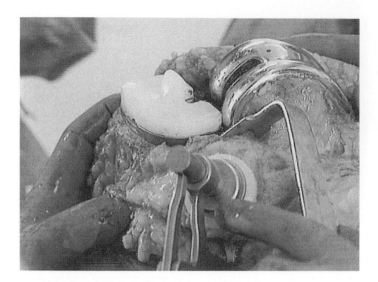

**Fig. 7.5**

With the components fully seated, all excess cement is removed from around the components in an effort to prevent particles from breaking free and getting trapped in the articulation. See also colour plate section.

entirety. In our own experience with the Total Condylar and posterior stabilized prostheses, we have routinely cemented the tibial component including the central stem.[13] In order to do so cement is pushed into the central stem hole in the tibia and the cement is manually pressurized on the tibial plateau (Fig. 7.4). It has always been our recommendation that the tibial component be completely cemented. "Hybrid" tibial fixation has little merit and is prone to unacceptable rates of loosening. Gunderson has shown a 9% tibial loosening rate with surface cementation versus no tibial component loosening with a fully cemented tibial component.[14] This result led those investigators to abandon the surface cementation technique. Bert further supports cemented stems with an *in vitro* study that shows that a 1 mm cement mantle surrounding the central stem improves stability of the tibial component.[15] Additionally, Ryd[16] and Albrektsson[17] have shown that, when compared to cementless fixation. the addition of cement to the implant has reduced micromotion. This reduction in micromotion greatly influences the final outcome because if there is little inducible displacement of a prosthesis at 6 weeks, there will be little inducible displacement after 1 year and little migration after 2 years.[18]

## Modes of cement failure

Though component loosening was the most frequent reported cause of failure with early designs, it is not accurate to blame it entirely on cement fixation. Early prosthetic designs with limited sizes and instrumentation did not appreciate kinematics, alignment, and soft tissue balancing. The original linked prostheses were highly constrained, placing stresses on the bone cement interfaces. This resulted in high rates of loosening. The introduction of less constrained surface replacing cemented prostheses, fabricated with greater attention towards knee kinematics, seems to have resolved some of the earlier problems. Despite the better than expected results with cemented TKR, there are still cases of aseptic loosening. There are those who believe that micromotion at the bone cement interface progresses to macromotion with eventual bone loss and component loosening. Others speculate that the underlying bone, when subjected to uneven stresses subsides leading to component loosening. This is particularly the case with varus malalignment of components. Subsidence is a problem of surgical technique and the underlying cancellous bone, not cement fixation.

The issue of constraint and increased stress at the bone–cement interface has carried over into PCL retaining and controversy. Advocates of PCL retention are concerned that the increased constraint with PCL substituting designs results in increased stresses on the bone–cement interface. In fact the interaction of the femoral cam and tibial spine, with the Insall Burstein Posterior Stabilized Knee (Zimmer, Warsaw, IN), imparts a compressive force on the tibia and negates tibial component liftoff.[19] Furthermore, metal backing of the tibial component has been shown to transmit the load better to the underlying bone.[20]

## Clinical results

The success of cemented TKR supports its continued use. Posterior cruciate ligament (PCL)-retaining designs, such as the Kinematic total knee prosthesis (Howmedica, Rutherford, NJ) have had a long-term success.[21] In a 5–9 year follow-up study of this prosthetic design, the investigators have reported a 90% good or excellent result. Though there were eight patellar complications in this study, there were no loose femoral or tibial components. Similarly, Scott in a review of his last 1000 consecutive primary TKR, with a PCL-retaining design, had no femoral or tibial components loosen.[22]

Retention of the PCL is not an objective to be obtained at all costs in cemented TKR. The drawbacks of a maltensioned PCL are currently being recognized. Surgeons who do not wish to retain the PCL have been attracted to PCL substitution. This particular design has shown that the spine–cam mechanism provides inherent posterior stability, along with good wear characteristics and excellent clinical results, without an increase in component loosening. In fact, a PCL-substituting design may have a more predictable articular pathway when compared to cruciate retaining designs.[23]

The Total Condylar prosthesis, which sacrificed the PCL, was one of the first modern knee prosthesis. Vince et al.,[24] along with Ranawat,[25] have reported excellent results with this prosthetic design, supporting the belief that cemented TKR is a durable and predictable procedure. Despite the success of the Total Condylar prosthesis, the posterior stabilized prosthesis was introduced.[19] The intent was to design a prosthesis that improved stair-climbing, increased range of motion, and prevented tibial subluxation. The early and midterm results were favorable. Aglietti and Buzzi[26] reported 90% good and excellent results at 3–8 year follow-up. Scott and coworkers[27] demonstrated 98% excellent and good results at 2–8 years. In 1992, Stern and Insall[28] reported on the long-term results of the posterior stabilized prosthesis. The 9–12 year results with an all polyethylene tibial component produced 87% good and excellent results, which were comparable to the long-term results with the Total Condylar prosthesis. Analyzing the failures in the posterior stabilized series, there were 5 infections, 3 loose femoral components (1.5%), and 6 loose tibial components (3%). Metal backing of the tibial component improved fixation. Colizza et al.,[29] in a 10–12 year follow-up study of the posterior stabilized prosthesis with a metal-backed tibial component, reported 96% excellent and good results. Despite the occurrence of two loose femoral components, there were no loose tibial components. The remaining two failures included one knee revised for recurrent hemarthosis of unknown etiology and the other for postoperative recurvatum. In both of these cases, the cemented components were well fixed. The results confirmed the advantage of prosthetic conformity in minimizing polyethylene wear without compromising fixation.

Several other designs have also yielded comparable results. Ranawat reviewed the 4–6 year results with the modular Press Fit Condylar PCL-substituting design (Johnson & Johnson, NJ).[30] He reported 93% excellent and good results with no cases of component loosening.

Speculating that the level of activity would influence the longevity of cemented TKR, Diduch et al. evaluated the long-term results and the functional outcome in patients who were 55 years of age or younger at the time of the index procedure.[31] All patients were rated good or excellent at an average follow-up of 8 years. The 18 year cumulative survivorship was 94%. This was an active group of patients who regularly participated in activities, which placed high stresses on the cement interfaces. Though there was one case of polyethylene wear, there were no cases of component loosening.

A comparison of current designs reveals that cemented TKA has a longer predicted survival than cementless implants. Rosenberg, in a clinical and radiographic comparison of cemented and cementless fixation with the Miller Galante Prosthesis (Zimmer, Warsaw, IN), found no cemented implanted failed do to loss of fixation, whereas 3 cementless implants failed owing to lack of tibial bone ingrowth.[32] Although an early comparison study of cemented and cementless Porous Coated Anatomic prostheses (Howmedica, Rutherford, NJ) demonstrated comparable results, cementless fixation has shown a precipitous decline in successful results with longer follow-up.[8–10,33]

Although some surgeons may seek other means of fixation, cemented TKR should be the gold standard against which alternative fixation techniques should be compared. A well-designed cemented prosthesis, implanted with meticulous surgical technique, has

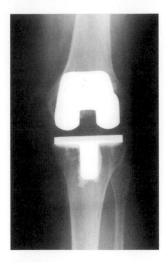

**Fig. 7.6**

The AP radiograph demonstrates a pristine cement mantle at 15 years.

proven to be predictable and durable with excellent long-term results (Fig. 7.6).

## References

1 Cook SD, Thomas, KA; Haddad RJ: Histologic analysis of retrieved human porous coated total joint components. *Clinical Orthopedics* **234**:90–101, 1988.

2 Engh GA, Parks NL, Ammeen DJ: Tibial osteolysis in cementless total knee arthroplasty. A review of 25 cases treated with and without tibial component revision. *Clinical Orthopedics* **309**:33–43, 1994.

3 Ezzet KA, Garcia R, Barrack RL: Effect of component fixation method on osteolysis in total knee arthroplasty. *Clinical Orthopedics* **321**:86–91, 1995.

4 Robinson EJ, Mulliken BD, Bourne RB *et al.*: Catastrophic osteolysis in total knee replacement. *Clinical Orthopedics* **321**:98–105, 1995.

5 Wasielewski RC, Parks N, Williams I *et al.*: Tibial insert undersurface as a contributing source of polyethylene wear debris. *Clinical Orthopedics* **345**:53–59, 1997.

6 Whiteside LA: Effect of porous coating configuration on tibial osteolysis after total knee arthroplasty. *Clinical Orthopedics* **321**:92–97, 1995.

7 Lewis PL, Rorabeck CH, Bourne RB: Screw osteolysis after cementless total knee replacement. *Clinical Orthopedics* **321**:173–177, 1995.

8 Dodd CAF, Hungerford DS, Krackow KA: Total knee arthroplasty fixation comparison of the early results of paired cemented versus uncemented porous-coated anatomic knee prostheses. *Clinical Orthopedics* **260**:66–70, 1990.

9 Moran CG, Pinder IM, Lees TA, Midwinter MB: 121 Cases in survivorship analysis of the uncemented porous coated anatomic knee replacement. *Journal of Bone and Joint Surgery* [Am] **73**:848–857, 1991.

10 Moran CG, Pinder IM, Midwinter MJ: Failure of the porous coated anatomic (PCA) knee. *Journal of Bone and Joint Surgery* [Br] **72**:1092, 1990.

11 Scuderi GR, Insall JN: Cement technique in primary total knee arthroplasty. *Techniques in Orthopedics* **6**(4):39–43, 1991.

12 Ryd L, Toksvig-Larsen S: Early prosthetic fixation of tibial components: an in vivo roentgenstereogrammetric analysis. *Journal of Orthopaedic Research* **11**:142–148, 1993.

13 Schai PA, Thornhill TS, Scott RD: Total knee arthoplasty with the PFC system. Results at a minimum of ten years and survivorship analysis. *Journal of Bone and Joint Surgery* [Br] **80**:850–858, 1998.

14 Gunderson R, Mallory TH, Herrington SM: Surface cementation of the tibial component in total knee arthroplasty. Presented at AAOS Annual Meeting, New Orleans, LA, 19–23 March, 1998.

15 Bert JM, McShane M: Is it necessary to cement the tibial stem to improve tibial implant stability in cemented total knee arthroplasty. Presented at the Knee Society Specialty Day, New Orleans, LA, 22 March, 1998.

16 Ryd L, Lindstrand A, Strenstrom A, Selvik, G: Porous coated anatomic tricompartmental tibial components. The relationship between prosthetic position and micromotion. *Clinical Orthopedics* **251**:189–197, 1993.

17 Albrektsson BEJ, Carlsson LV, Freeman MAR *et al.*: Proximally cemented versus uncemented Freeman–Samuelson Knee arthroplasty. A prospective randomized study. *Journal of Bone and Joint Surgery* [Br] **74**:233–238, 1992.

18 Toksvig-Larsen S, Ryd L, Lindstrand A: Early inducible displacement of tibial components in total knee prostheses inserted with and without cement. *Journal of Bone and Joint Surgery* [Am] **80**:83–89, 1998.

19 Insall JN, Lachiewicz PF, Burstein AH: The posterior stabilized condylar prosthesis: a modification of the total condylar design. *Journal of Bone and Joint Surgery* [Am] **64**:1317–1323, 1982.

20 Bartel DL, Bicknell VL, Wright TM: The effect of conformity, thickness and material on stresses in ultra-high molecular weight components for total knee replacement *Journal of Bone and Joint Surgery* [Am] **68**:1041–1051, 1986.

21 Emmerson KP, Moram CG, Pinder IM: Survivorship analysis of the kinematic stabilizer total knee replacement. A 10 to 14 year follow-up study. *Journal of Bone and Joint Surgery* [Br] **78**:441–445, 1996.

22 Scott RD: Posterior cruciate ligament retaining designs and results. In *Current concepts in primary and revision total knee arthroplasty*, ed. JN Insall, WN Scott, GR Scuderi, pp. 37–40. Lippincott-Raven, Philadelphia, 1996.

23 Stiehl JB, Komistek RD, Dennis DA, et.al: Fluroroscopic analysis of kinematics after posterior cruciate retaining knee arthroplasty. *Journal of Bone and Joint Surgery* [Br] **77**:884–889, 1995.

24 Vince KG, Insall JN, Kelly MA: The total condylar prosthesis: 10 to 12 year results of a cemented knee replacement. *Journal of Bone and Joint Surgery* [Br] **71**:793–797, 1989.

25 Ranawat CS, Boachie-Adjei, O: Survivorship analysis and results of total condylar knee arthroplasty. Eight to eleven year follow-up period. *Clinical Orthopedics* **226**:6–13, 1988.

26 Aglietti P, Buzzi R, Gaudenzi A: Patellofemoral functional results and complications with the posterior stabilized total condylar knee prosthesis. *Journal of Arthroplasty* **3**:17–25, 1988.

27 Scott WN, Rubinstein M, Scuderi G: Results of total knee replacement with a posterior cruciate substituiting prosthesis. *Journal of Bone and Joint Surgery* [Am] **70**:1163–1173, 1988.

28 Stern SH, Insall JN: Posterior stabilized results after follow-up of nine to twelve years. *Journal of Bone and Joint Surgery* [Am] **74**:980–986, 1992.

29 Colizza WA, Insall JN, Scuderi GR: The posterior stabilized total knee prosthesis. Assessment of polyethylene damage and osteolysis after a ten-year minimum follow-up. *Journal of Bone and Joint Surgery* [Am] **77**:1713–1720, 1995.

30 Ranawat CS, Luessenhop CP, Rodriguez JA: The press fit condylar modular total knee system: Four to six year results with a posterior substituting design. *Journal of Bone and Joint Surgery* [Am] **79**: 342–348, 1997.

31 Diduch DR, Insall JN, Scott WN *et al.*: Totalknee replacement in young active patients. *Journal of Bone and Joint Surgery* [Am] **79**:575–582, 1997.

32 Rosenberg AG, Barden RM, Galante JO: A comparison of cemented and cementless fixation with the Miller–Galante total knee arthroplasty. *Orthopedic Clinics of North America* **20**:97–111, 1989.

33 Nafei A, Nielsen S, Kristensen O, Hvid J: The press fit kinemax knee arhroplasty. High failure rate of noncemented implants. *Journal of Bone and Joint Surgery* [Br] **74**:243–246, 1992.

# Con: Johan Bellemans

## Cemented TKA

Many people today consider cemented TKA as the gold standard, based upon its published success rate. The prevalence of good and excellent results with cemented Total Condylar type TKAs have been reported to be 88–95%. With revision used as the endpoint, a survival rate of 95% at 10–15 years has been noted, in one recent report with the longest follow-up so far 91% at 21 years.[1-3]

PMMA bone cement can therefore be considered as an adequate anchoring substance for knee arthroplasty components, being able to withstand the applied loads for a relatively long period. Cementing knee arthroplasty components is a relatively easy and reproducible technique, and has the advantage that minor irregularities in the prepared bone surfaces can be filled, making a precise bone preparation less critical with regard to implant fixation.

Although the results of cemented knee arthroplasties are good, they certainly are not perfect. Loosening of one or more prosthetic components can occur, and is certainly noticeable when longer follow-up data are analyzed.[4-6]

Although the etiology of prosthetic loosening in TKA is complex—involving issues of technique, alignment, and prosthetic design—the agent utilized to fix the prosthetic device, PMMA, is been considered to be a major factor. Bone cement is prone to fatigue failure and is a poor transmitter of tensile and shear stress.[7,8] Although this is the biggest disadvantage of bone cement, it is not its only drawback (Table 7.1).

- Bone cement is brittle, it is a potential source for third-body wear, and it can cause massive osteolysis.[9-11]
- During its polymerization phase, cement is cytotoxic and heat necrosis of the underlying bone can occur.[12-15]
- In a study using transoesophageal echocardiography, bone cement has been suggested to contribute to the formation of venous clot and the intraopertive embolic insult by activation of the coagulation cascade.[16]
- Cadaver studies have shown that cement increases the risk for femoral stress shielding in TKA.[17]
- Furthermore, PMMA cement has been found to impair chemotaxis, phagocytosis, and killing ability of polymorphonuclear leucocytes, increasing the susceptibility to infection.[18-20]

The cementing technique itself is not free of problems: inadequate and asymmetric pressurization (tibial component), inadequate cement thickness (femoral component), periprosthetic cement extrusion (patellar components), inadequate porosity due to inadequate mixing, and inadequate cleaning of the bone surface with residual

**Table 7.1** Negative factors attributed to PMMA cement fixation

Fatigue failure
Poor transmission of tensile stress
Poor transmission of shear stress
Brittleness
Third-body wear
Osteolysis
Cytotoxicity
Heat necrosis of bone
Stress shielding
Wedge sign
Loosening
Cement extrusion and impingement
Impairment of chemotaxis
Inhibition of phagocytosis
Increased susceptibility to infection
Increased thromboembolic activation

blood or bone marrow contaminating the interface, all seem to be inevitable occurrences associated with cemented TKAs.[21,22]

## Uncemented TKA

Opponents of cemented TKA have argued that the disadvantages associated with the use of PMMA cement can be avoided by using cementless fixation.

This option has become increasingly attractive since published series of uncemented TKA have become available, showing that results at least equal to those using cement can be obtained both in the short and longer term.

- Scott *et al.*[23] have reported a 95% component survivorship at 7–11 years follow-up in 212 knees using cementless fixation of the Natural-knee system.
- Using revision as an end-point, Whiteside[24] has reported an overall survival rate of 94% at 10 years in 163 knees with the uncemented Ortholoc I knee.
- Buechel[25] published an overall survivorship rate of 95% at the 12 year interval for the cementless LCS-knee in 158 cases.
- Sorrells *et al.*[26] have reported a 93% survivorship at 13 years follow-up in 417 patients.

These reports cannot be disregarded and they do show that cementless TKA can be as successful as cemented total knees at the 10–15 years follow-up evaluation.

Opponents of uncemented TKA have argued that a number of negative papers have been published regarding uncemented knees, with a higher incidence of component loosening, radiolucencies, and osteolysis compared to cemented knees.

- Rosenberg et al. [27] reported a higher tibial component loosening rate in a comparative prospective study on the Miller–Galante uncemented versus cemented knee. Other uncemented knee designs such as the Porous-Coated Anatomic knee (PCA)[28–30] and the AGC knee,[31] have also been associated with increased loosening rates on the tibial components.
- A higher incidence of radiolucent lines has been reported by some authors at the interface of uncemented tibial components in the PCA and Miller–Galante system.[27,29] Other people, however, have seen no differences concerning radiolucent lines in studies comparing cemented versus uncemented fixation of identical implant types, or even a significantly higher number of radiolucent lines for the cemented group.[32,33]
- Osteolysis has been associated with uncemented TKA in a number of systems, such as a PCA knee, the Miller-Galante prosthesis, the Synatomic prosthesis, and the Arizona prosthesis,[34–36] but has also been reported for cemented knee components.[37–39]

The problems of loosening, radiolucent lines and osteolysis that were observed in several uncemented knee systems cannot be denied. They are, however, the consequence of not applying techniques or design features that are necessary for obtaining successful results with uncemented TKA. The criteria for successful uncemented TKA are now well established. They include

- the presence of an appropriate contact between the implant and the underlying bone
- rigid initial fixation of the prosthetic components
- the presence of an appropriate porous coating.

### Appropriate bone–implant contact

Several authors have shown that optimal integration of uncemented arthroplasty components requires the presence of an interface gap that is smaller than 0.5 mm.[40–42] Using modern instrumentation systems the operative accuracy for the femoral side has been reported to be 0.5–0.8 mm[43–45] and 1.0–2.4 mm for the tibial side.[44,46] Meticulous surgical technique and extremely accurate instrumentation are therefore of the utmost importance when performing uncemented TKA.

It is not surprising that many of the early uncemented knee systems were associated with increased loosening rates, especially at the tibial components, since they were inserted using instruments and surgical techniques that were not capable of reproducing the accuracy required for successful uncemented fixation, resulting in interface gaps larger than 0.5 mm. Using a precise surgical technique together with modern and more accurate instruments, these problems can be avoided.

The use of autologous bone grafts or hydroxyapatite coatings can further enhance the osseointegration process. Hofmann et al.[47] have reported on the use of cancellous bone paste on the cut surface of the tibia and the femur to augment ingrowth, using autograft bone obtained from the cut surface of the tibial wafer using the patellar reamer. Using this technique, excellent clinical results were noted at 7–11 years of follow-up, with consistent and abundant bone ingrowth in as high as 40% of the pore volume.[23,47]

The same effect has been noted for hydroxyapatite coatings based on their osteoconductive characteristics, making the bone–implant interface gap less critical. Soballe et al.[48] have shown that unloaded hydroxyapatite-coated titanium plugs became osseointegrated even in the presence of 1 mm interface gaps, whereas uncoated implants did not under these circumstances. These data ware confirmed in other studies using hip and knee arthroplasty components in animal models, showing significantly higher bone ingrowth and bone ongrowth for hydroxyapatite-coated implants on histomorphometric analysis.[49–51] Hydroxyapatite coatings therefore seem to be most beneficial in situations with relatively large (>0.5 mm) interface gaps between the implant and the bone.

An important concern, however, is the disintegration of hydroxyapatite coatings over time. Although some resorption or dissolution is of course essential to trigger the basic osteoconductive effect of hydroxyapatite coatings , fast or complete disintegration could theoretically lead to loss of integration and component loosening over time.[52–55] Long-term clinical data are therefore necessary to determine whether hydroxyapatite can serve as a substitute for precise surgical technique in obtaining a close implant–bone contact.

### Rigid initial fixation

Stable initial fixation is another prerequisite for successful integration of uncemented components. Excessive interface motion has been shown to lead to the formation of a fibrous connective tissue layer, and bone ingrowth has been noted in mechanically stable implants.[56,57] Achieving initial mechanical stability and thus minimizing micromotion is therefore a prime consideration in uncemented TKA. Relative displacement of less than 150 μm has been found to be consistent with osseointegration.[56,57]

Rigid initial fixation with micromotion less than 150 μm does not seem to be a problem for the femoral component in TKA, since it provides adequate intrinsic resistance to rigid body motion by virtue of its shape and box-like configuration. Press-fitting the anterior and posterior condylar surfaces increases the frictional forces and tends to immobilize the femoral component. The anterior and posterior surfaces tend to resist anteroposterior (AP) translation, flexion–extension tilt, and rotation. The routine use of metaphyseal lugs or pegs distally further prevents mediolateral tilt, mediolateral translation, and rotation.[58]

For the tibial component however, obtaining rigid fixation is more problematic. Tibial trays fixed with simple interference fit peg fixation have been shown to move 400–800 μm, with or without additional fixation of a central screw.[59,60] Tibial trays fixed with a central cylindrical stem alone, show an initial micromotion of 200–400 μm, which is still too high for reliable integration.

The addition of cruciate-shape blades to such a stem further inhibits micromotion, but even then micromotion in the region of 150–200 μm was further noted.[61] Volz et al.[60] and Miura et al.[62] have shown that when tibial trays are fixed with four screws, micromotion is 100–200 μm, which might be compatible with osseointegration. Adding a central stem to the four screws does not seem to improve micromotion in tibial bone with good quality, but can lead to substantially less micromotion in osteopenic bone.[63,64] The routine combination of four screws and a central stem for fixation of uncemented tibial components therefore seems to be the best choice for controlling micromotion.

The addition of interference pegs might be additionally beneficial, as has been shown by Natarajan and Andriacchi[65] who reported relative tangential displacements as high as 200 μm when subjecting tibial components to compressive loads. Such tangential displacement is the consequence of the variation in elastic modulus between the metal tibial tray and the underlying bone, and can be reduced substantially by the use of interference pegs. As stated above, these pegs do not influence the rigid body motion, which has to be controlled by screws and an additional stem. (Fig. 7.7).

In view of these data, it is again not surprising that an increased prevalence of radiolucent lines and an increased number of tibial component loosenings have been reported in many of the early and even current uncemented knee designs, as a consequence of the poor initial fixation options available for the tibial component in these systems, resulting in micromotion exceeding 150 μm (Fig. 7.8). Using components with an adequate initial fixation can, however, avoid these problems.

### Appropriate porous coating

The third prerequisite for successful uncemented TKA is the presence of an appropriate porous coating on the component surface. The effective pore size of the coating should be between 50 and 400 μm for reliable cementless integration.[66] The use of titanium rather than cobalt—chrome alloy or beads versus fiber structure appear not to be very important issues, but continuity of the coating is. Smooth metal bridges separating the porous coating are a pathway for debris migration, whereas a uniform continuous coating can effectively seal off the interface, even if that interface is occupied entirely by fibrous tissue. Protection of the implant–bone interface by the fibrous tissue mantle that penetrates the porous coating is a well-documented phenomenon.[67–69] Further evidence concerning

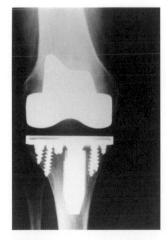

**Fig. 7.7**

Rigid component fixation and precise surgical fit are two important prerequisites for successful uncemented TKA.

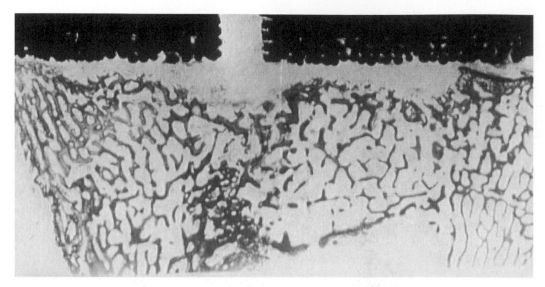

**Fig. 7.8**

Many "first generation" cementless knees were inserted with poor initial fixation, leading to the formation of a fibrous connective tissue layer and an increased risk for loosening. See also colour plate section.

this was provided by Whiteside,[70] who reported a 0% incidence of osteolysis in the uncemented Ortholoc knee when a continuous porous coating was applied, versus a 17% incidence of osteolytic lesions when a porous coating interrupted by smooth metal bridges was used on the same system.

With a limited distribution of porous coating, particles can enter the implant–bone interface and metaphyseal bone by way of the unbonded interface between the smooth metal and bone. The development of osteolysis is not a direct function of the absence of cement, but is related to other variables associated with first-generation total knee replacements, such as polyethylene quality and articular surface design.[71] It is therefore not surprising that osteolysis has also been noted with cemented components.[37-39] For the same reason it is not surprising that many of the early cementless knees, with a high potential for debris generation owing to poor articular surface design and polyethylene quality, in combination with the presence of smooth metal bridges separating the porous coating, have been associated with osteolysis. This can, however, be minimized when modern designs with more confirming surfaces in combination with an appropriate continous porous coating are used.

## Conclusion

Several authors have shown that uncemented TKA can be as successful as cemented TKA at the 10–15 years follow-up.

The prerequisites for successful uncemented TKA are now well established, and include the presence of an appropriate contact between the implant and the bone, rigid initial fixation of the prosthetic components, and an appropriate continuous porous coating. When these criteria are not fulfilled, uncemented TKA is contraindicated. Failure to comply with these criteria has lead to a number

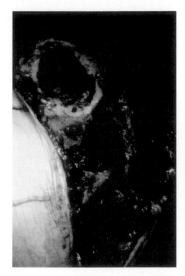

**Fig. 3.17 (b)** At time of revision, there is marked central cavitary bone loss.

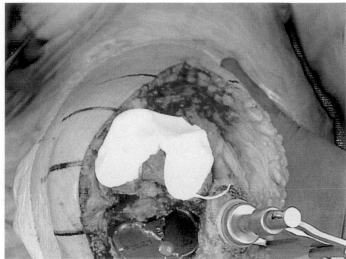

**Fig. 7.2** The doughy cement is placed in a "horseshoe" fashion around the distal femur.

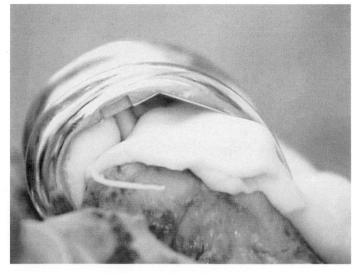

**Fig. 7.3** Cement is placed on the posterior condyles of the femoral component prior to impaction.

1

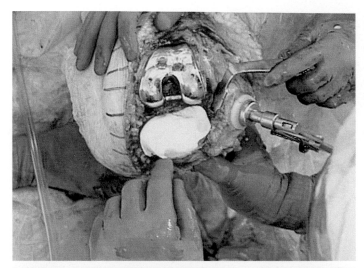

**Fig. 7.4** Since the entire tibial component is cemented, cement is placed on the proximal tibial surface (a) as well as pushed into the central fixation hole (b).

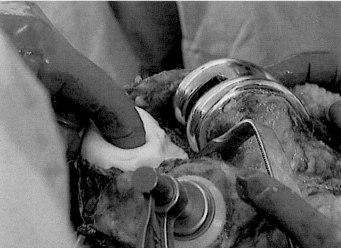

**Fig. 7.4 (b)**

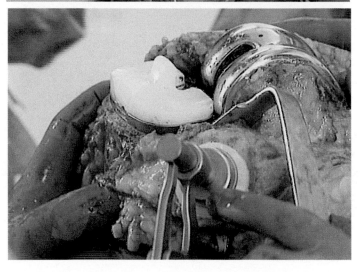

**Fig. 7.5** With the components fully seated, all excess cement is removed from around the components in an effort to prevent particles from breaking free and getting trapped in the articulation.

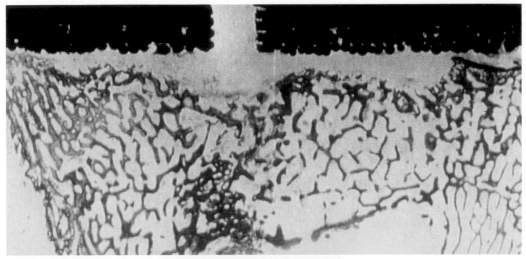

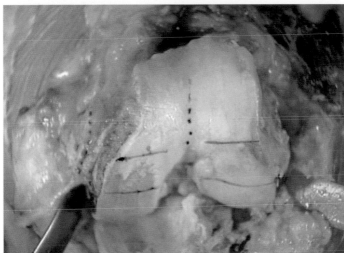

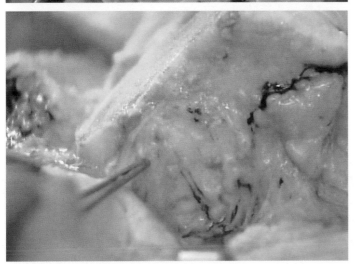

**Fig. 7.8** Many "first generation" cementless knees were inserted with poor initial fixation, leading to the formation of a fibrous connective tissue layer and an increased risk for loosening.

**Fig. 9.1** Fixed femoral landmarks for determining femoral rotation include the AP axis and the epicondylar axis.

**Fig. 9.2** The center of the lateral epicondyle is the most prominent point.

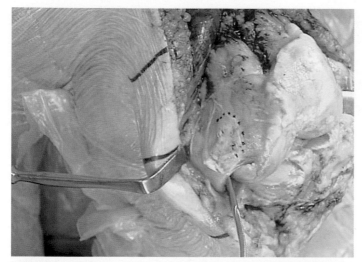

**Fig. 9.3** The sulcus is the center of the medial epicondyle.

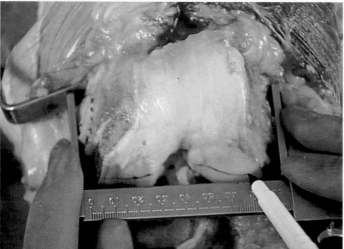

**Fig. 9.4** The epicondylar axis is determined by a line connecting the medial and lateral epicondyles.

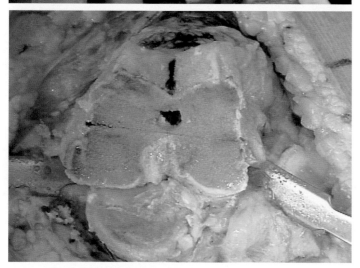

**Fig. 9.5** Once the epicondylar axis is identified, the femoral component rotation is set.

of negative reports in the past concerning cementless fixation of knee arthroplasty components.

It has now repeatedly been shown that surgeons who do use the techniques necessary for uncemented TKA, together with an appropriate design, can achieve the same excellent results as with cemented TKA, giving their patients the benefit of a biological and durable, cement-free interface.

## References

1   Ranawat C, Flynn W, Saddler S *et al.*: Long-term results of the total condylar knee arthroplasty: a 15-year survivorship study. *Clinical Orthopaedics and Related Research* **286**:94–102, 1993.

2   Stern S, Insall J: Posterior stabilized prosthesis. Results after follow-up of nine to twelve years. *Journal of Bone and Joint Surgery* [Am] **74**:980–986, 1992.

3   Font-Rodriguez D, Scuderi G, Insall J: Survivorship of cemented total knee arthroplasty. *Clinical Orthopaedics and Related Research* **345**:79–86, 1997.

4   Bartz R, Sheth D, Rowder N *et al.*: Early loosening of the tibial component of the posterior stabilized Insall–Burstein knee prosthesis. *Proceedings of the 66$_{th}$ Annual Meeting of the American Academy of Orthopaedic Surgeons*, p. 49, 1999.

5   Rand J, Ilstrup JD: Survivorship analysis of total knee arthroplasty. Cumulative survival of 920 total knee arthroplasties. *Journal of Bone and Joint Surgery* [Am] **73**:397–409, 1991.

6   Moreland J: Mechanisms of failure in total knee arthroplasty. *Clinical Orthopaedics and Related Research* **226**:49–64, 1988

7   Lewis G: Properties of acrylic bone cement: state of the art review. *Journal of Biomedical Materials Research* **38**:155–182, 1997.

8   Spector M: Biomaterial failure. *Orthopaedic Clinics of North America* **23**:211–217, 1992.

9   Jones L, Hungerford D: Cement disease. *Clinical Orthopaedics and Related Research* **225**:192–203, 1987.

10  Isaac G, Wroblewski B, Atkinson J, Dowson D: Source of the cement within the Charnley hip. *Journal of Bone and Joint Surgery* [Br] **72**:149–150, 1990.

11  Jasty M, Jiranek W, Harris W: Acrylic fragmentation in total hip replacements and its biological consequences. *Clinical Orthopaedics and Related Research* **285**:116–128, 1992.

12  Oates K, Barrera D, Tucker W *et al.*: In vivo effect of pressurization of polymethyl methacrylate bone cement. Biomechanical and histologic analysis. *Journal of Arthroplasty* **10**:373–381, 1995.

13  Savarino L, Stea S, Ciagetti G *et al.*: Microstructural investigation of bone–cement interface. *Journal of Biomedical Materials Research* **29**:701–705, 1995.

14  Kindt-Larsen T, Smith D, Jensen J: Innovations in acrylic bone cement and application equipment. *Journal of Applied Biomaterials* **6**:75–83, 1995.

15  Liu Y, Park J, Njus G, Stienstra D: Bone particle-impregnated bone cement: an in vitro study. *Journal of Biomedical Materials Research* **21**:247–261, 1987.

16  Berman A, Parmet J, Harding S *et al.*: Emboli observed with use of transesopheal echocardiography immediately after tourniquet release during total knee arthroplasty with cement. *Journal of Bone and Joint Surgery* [Am] **80**:389–396, 1998.

17  Seki T, Tashiro T, Omori G *et al.*: Microstrain on the cortex and within the bone of the distal femur with cemented and uncemented femoral components in total knee arthroplasty. *Proceedings of the 44th Annual Meeting of the Orthopaedic Research Society*, p. 699, 1998.

18  Petty W: The effect of methylmetacrylate on bacterial phagocytosis and killing by human polymorphonuclear leukocytes. *Journal of Bone and Joint Surgery* [Am] **60**:752–757, 1978.

19  Petty W: The effect of methylmetacrylate on chemotaxis of polymorphonuclear leukocytes. *Journal of Bone and Joint Surgery* [Am] **60**:492–498, 1978.

20  Hanssen A, Rand J: Evaluation and treatment of infection at the site of a total hip or knee arthroplasty. *Journal of Bone and Joint Surgery* [Am] **80**:910–922, 1998.

21  Otani T, Fujii K, Ozawa M *et al.* 1998 Impingement after total knee arthroplasty caused by cement extrusion and proximal tibiofibular instability. *Journal of Arthroplasty* **13**:589–591.

22  Sambatakakis A, Wilton T, Newton G: Radiographic sign of persistent soft-tissue imbalance after knee replacement. *Journal of Bone and Joint Surgery* [Br] **73**:751–756, 1991.

23  Scott D, Hofmann A, Thach T *et al.* Seven to eleven year experience with cementless fixation using the Natural knee. *Proceedings of the 64th Annual Meeting of the American Academy of Orthopaedic Surgeons*, p. 353, 1997.

24  Whiteside L: Cementless total knee replacement. 9 to 11-year results and 10-year survivorship analysis. *Clinical Orthopaedics and Related Research* **309**:185–192, 1994.

25  Buechel F: Cementless meniscal bearing knee arthroplasty: 7 to 12-year outcome analysis. *Orthopaedics* **17**:833–836, 1994.

26  Sorrells B, Voorhorst P, Greenwald S: The long-term clinical use of a rotating platform mobile bearing TKA. *Proceedings of the 66th Annual Meeting of the American Academy of Orthopaedic Surgeons*, p. 228, 1999.

27  Rosenberg A, Barden R, Galante J: Cemented and ingrowth fixation of the Miller–Galante prosthesis. Clinical and roentgenographic comparison after 3 to 6 years follow-up studies. *Clinical Orthopaedics and Related Research* **260**:71–79, 1990.

28  Moran C, Pinder I, Lees T, Midwinter M: Survivorship analysis of the uncemented porous-coated anatomic knee replacement. *Journal of Bone and Joint Surgery* [Am] **73**:848–857, 1991.

29  Collins D, Heim S, Nelson C, Smith P: Porous-coated anatomic total knee arthroplasty: A prospective analysis comparing cemented and cementless fixation. *Clinical Orthopaedics and Related Research* **267**:128–136, 1991.

30  Eskola A, Vahvanen V, Santavita S *et al.*: Porous-coated anatomic knee arthroplasty. Three year results. *Journal of Arthroplasty* **7**:223–228, 1992.

31  Nielsen P, Hansen E, Rechangel K. Cementless total knee arthroplasty in unselected cases of osteoarthritis and rheumatoid arthritis. A 3 year follow-up study of 103 cases. *Journal of Arthroplasty* **7**:137–143.

32  Rand J: Cement or cementless fixation in total knee arthroplasty. *Clinical Orthopaedics and Related Research* **273**:52–62, 1991.

33  McCaskie, Deehan D, Green T *et al.*: Randomised, prospective study comparing cemented and cementless total knee replacement. *Journal of Bone and Joint Surgery* [Br] **80**:971–975, 1998.

34  Lewis P, Rorabeck C, Bourne R: Screw osteolysis after cementless total knee replacement. *Clinical Orthopaedics and Related Research* **321**:173–177, 1995.

35  Peters P, Engh G, Dwyer K, Vinh T: Osteolysis after total knee arthro-
    plasty without cement. *Journal of Bone and Joint Surgery* [Am]
    **74**:864–876, 1992.

36  Kim Y, Oh J, Oh S: Osteolysis around cementless porous-coated
    anatomic knee prosthesis. *Journal of Bone and Joint Surgery* [Br]
    **77**:236–241, 1995.

37  Robinson E, Mulliken B, Bourne R, Rorabeck C, Alvarez C:
    Catastrophic osteolysis in total knee replacement. A report of 17
    cases. *Clinical Orthopaedics and Related Research* **321**:98–105, 1995.

38  Ries M, Guiney W, Lynch F: Osteolysis associated with cemented total
    knee arthroplasty. A case report. *Journal of Arthroplasty* **9**:555–558,
    1994.

39  Ezzet K, Garcia R, Barrack R: Effect of component fixation method on
    osteolysis in total knee arthroplasty. *Clinical Orthopaedics and
    Related Research* **321**:86–91, 1995.

40  Carlsson L, Rostlund T, Albrektsson B, Albrektsson T: Implant fixation
    proved by close fit cylindrical implant-bone interface studies in
    rabbits. *Acta Orthopaedica Scandinavica* **59**:272–275, 1988.

41  Sandborn P, Cook S, Spires W, Kester M: Tissue response to porous
    coated implants lacking initial bone apposition. *Journal of
    Arthroplasty* **3**:337–346, 1988.

42  Dalton J, Cook S, Thomas K, Kay J: The effect of operative fit and
    hydroxyapatite coating on the mechanical and biological response
    to porous implants. *Journal of Bone and Joint Surgery* [Am]
    **77**:97–110, 1995.

43  Otani T, Whiteside L, White S: Cutting errors in preparation of femoral
    components in total knee arthroplasty. *Journal of Arthroplasty*
    **8**:503–510, 1993.

44  Dueringer K, Stalcup G: *Bone cut accuracy and flatness from milling and
    sawing. A comparative study.* Zimmer Inc., 1995.

45  Lennox D, Cohn B, Eschenroeder H: The effects of inaccurate bone
    cuts on femoral component position in total knee arthroplasty.
    *Orthopedics* **11**:257–260, 1998.

46  Toksvig-Larsen S, Ryol L: Surface flatness in orthopedic bone cutting.
    *Transactions of the Orthopaedic Research Society* **15**:564, 1991.

47  Hofmann A, Murdock L, Wyatt R, Alpert J: Total knee arthroplasty: 2
    to 4 year experience using an assymetric tibial tray and a deep
    trochlear-grooved femoral component. *Clinical Orthopaedics and
    Related Research* **269**:78–88.

48  Soballe K, Overgaerd S: The current status of hydroxyapatite coating of
    prostheses. *Journal of Bone and Joint Surgery* [Br] **78**:689–691,
    1996.

49  Geesink R: Experimental and clinical experience with hydroxyapatite
    coated hip implants. *Clinical Orthopaedics and Related Research*
    **291**:239–242, 1989.

50  Munting E: The contribution and limitation of hydroxyapatite coating
    to implant fixation. *International Orthopaedics* **20**:1–6, 1996.

51  Bellemans J: Osseointegration in porous coated knee arthroplasty.
    The sheep stifle joint as in vivo evaluation model, pp. 56–127.
    PhD Dissertation, Katholieke Universiteit Leuven, Belgium,
    1997.

52  Bauer T: The histology of HA-coated implants. In *Hydroxyapatite coat-
    ings in orthopaedic surgery*, ed. R Geesinck, M Manley, pp. 305–318.
    Raven Press, New York, 1993.

53  Bloebaum R, Beeks D, Dorr L: Complications with hydroxyapatite par-
    ticulate separation in total hip arthroplasty. *Clinical Orthopaedics
    and Related Research* **298**:19–26, 1994.

54 Le Geros R, Dalculsi G, Orly I *et al.*: Formation of carbonate apatite on calcium phosphate materials: dissolution/precipitation processes. In *Bone-bonding biomaterials*, pp. 201–212. Read Healthcare Communications, Leiderdorp, 1992.

55 Soballe K, Hansen E, Brockstedt-Rasmussen H *et al.*: Hydroxyapatite coating enhances fixation of porous coated implants: a comparison in dogs between press fit and non interference fit. *Acta Orthopaedica Scandinavica* **61**:299–306, 1990.

56 Burke D: Dynamic measurements of interface mechanics in vivo and the effect of micromotion on bone ingrowth into a porous coated surface device under controlled loads in vivo. *Transactions of the Orthopaedic Research Society* **16**:103, 1991.

57 Pilliar R, Lee J, Maniatopoulos C: Observations on the effect of movement on bone ingrowth into porous-surfaced implants. *Clinical Orthpaedics and Related Research* **208**:108–113, 1986.

58 Rosenberg A, Galante J: Cementless total knee arthroplasty. In *Knee surgery*, ed. F Fu, C Harner, K Vince, Vol. II, pp. 1367–1383. Williams and Wilkins, Baltimore, 1994.

59 Shimagaki H, Bechtold J, Sherman R, Gustilo R: Stability of initial fixation of the tibial component in cementless total knee arthroplasty. *Journal of Orthopaedic Research* **8**:64–71, 1990.

60 Volz R, Nisbet J, Lee W, McMurtry M: The mechanical stability of various noncemented tibial components. *Clinical Orthopaedics and Related Research* **226**:38–42, 1988.

61 Walker P, Hsu P, Zimmerman R: A comparative study of uncemented tibial components. *Journal of Arthroplasty* **5**:245–253, 1990.

62 Miura M, Whiteside L, Easley J, Amador D: Effects of screws and a sleeve on initial fixation in uncemented total knee tibial components. *Clinical Orthopaedics and Related Research* **259**:160–168, 1990.

63 Lee R, Volz R, Sheridan D: The role of fixation and bone quality on the mechanical stability of tibial knee components. *Clinical Orthopaedics and Related Research* **273**:177–183, 1991.

64 Yoshii J, Whiteside L, Milliano M, Write S: The effect of central stem and stem length on micromovement of the tibial tray. *Journal of Arthroplasty* **7**:433–438, 1992.

65 Natarajan R, Andriacchi T: The influence of displacement incompatibilities on bone growth in porous tibial components. *Transactions of the Orthopaedic Research Society* **13**:331, 1988.

66 Bobyn J, Pilliar R, Cameron W, Weatherly G, Kent G: The optimum pore size for the fixation of porous-surfaced metal implants by the ingrowth of bone. *Clinical Orthopaedics and Related Research* **150**:263–270, 1980.

67 Engh C, Zettl-Schaffer K, Kukita Y *et al.*: 1993 Histological and radiographic assessment of well functioning porous-coated acetabular components. *Journal of Bone and Joint Surgery* [Am] **75**:814–824.

68 Ward W, Johnson K, Dorey F, Eckardt J: Extramedullary porous coating to prevent diaphyseal osteolysis and radiolucent lines around proximal tibial replacements. *Journal of Bone and Joint Surgery* [Am] **75**:976–987, 1993.

69 Bobyn J, Jacobs J, Tanzer M *et al.*: 1995 The susceptibility of smooth implant surfaces to peri-implant fibrosis and migration of polyethylene wear debris. *Clinical Orthopaedics and Related Research* **311**:21–39.

70 Whiteside L: 1995 Effect of porous coating configuration on tibial osteolysis after total knee arthroplasty. *Clinical Orthopaedics and Related Research* **321**:92–97.

71 Schmalzried T, Callaghan J: Wear in total hip and knee replacements. *Journal of Bone and Joint Surgery* [Am] **81**:115–136, 1999.

## Questions and answers

*Moderator:* Dr. Scuderi, you use Simplex cement in a doughy state. There are many surgeons who use cement in a more liquid state and pressure inject it into the bone. Why do you think that doughy cement is better? Is there a real downside to pressure injected cement?

*Dr. Scuderi:* Doughy cement is easy to handle and can be manually pressurized into the cancellous bone. This creates a penetration depth of about 2 mm. Pressure injected cement will penetrate deeper into the bone, which may be acceptable, but if the knee becomes infected, there is greater bone loss when all the cement is removed.

*Moderator:* Drs. Scuderi and Insall, you cement the femur first and the tibia second. Doesn't that result in situations where you may have extruded cement behind the tibial component that you cannot physically see or remove because the femoral component is blocking your access?

*Dr. Scuderi:* The key to removing all the cement is exposure. When I cement the tibial component, the tibia is subluxed anteriorly and externally rotated, permitting complete exposure to the back of the knee.

*Moderator:* Dr. John Hart in Australia has presented data showing that whether or not you cement the stem has no relationship to long-term loosening or radiolucent lines. Do you think that cementing the stem (or not) may be more prosthesis dependent, rather that a blanket across-the-board idea?

*Dr. Scuderi:* If you are referring to cementing the tibial stem, there is some difference between stem designs, such as the I-beam and cruciate designs, but I believe that the stem of the core prosthesis should be cemented. Surface cementing has shown not to be as durable as completely cementing the tibial component. Gunderson has reported a 9% tibial loosening rate with the surface cement technique vesus no tibial loosening with a fully cemented tibial component[15]. This is further supported by the work of Bert[4] and Ryd[27].

*Moderator:* Is there a chance of over-pressurizing the cement when dealing with severely osteopenic bone? How do you prevent this, and what is the downside of over pressurization?

*Dr. Scuderi:* Care must be taken with osteopenic bone, such as that seen with rheumatoid arthritis. Initially the bone is carefully cleaned with pulsatile lavage and then while the cement is in a doughy state, it is manually pressed into the cancellous bone. The only downside to over-penetration is if it needs to be removed during an infected case.

*Moderator:* With our current generation of instruments the cut are usually so "true" that we may almost be press-fitting the femoral component. Why not go all the way and not cement it at all?

*Dr. Scuderi:* Instrument systems have improved bone preparation, in fact the cuts are almost perfect with a line to line fit. This has caused some surgeons to experiment with cementless femoral fixation. This is not a new concept, since it sprouted from the PCA era. Hybrid fixation was introduced in the 1980s in hopes of gaining the theoretical advantage of bone ingrowth in the femoral component and avoiding the pitfalls of cementless tibial fixation. The early short-term reports were promising, but long-term follow-up has not been successful. At an average follow-up of 7.4 years (range 5–10 years), Campbell and coworkers reported a 13.8% revision rate and a 85% survivorship with this type of fixation using the Press-fit Condylar prosthesis.[6] The main cause of failure was femoral component loosening. This information supports my belief that hybrid fixation is unreliable and is not as durable as completely cemented total knee replacement.

*Moderator:*.It has been shown that the monomer in cement can decrease leukotactic and phagocytitic rates in white cells. Do you therefore routinely add antibiotics to your cement for patients who are immunocompromised (e.g., patients taking systemic steroids) so as to aid in preventing infection?

*Dr. Scuderi:* I do not routinely add antibiotics to my cement in primary total knee replacements. My concern is that the addition of antibiotics into the cement will alter the mechanical properties of the cement.

*Moderator:* Do you think that there is any place for an uncemented total knee replacement?

*Dr. Scuderi:* Unless a patient has an allergy to PMMA, I do not think there is a place for uncemented total knee replacement. The long-term survivorship of cementless total knee replacement has not been comparable to the success and durability of cemented total knee replacement.

*Moderator:* If cemented and uncemented knees do equally well, Dr. Bellemans, why should a surgeon opt to use an uncemented implant, especially since it is more expensive?

*Dr. Bellemans:* A lot of factors determine the price of total knee implants. It is for example strange to notice that sometimes cemented components from company A are more expensive than uncemented components from company B. Generally speaking, however, the price for uncemented components is higher, because of the application of the porous texture. Whether this price difference is still present once the prosthesis has been inserted, is much less clear. Indeed, the additional cost of the PMMA cement, the additional equipment required for cement preparation, and the cost of extra operating room time are factors that need to be taken into account. I therefore believe that the real price difference between cemented and uncemented knees is much less than generally believed. The advantage of using uncemented components is that one extra step is eliminated from the whole procedure, i.e., the cementing procedure. As I explained before, a number of negative factors have indeed been associated with the use of PMMA cement, and although these factors may indeed not lead to frequent or important negative clinical consequences, why should we take the risk if this extra step is frequently unnecessary? I therefore am not stating that everybody should use uncemented knees, my only point is that when you are confident that you have met all the criteria for successful uncemented TKA, you can achieve as good results as with cemented TKA, with the additional benefit of having a biological interface, without having to worry about cement issues.

*Moderator:* Do you believe in hybrid knees, Dr. Bellemans, and if so why? And if not why?

*Dr. Bellemans:* I do indeed believe that hybrid knees, using an uncemented femoral component and cementing the tibial component, are a valid option.

The reason is that the prerequisites for optimal integration of uncemented components are much more easily achieved for the femoral component than for the tibial component. Because of the box-shape configuration of the femoral component, rigid initial fixation is relatively easily achieved by press-fitting between the anterior and posterior condylar surfaces and by using metaphyseal pegs. Secondly, intimate contact between the implant and the bone is easier to achieve on the femoral side than on the tibial. These are the two reasons why it makes sense to cement the tibial component alone whenever the surgeon is not confident that the necessary requirements for optimal uncemented integration are obtained on the tibial side.

*Moderator:* Dr. Bellemans, do you believe that you can really insert a patellar component without cement? Do you and why, or why not?

*Dr. Bellemans:* For the same reasons as in the previous question, I believe that using an uncemented patellar component is indeed a controversial issue, much more than for the femoral and tibial components. Appropriate contact between the implant and the patellar bone can usually be achieved, but rigid initial fixation is much more problematic. The use of aggressive fixation pegs or other devices on the patellar component is impossible because of the limited availability of bone stock and the inherent risk of patellar fracture. A second concern is the use of metal backing to obtain osseous integration. Metal backing inevitably leads to thinner polyethylene especially on the periphery of the implant, and we all know that this may lead to rapid edge wear (Bayley *et al.* 1988). For these two reasons I personally do not use uncemented patellar components. Having said this, however, a number of published studies show satisfactory clinical and histological results with uncemented metal-backed patellar components (Buechel *et al.* 1989, Lagae *et al.* 1997, Bloebaum *et al.* 1998). Placing the patellar component deep into the patellar bone (countersinking) thus seems to be an important factor.

## Reference

Bayley J, Scott R, Ewald F, Holmes G: Failure of metal-backed patellar component of the total knee replacement. *Journal of Bone and Joint Surgery* **70**A:668–674, 1988.

Bloebaum R, Bachus K, Jensen J, Scott D, Hofmann A: Porous-coated metal-backed patellar components in total knee replacement. *Journal of Bone and Joint Surgery* **80**A, 518–528, 1988.

Buechel F, Rosa R, Pappas J: A metal-backed, rotating-bearing patellar prosthesis to lower contact stress. A 11-year clinical study. *Clinical Orthopaedics and Related Research* **248**, 34–49, 1998.

Lagae K, Roos J, Victor J: Metal-backed patellae: history and clinical follow-up. *Acta Orthopaedica Belgica*, **63**–S1, 98, 1997.

# 8

*The initial "total" knee prostheses were not really total: they merely resurfaced the femoral and tibial surfaces, making no provision for arthroplasty of the patellofemoral surfaces. In the mid 1970s, however, surgeons began resurfacing the patella with polyethylene implants and having it articulate with a metallic trochlear surface on the femoral component. Not all surgeons have gone this route, however, and many still feel that better results can be obtained by not resurfacing the patella.*

# The patella need not be resurfaced during total knee replacement

## Pro: Frank Hagena

Resurfacing of the patella is still the most controversial problem in total knee arthroplasty (TKA). The first generation of knee arthroplasties did not provide a replacement of the patellar surface at all. With the increase of survival rates peripatellar complaints were also increasing, and an anterior flange of the femoral condyles was introduced.

The next step of development in TKA was to make retropatellar resurfacing possible, leading to better results with an improvement of function and reduction of pain.

Long-term studies after TKA without patellar resurfacing (PR) demonstrate that good clinical results can be obtained but a considerable amount of anterior knee pain or peripatellar pain is recorded. Mild retropatellar pain was recorded in 19% of 79 knees followed for 7.5 years on average (range 2.4–15.5 years) without any revision surgery. In comparison to the contralateral knee that was replaced in bilateral cases, the patients preferred the resurfaced ones in 46% and the nonPR knee only in 7.7%. However, this might has been related to the selection that was performed for those cases in which a retention of the surface was used for cases of lesser disease, and the worse cases were resurfaced.[1] Fern *et al.*[2] identified patients suffering from retropatellar pain after TKA in rheumatoid patients. Out of 119 TKA nonPR (Insall–Burstein I) knees they found 13.5% of patients with mild pain and another 13.5% with severe pain. The presence of pain directly related to those knees with a patellar height of 15 mm as related to the joint line. That is to say, a low-riding patella seemed to cause pain. In contrast to this, we could show that the alteration of the joint line, especially into the patella alta position after semiconstrained TKA, leads to a tremendous deterioration of the patella followed by anterior knee pain.[3]

The development of new TKA designs and the introduction of accurate instrumentation have reduced surgical errors, and concomitantly the replacement of the retropatellar surface has become very popular. These instruments and implants, however, did not prevent complications after a tricompartmental TKA that included PR.

D.C. Ayers *et al.*[4] summarized that the rate of complications resulting from patellofemoral resurfacing has ranged from 5% to 50% and such complications have accounted for as many as half of the total revisions performed. The literature gives examples of many severe complications after replacing the retropatellar surface with a prosthesis. Complications after resurfacing the patella in TKA can be related to patient factors, design factors, surgical technique, and material properties:

- Patient factors are diminished bone stock and osteoporosis. Osteoporosis diminishes the change of achieving long-term stability of the implant in the patella. Causes of osteoporosis can include steroids, rheumatoid arthritis, and disuse. Post-traumatic knees demonstrate disturbance and major defects of the patellae in many cases.
- Design factors of most TKAs produce kinematic patho-mechnisms of the femoropatellar joint. Rotational movements of the normal patellae are restricted by the design of the condyles. Even more, overstuffing of the patella increases retropatellar force and pathological translation loads causing lateralization, subluxation, or even dislocation of the patella. Increased strain to the lateral retinaculum and capsule increase the potential risk of wear of the retropatellar resurfacing. Obviously the prosthetic design has an influence on patellar function and complications.[5-11]

  Research has been carried out to optimize the surgical procedure in terms of improving the bone resection; however, the surgical technique of patella resurfacing is not as standardized as many other aspects of arthroplasty.

  In many ways the surgeon has so far been left alone to resect the patella and position the patellar implant. Malposition, tilt, impingement of the patella, and inappropriate resection weakening the patellar bone or increasing the patella thickness are the results.
- The material properties in terms of PR have been discussed especially after the experiences with metal-backed patellae.[4,12-14] The list of complications is indeed very long.[15-26]

**Fig. 8.1**

The non-resurfaced patella
5 yrs postop. (a, b) Skyline
view in 60° and 90° flexion
with good congruity between
the patella and the condylar
flange, (c) lateral view of the
patella after TKR with adaption
to the femoral component.

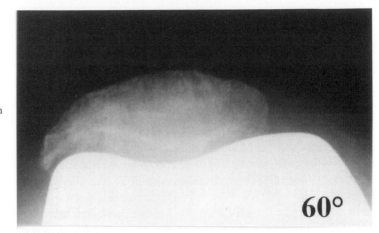

a

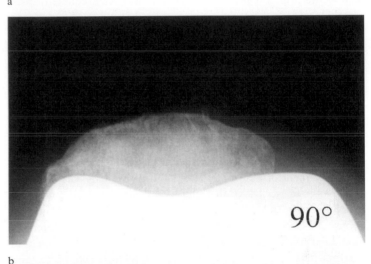

b

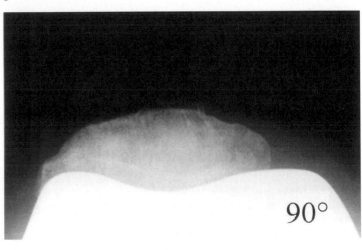

c

## Complications after patella resurfacing

The recognized complications include wear, loosening or dislocation of the implant, fractures, osteonecrosis of the patella, soft tissue formations ("meniscoid"), increase of infections, anterior knee pain, and patellectomy following implant-failures. The incidence of complications after resurfacing the patella ranges from 1.5% to 30%.[5,12,27–29]

Patellar complications reduce the survival rate of TKA considerably. Diduch et al.[30] evaluated a total of 114 TKA at an average of 8 years follow-up; 32 of them had been followed for more than 10 years. Using revision as the failure end-point, the survival rate after 18 years was 94.3%. When revision and patella fractures were used as the failure end-point, the survival rate dropped to 89.7% at 18 years. In conclusion, the failure rate due to patellar fractures is as high as the overall revision rate related to any other course (sepsis, aseptic loosening, wear, component malposition).

The complications of the patella and of the patellar replacement itself depend not only on the state of the patella but also on the condylar implant and the femoropatellar joint. They are also related to the tibiofemoral joint and its biomechanics after TKA, as studied by Chew et al.[31] and Stiehl et al.[32]

Unresurfaced patellae can undergo secondary degeneration; the incidence of this is higher in rheumatoid arthritic (RA) than in osteoarthritic (OA) knees. After 5 years follow-up, this has been observed in 10% of RA patients and only 1.5% of OA patients.[10]

Impingement of the patella after PR in RA patients was observed in 7% (3 of 50 TKA) in Total Condylar posterior stabilized Insall–Burstein (IB) TKA with a follow-up period ranging from 5 to 13 years.[33] Crepitus at the femoropatellar joint does not alter the functional result, but it may be related to mild anterior knee pain. In a prospective study of 118 IB II PS TKAs a fracture rate of 3% and mild to severe patellofemoral pain was documented at a mean follow-up of 4.0 years.[34] None of these clinical symptoms had to be revised.

Pathomechanism leading to patellofemoral failure after retropatellar resurfacing are malposition of the implant, alterations of the joint line, instability and subluxation, loosening, wear, and fracture of the implant.

Wear of the retropatellar resurfacing may lead to loosening of the TKA and considerable synovitis after TKA. Wear of the retropatellar resurfacing was felt to be the of cause of aseptic loosening after cementless Ortholoc I TKA in 3.1% (5 knees) of a total of 163 re-examined knees with a follow-up time of 9–11 years. This wear of the patellar component lead to increased reaction and failure of the tibial component also.[35]

Increased wear and third-body wear was increased after the use of metal-backed patellae leading to a higher incidence of revision: 9.5% of the 252 TKAs after 3–8 years.[36] The 10 year survival rate of metal-backed PR is estimated to be 64.8% for a cemented PFC and 63.5% for an uncemented PFC TKA.[37]

### Loosening of the patella implant

Aseptic loosening of the retropatellar implant is in general a rare case leading to revision. Nevertheless, it should be noted that cementless fixation may have a higher incidence of aseptic loosening. This fact is dependent on the implant design and retropatellar stresses.[38] Factors which may increase the risk of loosening of the patellar implant are malalignment, malrotation, unbalanced soft tissue and malpositioning of the patellar implant. Overall, the literature suggest a loosening of 3% of cemented patellar implants.[39]

Patellar fractures following TKA with PR are related to:

- excessive retropatellar stress
- over-resection of the patella
- under-resection of the patella
- devascularization of the patella
- reduced bone stability due to the design of the patellar implant or to the surgical technique.

It is well accepted that not all kinds of fracture need to be revised, but it may weaken the extensor mechanism and the quadriceps muscle strength.

Revision surgery after failed patellar resurfacing may lead to an unsolved problem. The modular TKA systems available offer good components to manage even deleterious situations at the time of first or second revision.

In some cases the patellar resurfacing may remain *in situ* at the time of revision if the implant is stable, if there is only a small amount of wear, and if it is congruent to the revision arthroplasty. Also the application of a biconvex patella can salvage the defect.[40,41] But the bone loss after failed PR often leaves only a bony shell that is not strong enough to hold an implant at time of revision. This remnant is too small and the blood supply is compromised, so a grafting of this patellar shell is not possible. Functional results of these cases are inferior to those in which a reimplantation can be performed.[42-44]

The economic question is an important one. The costs for a patella replacement itself averages 20% of the total amount of a tricompartmental TKA. Saving this money without diminishing the excellent results of the surgery may allow the clinic to care for more patients. When the rate of revisions for patellar disorders is statistically indistinguishable, it is inevitable that the costs for revision of the patellofemoral joint is much higher than for those cases that did not have a PR at the time of the index operation.

### Does TKA present good results without PR?

If we ask experienced knee surgeons whether to use PR routinely or not, we will get contradictory answers. Some of them always resurface the patella, some never use a patellar implant, and some just do it in selected cases.

My considerations for not resurfacing the patella on TKA are:

- no obvious deterioration of the retropatellar surface at time of surgery
- congruency with the femoral flange
- correct tracking of the patella
- young patients.

Following 47 consecutive cases after TKA with a follow-up time of up to 48 months, Marcacci et al.[45] reported 87.1% good to excellent results (according to the HSS score) without PR. Osteoarthritis was the indication in all these overweight patients. Only mild anterior knee pain was experienced during this period. No complications were observed. They concluded that TKA without substitution of the patella seemed to guarantee good results in patients with primary gonarthrosis, as long as patellar reconstruction was performed correctly so that femoropatellar alignment, tibiofemoral axis alignment, and accurate positioning of the prosthetic components were achieved.

RA has been considered to be an indication for PR.[10,46,47] These publications were contradicted by other reports stating that there was nothing to indicate that RA patients would have an inferior result if they did not have PR, and that the indication for PR should not be made on the basis of the diagnosis alone.[6,48]

Using a blood-supply-preserving lateral approach and a biomechanically adequate implant, TKA without PR gives excellent long-term results.[49] This is also true in active and overweight patients.[45]

## Is there any difference if PR is perfomed?

In a randomly allocated study there was no statistical difference.[50] These results were supported by another study of 17 bilateral TKAs. After a mean follow-up of 2 years no difference at all between the knees was documented.[51]

In their randomized prospective study of 100 TKAs with PR and nonPR, Bourne et al.[52] could not demonstrate a difference at 2 years follow-up in terms of the functional score results. Though the nonPR group showed statistically less pain and a better outcome in terms of knee flexor torques than the PR group, two of the nonPR knees had to be revised because of anterior knee pain.

An even more reliable study was performed by Keblish et al.[53] In a prospective study of 52 patients with bilateral TKA (104 knees) with movable bearings, the patella was resurfaced on one side and not on the other in performing a patellaplasty. The identical procedures were performed by one surgeon. After a mean follow-up time of 5.24 years (range 2–10 years) there was no difference between both sides in subjective preference, stair-climbing, or the incidence of anterior knee pain. Radiographs showed no differences in prosthetic alignment, femoral condylar height, patellar congruency, or joint line position. The authors concluded that selective retention of the patellar surface is an acceptable option.

A similar study was performed including patients with severe degenerative changes of the patella for comparison of resurfacing versus nonresurfacing. In this prospective study of 25 TKAs with PR on the right knee but not on the left, who were followed for 40 months, over 50% of the patients could not tell which side was better.[6]

### Is there an increased rate of revision if the patella is not resurfaced?

In a study of 647 TKAs without PR using a "more contemporary" design of condylar implant, Shoji[54] demonstrated that a secondary PR was needed only in 1.5% of cases. Comparing these patients with 372 TKAs where an implant had been inserted, there was no difference in terms of clinical outcome.

Revision surgery after PR is even more difficult in case of failed patellar components and extensor mechanism failures.[55]

Contraindications for PR, to avoid the high risk of fracture, are a very small patella or a patella of less than 20 mm thick.

In summarizing the pro and cons for routine PR in TKA (Table 8.2), we have to acknowledge that the cumulative revision rate is not significantly different between TKA with and without a patellar component. It seems that the need for a secondary patellar replacement in nonPR cases was balanced by the need for revision of failed patellar components in PR cases. Secondary failures after 9 years averaged

**Table 8.1** Complications after patella resurfacing

Wear
Loosening of the implant
Dislocation of the implant
Fractures
Osteonecrosis of the patella
Soft tissue formations ("*meniscoid*")
Increase of infections
Anterior knee pain
Patellectomy following implant-failures

**Table 8.2** Recommendations for indication of patella retention or resurfacing

| NonPR | PR |
| --- | --- |
| Weak bone stock | Intact bony stability |
| Congruous FP joint | FP—incongruency |
| Small patella | Preoperative patella pain |
| Young patients/OA | Patient's wish |
| FP—alignment not secured | |

7% for nonPR in RA and in OA, and for PR 8% in RA and 12% in OA respectively, in the Swedish National Register.[56] The most common reason for failure is instability with subluxation of the patella. Up to 75% can be attributed to technical errors, i.e., alignment and rotation.[19,21] The multiple failure rates and the various surgical difficulties in the hands of less experienced surgeons lead to the conclusion that PR is indicated only in rare cases. There are on the other hand a few patellae that require resurfacing, promising better results if a tricompartmental replacement of the knee is performed. It is not a "black and white" decision. We strongly advocate retention of the patella the in the majority of TKAs, with PR in selected cases.

# References

1   Levitzky KA, Harris WJ, McManus J, Scott RD: Total knee arthroplasty without patelllar resurfacing. Clinical outcomes and long-term follow-up evaluation. *Clinical Orthopedics* **286**:116–121, 1993.

2   Fern ED, Winson IG, Getty CJ: Anterior knee pain in rheumatoid patients after total knee replacement. Possible selection criteria for patellar resurfacing. *Journal of Bone and Joint Surgery* [Br] **74**:745–748, 1992.

3   Hofmann GO, Hagena FW: Pathomechanics of the femoropatellar joint following total knee arthroplasty. *Clinical Orthopedics* **224**:251–259, 1987.

4   Ayers DC, Dennis DA, Johanson NA, Pelligrini VC: Common complications of total knee arthroplasty. *Journal of Bone and Joint Surgery* [Am] **79**:278–311, 1997.

5   Boyd AD jr, Ewald FC, Thomas WH *et al.*: Long-term complications after total knee arthroplasty with or without resurfacing of the patella. *Journal of Bone and Joint Surgery* [Am] **75**:674–681, 1993.

6   Enis JE, Gardner R, Robledo MA *et al.*: Comparison of patellar resurfacing versus nonresurfacing in bilateral total knee arthroplasty. *Clinical Orthopedics* **260**:38–42, 1990.

7   Insall JN, Scott WN, Ranawat CS: The total condylar knee prosthesis: a report of two hundred and twenty cases. *Journal of Bone and Joint Surgery* [Am] **61**:173–180, 1979.

8   Matsuda S, Ishinishi T, White SE, Whiteside LA: Patellofemoral joint after total knee arthroplasty. Effect on contact area and contact stress. *Journal of Arthroplasty* **12**:790–797, 1997.

9   Ranawat CS: The patellofemoral joint in total condylar knee arthroplasty: pros and cons based on five- to ten-year follow-up observations. *Clinical Orthopedics* **205**:93–99, 1986.

10  Scott RD, Reilly DT: Pros and cons of patellar resurfacing in total knee replacement. *Orthopedic Transactions* **4**:328–331, 1980.

11  Theiss SM: Patellofemoral design affects early results. *Orthopedics* Spec Ed **3**:24, 1994.

12  Kitsugi T, Gustillo RB, Bechtold JE: Results of non-metal-backed, high-density polyethylene, biconvex patellar prosthesis. *Journal of Arthroplasty* **9**:151–162, 1994.

13  Laskin RS, Bucknell A: The use of metal-backed patellar prostheses in total knee arthroplasty. *Clinical Orthopedics* **260**:52–55, 1990.

14  Wright TM, Bartel DL: The problem of surface damage in polyethylene total knee components. *Clinical Orthopedics* **205**:67–74, 1986.

15  Briad JL, Hungerford DS: Patellofemoral instability in total knee arthroplasty. *Journal of Arthroplasty* **4**(Suppl): 87–97, 1989.

16  Clayton ML, Thirupathi R: Patellar complications after total condylar arthroplasty. *Clinical Orthopedics* **170**:152–155, 1982.

17  Grace JN, Rand JA: Patellar instability after total knee arthroplasty. *Clinical Orthopedics* **237**:184–189, 1988.

18  Grace JN, Sim FH: Fracture of the patella after total knee arthroplasty. *Clinical Orthopedics* **230**:168–175, 1988.

19  Insall JN, Lachiewicz PF, Burstein AH: The posterior stabilized condylar prosthesis: a modification of the condylar design. Two to four-year clinical experience. *Journal of Bone and Joint Surgery* [Am] **64**:1317–1324, 1982.

20  Leblanc J: Patellar complications in total knee arthroplasty. *Orthopedics Review* **18**:296–304, 1989.

21  Merkow RL, Soudry M, Insall JN: Patellar dislocation following total knee replacement. *Journal of Bone and Joint Surgery* [Am] **67**:1321–1327, 1985.

22  Mochizuki RM, Schurman DJ: Patellar complications following total knee replacement. *Journal of Bone and Joint Surgery* [Am] **67**:879–883, 1979.

23  Reithmeier E, Plitz W: A theoretical and numerical approach to optimal positioning of the patellar surface replacement in a total knee endoprosthesis. *Journal of Biomechanics* **23**:883–892, 1990.

24  Roffman M, Hirsh DM, Mendes DG: Fracture of the resurfaced patella in total knee replacement. *Clinical Orthopedics* **148**:112–118, 1980.

25  Scott RD, Turoff N; Ewald FC: Stress fractures of the patella following duopatellar total knee arthroplasty with patellar resurfacing. *Clinical Orthopedics* **170**:147–151, 1982.

26  Sutherland CJ: Patellar component dissociation in total knee arthroplasty: A report of two cases. *Clinical Orthopedics* **228**:178–181, 1988.

27  Brick GW, Scott RD: The patellofemoral component of the total knee arthroplasty. *Clinical Orthopedics* **236**:163–178.

28  Healy WL, Wasilewski SA, Takei R. *et al.*: Patellofemoral complications following total knee arthroplasty. Correlation with implant design and patient risk factors. *Journal of Arthroplasty* **10**:197–201, 1995.

29  Insall JN, Ninazzi R, Soudry M: Total knee arthroplasty. *Clinical Orthopedics* **92**:13–22, 1985.

30  Diduch DR, Insall JN, Scott WN *et al.*: Total knee replacement in young, active patients. Long-term follow-up and functional outcome. *Journal of Bone and Joint Surgery* [Am] **79**:575–582, 1997.

31  Chew JTH, Stewart NJ, Hanssen AD *et al.*: Differences in patellar tracking and knee kinematics among three different total knee designs. *Clinical Orthopedics* **345**:87–98, 1997.

32  Stiehl JB, Dennis DA, Komistek RD, Keblish PA: In vivo kinematic analysis of a mobile bearing total knee prosthesis. *Clinical Orthopedics* **345**:60–66, 1997.

33  Aglietti P, Buzzi R, Segoni F, Zacherotti G: Insall–Burstein posterior-stabilized prosthesis in rheumatoid arthritis. *Journal of Arthroplasty* **10**:217–225, 1995.

34  Larson CM, Lachiewicz PF: Patellofemoral complications with the Insall–Burstein II posterior-stabilized total knee arthroplasty. *Journal of Arthroplasty* **14**:288–292, 1999.

35  Whiteside LA: Cementless total knee replacement. Nine- to 11-year results and 10-year survivorship analysis. *Clinical Orthopedics* **309**:185–192, 1994.

36  Cameron HU, Jung YB: Noncemented, porous ingrowth knee prosthesis: The 3- to 8-year results. *Canadian Journal of Surgery* **36**:560–564, 1993.

37 Duffy GP, Trousdale RT, Stuart MJ: Total knee arthroplasty in patients 55 years old or younger. 10- to 17-year results. *Clinical Orthopedics* **356**:22–27, 1998.

38 Firestone TP, Teeny SM, Krackow KA, Hungerford DS: The clinical and roentgenographic results of cementless porous-coated patellar fixation. *Clinical Orthopedics* **273**:184–191, 199

39 Wright J, Ewald FC, Walker PS, Thomas WH, Poss R, Sledge CB: Follow-up note of total knee arthroplasty with the Kinematic prosthesis. *Journal of Bone and Joint Surgery* [Am] **70**:1003–1009, 1990.

40 Gomes LSM, Bechtold JE, Gustilo RB: Patellar prostesis positioning in total knee arthroplasty. A roentgenographic study. *Clinical Orthopedics* **236**:72–81, 1988.

41 Rand JA, Gustilo RB: Technique of patellar resurfacing in total knee arthroplasty. *Techniques in Orthopedics* **3**:57–66, 1988.

42 Barrack RL, Matzkin E, Ingraham R *et al.*: Revision knee arthroplasty with patella replacement versus bony shell. *Clinical Orthopedics* **356**:139–143, 1998.

43 Pagnano MW, Scuderi GR, Insall JN: Patellar component resection in revision and reimplantation total knee arthroplasty. *Clinical Orthopedics* **356**:134–138, 1998.

44 Spitzer AI, Vince KG: Patellar considerations in total knee replacement. In *The Patella,* ed. GR Scuderi, p. 309–33. Springer-Verlag, New York, 1995.

45 Marcacci M, Iacono F, Zaffagnini S *et al.*: Total knee arthroplasty without patellar resurfacing in active and overweight patients. *Knee Surgery, Sports Traumatology, Arthroscopy* **5**:258–261, 1997.

46 Sledge CB, Ewald FC: Total knee arthroplasty experience at the Robert Breck Brigham Hospital. *Clinical Orthopedics* **145**:78–84, 1979.

47 Steinberg J, Sledge CB, Noble J, Sirrat CR: A tissue-culture model of cartilage breakdown in rheumatoid arthritis. Quantitive aspects of proteoglykan release. *Biochemical Journal* **180**:403–408, 1979.

48 Shoji H, Yoshino S, Kajino A: Patellar replacement in bilateral total knee arthroplasty. *Journal of Bone and Joint Surgery* [Am] **71**:853–856, 1989.

49 Arnold MP, Friederich NF, Widmer H, Müller W: Patellar substitution in total knee prosthesis—is it important? *Orthopäde* **27**:637–641, 1998.

50 Feller JA, Bartlett RJ, Lang DM: Patellar resurfacing versus retention in total knee arthroplasty. *Journal of Bone and Joint Surgery* [Br] **78**:226–228, 1996.

51 Greenky B, Hostein E, Scott R *et al.*: Bilateral knee replacment with and without patella resurfacing. *Orthopedics Transactions* **15**:726–731, 1991.

52 Bourne RB, Rorabeck CH, Vaz M *et al.*: Resurfacing versus not resurfacing the patella during total knee replacement. *Clinical Orthopedics* **321**:156–161, 1995.

53 Keblish PA, Varma AK, Greenwald AS: Patellar resurfacing or retention in total knee arthroplasty. A prospective study of patients with bilateral replacements. *Journal of Bone and Joint Surgery* [Br] **76**:930–937, 1994.

54 Shoji H, Shimozaki E: Patella clunk syndrome in total knee arthroplasty without patellar resurfacing. *Journal of Arthroplasty* **11**:198–201, 1996.

55 Laskin RS: Management of the patella during revision total knee replacement arthroplasty. *Orthopedic Clinics of North America* **29**:355–360, 1998.

56 Robertsson O, Knutson K, Kewold S, Lidgren L: Knee arthroplasty for osteoarthrosis and rheumatoid arthritis 1986–1995. Validation and

outcome in the Swedish National Register. Scientific Exhibition, AAOS, Anaheim, 1999.

# Con: Jonathan Noble

Whether or not to resurface the patella has been and remains a contentious issue.[1] We must examine the history of the subject to discover why prejudices have arisen, and then examine current evidence upon this issue. Rand[2] has indicated that extensor mechanism problems are the commonest cause of reoperation after Total Condylar knee replacement. He described wear and/or loosening of the patellar component, patellofemoral instability, fracture, and soft tissue impingement as well as the dreaded patellar ligament rupture. Moreover, he warned of a high complication and failure rate in procedures to individually revise the patellar component.[3] When we read of 13/56 subluxation (23%) and 15/56 patients complaining of patellofemoral pain (27%) there is clearly something amiss.[4] Are these reports representative of experience in general, or not? After all, Levitsky et al.[5] have pointed out that good results without resurfacing are possible in "selected cases." Scott and Reilly[6] advised that patellar resurfacing be avoided in cases with normal articular cartilage. We consider that a near-normal patellar articulation is rare in any patient whose knee pain is severe enough to warrant TKA. This is supported by an autopsy study[7] that reported a 79% incidence of patellofemoral OA in a random group of subjects, comparable in age distribution to those typical of a series of TKA patients. In their development of a unicompartmental arthroplasty the Oxford group attach little importance to the condition of the patellofemoral joint.[8]

In 1982 Armstrong and Mow[9] concluded that the visual and histological appearance of cartilage is a poor indicator of its ability to function in an intact joint. Obeid et al.[10] found that "unaffected" cartilage at unicompartmental replacement was significantly thinner and softer than control cartilage and concluded that it was mechanically inferior to normal cartilage despite appearing to be sound.

So what does a historical review reveal? Hinged knee arthroplasty without patellar resurfacing had a high incidence of retropatellar pain after operation.[11] The polycentric school of design also ignored the patellofemoral joint and Gunston[12] reported a 39% incidence of patellofemoral pain. This persisted with subsequent designs such as the Spherocentric,[13] the Attenborough,[14] the Geomedic,[15,16] and the Ducondylar.[17,18]

The literature further reveals that when the patella was not resurfaced, irrespective of the arthroplasty used, the average incidence of patellofemoral pain was in the order of 25%.[19-26] Of these, however, only the posterior stabilized (PS)[23] approaches modern practice.

Pain is not the only parameter on which to base judgement. Function, and for some an easy independence in the activities of daily living, is also vital. Soudry[27] compared Total Condylar arthroplasty, with and without patellar resurfacing, finding similar results for pain relief, but that 33% of patients with an unresurfaced patella could not climb stairs unaided. This was in marked distinction to our own series over a similar time period using the same prosthesis, but all with PR,[1] in that only 16% were unable to climb stairs, despite 65% of our group suffering from RA. A useful contribution to the controversy was the report by Enis et al.,[28] who reported 25 patients with bilateral Townley prostheses, one resurfaced, the other not. The majority of these patients reported the resurfaced knee to be stronger and more comfortable, especially in relation to stair-climbing. Continuing to scavenge the published literature, we encounter two topics of great interest. The first, in relation to metal backing, is now probably incontestable. The second, in relation to rheumatoid disease, is accepted by many, but not all. In 1990 Laskin[29] reported optimistically on the addition of metal backing to patellar prostheses, concluding that "the combination of implant design and implantation technique may have eliminated serious problems seen with other metal backed patellar implants." Subsequent experience has revealed that adding metal reduces the thickness of available high-density polyethylene, with serious consequences, and metal backing generally is no longer acceptable.[4,30-33] However, Laskin and Bucknell[29] believe that the problems of failure with metal backing can be solved by converting the implant design from an onlay to an insert. This is merely to replace the need to accommodate metal at the expense of plastic, by now doing so at the expense of bone stock. As Insall and Kelly[34] pointed out, few serious complications have been associated with the use of all-plastic patellae. In a study of 1837 TKAs 843 had undergone metal-backed patellar resurfacing and 994 received an all-polyethylene patellar component.[35] Those cases with a metal-backed prosthesis had a 2.9% infection rate, as opposed to 1.6% in the all-plastic group. This difference was statistically significant and assumed to be due to the greater risk of there being debris with the metal-backed group into which bacteria can seed. In 1997 Scott, Thornhill and colleagues,[36] reviewing 1378 PFC knees 5-9 years postoperatively found that 95% were pain-free, but 17 complications required re-operation (4.5%). If those cases whose problems were attributable to metal backing of the patella surface were excluded, this figure was reduced from 4.5% to 2.9%. We advocate PR but believe that the work by Petrie and colleagues[35] is yet one more pointer away from metal backing to the patella component, as is that of Scott's group.[36]

There are surgeons who quite simply and unashamedly do not resurface patellae.[37,38] There are others who see no reason not to, on all occasions, providing there is sufficient bone stock to accommodate a patellar prosthesis and its fixation method.[1]

Picetti et al.[39] reported the results of 100 TKAs performed without resurfacing the patella. On the basis of postoperative anterior pain they recommended resurfacing the patella for all cases of rheumatoid disease with a height in excess of 5.3 ft (1.6 m)or a weight of more than 132 lbs (60 kg). One can but conclude from their paper that failure to resurface is only satisfactory in the less demanding cases. For many the matter is one of choice, and case selection. Boyd *et al.*[40] compared, at a mean 6.5 years follow-up, 396 knees where the patella had been resurfaced with 495 where it had not, the separations having been made at the time of surgery, based on the appearance of the retropatellar surface. They concluded by recommending resurfacing for both inflammatory and degenerative arthritis.

In a tissue culture model Steinberg *et al.*[41] showed that active rheumatoid synovium can function only in the presence of active chondrocytes, and therefore removing all articular surfaces removes any potential trigger for active synovitis. In a subsequent study Read *et al.*[42] showed that the synovium from active OA can react with chondrocytes in a similar manner. It is well known that significant erosion of the unresurfaced patella by a prosthesis, can make resurfacing difficult owing to loss of bone stock. Soudry *et al.*[27] found that 65% of unresurfaced patellae exhibit progressive erosion on follow-up. Although Berry and Rand[3] have warned that isolated patellar component revision is associated with a high complication rate, at least part of their pattern was associated with patellar metal backing, now a discredited prosthesis. However, revising the unresurfaced patella to one with a plastic button or dome is also associated with problems. A well-executed primary patellar resurfacing will therefore largely mitigate against subsequent problems.

## Good results with patellar resurfacing

The survivorship of the PFC system, after 10 or more years in Schai *et al.*'s series,[43] was 90%. Had metal-backed patellar prostheses not been used in the majority of their cases then the figure would have been higher.

With over 700 PFC knees since 1990, we have had few postoperative problems requiring further surgery. Several patients have had a soft tissue resection for soft tissue interposition between patellar and femur, generally with an improvement in symptoms. A few cases have exhibited signs of fragmentation on radiography, none so far requiring revision. Three loose patellae have been revised, two with satisfactory results. None of these features have been related to whether or not lateral patellofemoral release was undertaken. Our incidence for lateral release is now less than 10%, whereas in our original series of Total Condylar knees it was 40%.[1] However, we noted that over 10 years RD Scott seemed to become more enthusiastic in his use of lateral release.[44,45]

The most severe case of avascular necrosis and bone fragmentation which I have ever encountered was a young woman with rheumatoid disease and a failed synovectomy. At PFC arthroplasty her patellar surface was remarkably well preserved and she became the first case in whom my failure to resurface was not related to massive loss of bone stock. No lateral release was carried out. The patella essentially disintegrated to little more than an anterior cortical shell within 2 years.[47]

It has been suggested that lateral parapatellar release[19,38,45,48] and infrapatellar fat pad excision[49] increase the incidence of patellar fracture by decreasing the patella's blood supply. This is not my experience.

In a further study Ranawat and his colleagues[50] reported 95% excellent or good results from patellar resurfacing at 2 or more years after surgery, with the Total Condylar prosthesis. In their discussion they emphasized that there had been no subluxation, dislocations, or fractures, although 1 of the 241 cases had patellar component loosening. They attributed these excellent results to quadriceps realignment, minimal patella bone excision with subchondral bone preservation, and preservation of the fat pad. Ranawat[51] reported again on 100 knees in 77 patients, more than half with rheumatoid disease, followed for 5–10 years after a Total Condylar prosthesis. There were no dislocations although 14 patellae were "tilted" on radiography. There was 1 case of loosening and 1 of osteonecrosis, with over 90% having good to excellent results. Clearly these results are very similar to our own[1] with the same prosthesis. So we might conclude that preserving the fat pad and the subchondral bone and avoiding lateral release are the keys to avoiding problems with patellofemoral resurfacing.

Ritter and Campbell[52] showed that the incidence of patellar fracture after resurfacing was significantly reduced by performing lateral patellofemoral release. In our series[1] of similar case material to that reported by Ranawat[50] care was taken to remove subchondral bone, the fat pad was invariably removed to facilitate exposure, and 40.2% of the patients had a lateral patellofemoral release. We had just 1 fracture and that followed a direct fall. In the same series of 204 Total Condylar knee replacements we had one patellar ligament rupture, 3 weeks postoperatively. This was undoubtedly due to a vigorous physiotherapist forcing passive flexion. Since that case, in 1981, we have had 1 more case of patellar ligament rupture, in a tight valgus knee due to the operating surgeon's reluctance to carry out a rectus (Insall) snip at exposure. Our own improvised repair was highly successful.[46] Thus in our experience of approximately 1500 knee arthroplasties (total, revision, unicondylar, and patellofemoral) there have been two patellar ligament ruptures. Both were due to technical errors and should not be attributed to lateral release, patellofemoral resurfacing, or fat pad excision.

Reverting to a 3–8 year follow-up of 204 Total Condylar knees only 2 patients (3 knees) had significant anterior knee pain and both were associated with patellar maltracking. One of these patients had undergone several knee operations before we revised a Manchester knee replacement to a Total Condylar. She required a Hauser procedure with both knees to achieve patellar stability.[53] The other woman had poor bone stock originally and the prosthesis had to be removed. It should not have been inserted in the first place. Again the fault lies with surgical judgement and not with the intrinsic technique and procedure. Two other patients had asymptomatic loosening and 2 more had some radiographic fragmentation, but remained pain-free and functionally satisfactory. Interestingly none of these patients had undergone lateral release.

Function generally was gratifying in this series, 65% of whom had RA. All patients were able to arise from a chair, although only 31.5% could do so normally. Eighty-four per cent of the patients were able to climb stairs although many required some form of aid. Ninety-seven per cent felt that they had been significantly helped by surgery. It is interesting that some of the best long-term results with PR have been with the original Total Condylar knee replacement with which the patellar prosthesis is a simple dome, as opposed to a more conforming shape. Whiteside and his colleagues[54] have recently shown in cadaveric experiments that conforming patellae had higher contact stresses, at flexion angles greater than 90°. Clearly one of the questions to be answered will be the effect of the now commonplace 110° or more of flexion on long-term patellar component wear and fixation.

A subsequent study of the same case group has revealed a 98% survivorship of the prostheses at 8–13 years[55] and this is holding up with our 10–19 year review.[56] The localization of anterior pain after total knee replacement is difficult and not necessarily attributable to the patella (or its replacement).[57] Maltracking of the patella is probably the commonest and most potent cause of wear, mechanical difficulties, and pain after knee replacement.[58] Conversely, in an interesting review of this topic in the German literature[59] one is left with several impressions. Firstly, many good, pain-free, long-term results exist in patients with whom there is tilt of a resurfaced patella. Secondly, such departures from perfection may well be mitigated against by ensuring a correct rotational alignment of and between femoral and tibial components. With hindsight the authors have extended indications for PR.

One of the key issues still to be resolved is the influence of patellofemoral geometry and of patellar tilt on outcome. It is interesting that in a report on this subject Bindelglass et al.,[60] studying a variety of 234 primary total knees, found that the incidence of central tracking, on a 45° Merchant view, was 55%. Thirty one per cent tilted and 14% subluxed. They concluded that neither pain scores nor fixation were effected by patellar tracking, nor particularly influenced by lateral release at surgery. They did, however, comment that this did not bode well for wear "in a metal-backed patella." By contrast, it is interesting to note the excellent results in terms of both pain relief and freedom from complications with the quite restrained patellar dome to a fairly deep symmetrical femoral groove with the old Total Condylar design.[1,51] Recently the Brigham group[61] have reported their 5–8 year follow-up results with 518 cemented

Kinemax knees with patellar resurfacing. The femoral geometry remained symmetrical, although the patellar component was now oval. There were 4 (0.76%) complications, 1 a fracture after a fall and another 1 attributable to patient selection.

In a 4–10 year review of 186 consecutive anatomic modular knee arthroplasties reported by Bugbee et al.[62] there were only 2 component revisions and no complications related to patellofemoral articulation. Clearly the current generation of total knee replacements are standing up well to the tests of time. It is equally clear that well-executed PR is followed by very low incidence of patellofemoral complications, although patellar scores at 10 years are lower in obese patients.[63]

In arguing the case for patellar resurfacing it may first seem that the Swedish Knee Arthroplasty Register on 4381 primary operations for rheumatoid disease is not supportive. There was no significant difference in revision rates between knees with and without PR.[64] The study, admirable as it is, nevertheless contains multiple variables. Taking the data at face value, the very fact that the Swedish complication rate was no higher with PR is in fact persuasive for replacement. We suspect that the patella was resurfaced generally in worse cases and despite this the complication rate was no higher, so we are encouraged by our Swedish colleagues.

## Provisional conclusions

- The balance of evidence from a review of the literature is that there is a higher incidence of anterior knee pain in nonPR knees than in PR knees.
- Even in series where pain scores have been similar for PR and nonPR knees, those without patellar resurfacing have had more difficulty getting up and down from chairs and especially on stairs.
- Literature review must, however, be viewed cautiously. Implicit are all the weaknesses of retrospective studies with a mixture of surgeons and prostheses, as well as variable durations of follow-up.
- Looking specifically at patellar pain, the scoring systems used must be viewed critically. Some give little cognisance to pain or function during activities such as stair-climbing.
- Our own experience leads me to question the attribution of problems such as patellar fracture, avascular necrosis (AVN) or patellar ligament rupture, or to fat pad removal or lateral release, let alone resurfacing itself.
- Taking an overview of the literature, re-operation rates are higher with nonPR knees than after PR. Alternatively, the results of revision with PR are mixed, with some quite high failure and complication rates.
- There are strong theoretical grounds for advocating routine PR in rheumatoid cases.

- The weakness of case selection (by eye) with OA is that the incidence of failure from not resurfacing patellae is not proportional to how good or bad the patellar cartilage looked at surgery. Studying cartilage pathology calls into question the very concept of normal patellar cartilage.
- PR is as good as the technique and case selection applied to it. Filling in concave bony shells with cement and plastic is as unwise as creating them and then inlaying metal. The operation is a plastic onlay to a flat cancellous bone surface, cut to the appropriate thickness, in the correct three-dimensional alignment.
- The debate can not be finally concluded until we have properly controlled prospective studies, to which we now turn.

## Prospective studies

There are three studies where in bilateral cases one patella was resurfaced, the other not. The retrospective study by Enis[28] of 25 bilateral Townley knees revealed a majority preference for the resurfaced side. In a more recent prospective study Kajino et al.[65] reported 26 bilateral simultaneous rheumatoid cases, in whom PR was randomly allocated to one side. At a 4–7.5 year follow-up, scores for pain, function, range of movement, stability, and correction of deformity revealed no significant difference between the two sides. However, pain on standing and on stairs was worse without PR. There is, however, one study which is prospective and which I can not ignore despite my own preferences. Keblish et al.[66] reported on 59 patients (118 knees) who underwent LCS mobile bearing arthroplasty, with a patella mobile bearing used on just one side. A patellar debridement was undertaken on the other unresurfaced side and we are not told how the cases were randomly (if they were) allocated. Neither is it explained how only 30 of the 52 surviving patients (58%) were available for review. Although the 30/52 patients were given an in-depth interview regarding subjective preference, stair-climbing, etc, I note that clinical evaluation was on a modified Hospital for Special Surgery scoring system, to which reference has already been made. Despite these flaws the report is notable for its absence of any need for revision, at a mean of 5.24 years, for a patellofemoral problem, in either group. One wonders what happened to the 42% who disappeared from this series, but there may be something special about mobile bearings and the patella.

Bourne et al.[67] published a prospective, randomized trial of 100 OA patients treated with the Anatomic Medullary knee, reviewed at 2 years. The knee scores were good in both groups but significantly better in the nonPR group. Two of that group had to undergo subsequent resurfacing and successfully so, giving a 4% reoperation rate within 2 years. Bourne et al. did well to point to the brevity of follow-up and to advise us to keep an open mind. I understand that at

5 years the reoperation rate in the unresurfaced group is now 8% and Bourne and Rorabeck now resurface all patellae unless they are less than 10 mm in thickness.

Barrack et al.[68] carried out a prospective study of 118 Miller–Galante knees, 58 of which were resurfaced and 60 were not, by random allocation. Their mean follow-up was 2.5 years (range 2–4 years). The Knee Society scores for pain, function, and patient satisfaction were similar. Almost twice as many of the unresurfaced knee patients complained of anterior knee pain, but this was not statistically significant. However, as yet none of the resurfaced cases have undergone further surgery, whereas 10% of the unresurfaced group have, and that is within only 2–4 years.

Lastly, I have been privileged to view a paper accepted for publication by Newman and his colleagues,[69] whose content has recently been presented to a number of learned societies. They have reported the results at 5 years of a randomized prospective study, in which there were three groups: PR (A), nonPR (B), and surgeon's choice (C). It is noteworthy that they report (unlike Bourne or Barrack) at 5 years, in that Boyd et al.[40] pointed out that most complications occur 3–4 years after initial surgery. These were all primary replacements, exclusively in OA. Allocation to groups A, B, and C was random, and the case-mix across the three groups was very similar, although group C had fewer (18%) lateral releases than A (24%) or B (27%). They also employed a clinical Patella Score and a Patella Wear Score, as well as the Bristol Knee Score. Of the 37 still alive in group A no further surgery had been necessary. Of the 34 in group B, 6 had undergone PR, whereas one of the remaining 34 patients in group C had a resurfacing revised. There are a further 4 patients in group B (unresurfaced) with significant patellofemoral symptoms, who as yet have not undergone surgery. This is reflected in the lower patella scores for groups B and C and this is despite the 6 worst group B cases by now being revised. It is also interesting to note that within the limits of their small numbers the preoperative state of articular cartilage and alignment were not obvious determinants of failure. From their evidence, and indeed a general literature review, it seems that it is not possible to predict or preselect those OA cases who do or do not require resurfacing. However, as Newman et al.[70] reported "resurfaced patellae tolerated minor degrees of maltracking far better than unresurfaced patellae and gave more comfortable knees when the extensor mechanism was perfectly aligned."

## Final conclusions

It has been interesting to note that both the Ontario group[67] and the Japanese group[65] appear to have changed their minds in favor of resurfacing as follow-up advanced. Overall, therefore, there is a greater incidence of patellofemoral pain without PR and from the early Total Condylar reports onwards a very high level of good and excellent results with PR, as epitomized by the older reports of Ranawat[17,49-51] (Ranawat 1986), (Ranawat *et al.* 1976), (Ranawat *et al.* 1981), (Ranawat *et al.* 1984) and Rae *et al.*[1] through to the more recent report by Wright and colleagues.[61]

Perhaps most importantly, the incidence of the need for reoperation is the final determinant making resurfacing the safe, sensible, and sound option. Looking to 5–10%, or worse, quite early reoperation rates without PR neither can nor should be sustained. Despite such unequivocal advocacy for PR we must accept the occasional difficulties and failures implicit with PR when it does fail, although many are avoidable.

# References

1   Rae PJ, Noble J, Hodgkinson JP: Patellar resurfacing in total condylar knee arthroplasty. *Journal of Arthroplasty* **5**:259–265, 1990.
2   Rand JA: The patello-femoral joint in total knee arthroplasty. *Journal of Bone and Joint Surgery* [Am] **76**:612–620, 1994.
3   Berry DJ, Rand JA: Isolated patellar component revisions of total knee arthroplasty. *Clinical Orthopaedics and Related Research* **286**:110–115, 1993.
4   Johnson DF, Eastwood DM: Patellar complications after knee arthroplasty. A prospective study of 56 cases using the Kinematic prosthesis. *Acta Orthopaedica Scandanavica* **63**:74–79, 1992.
5   Levitsky KA, Harris WJ, McManus J and Scott RD: Total knee arthroplasty without resurfacing. Clinical outcomes and long-term follow-up evaluation. *Clinical Orthopaedics and Related Research* **286**:116–121, 1993.
6   Scott RD, Reilly DT: Pros and cons of patellar resurfacing in total knee replacement. *Orthopaedic Transactions* **4**:328, 1980.
7   Noble J, Hamblen DL: The pathology of the degenerate meniscus lesion. *Journal of Bone and Joint Surgery* [Br] **57**:180–185, 1975.
8   Murray DW, Goodfellow JW, O'Connor JJ: The Oxford medial unicompartmental arthroplasty. A 10 year review. *Journal of Bone and Joint Surgery* [Br] **80**:983–989, 1998.
9   Armstrong CG, Mow VC: Variations in intrinsic mechanical properties of human articular cartilage with age, degeneration and water content. *Journal of Bone and Joint Surgery* [Am] **64**:88–94, 1982.
10  Obeid EMH, Adams MA, Newman JP: Mechanical properties of articular cartilage in knees with unicompartmental osteoarthritis. *Journal of Bone and Joint Surgery* [Br] **76**:315–319, 1994.
11  Craig DM, Lettin AWF, Scales JT: Stanmore total knee replacement. *Journal of Bone and Joint Surgery* [Br] **65**:225, 1983.
12  Gunston FH: Ten year results of polycentric knee arthroplasty. *Journal of Bone and Joint Surgery* [Br] **62**:133, 1980.
13  Kauffer H, Matthews L: 1981 Spherocentric arthroplasty of the knee. *Journal of Bone and Joint Surgery* [Am] **63**:545–559.
14  Simison AJM., Noble J, Hardinge K: Complications of the Attenborough knee replacement. *Journal of Bone and Joint Surgery* [Br] **68**:100–105, 1986.
15  Insall J, Ranawat CS, Aglielli P, Shine J: A comparison of four models of total knee replacement prosthesis. *Journal of Bone and Joint Surgery* [Am] **58**:754–765, 1976.

16 Riley LH, Hungerford DS: Geomedic total knee replacement for treatment of the rheumatoid knee. *Journal of Bone and Joint Surgery* [Am] **60**:523–527, 1978.

17 Ranawat CS, Insall J, Shine J: Duo-condylar knee arthroplasty. *Clinical Orthopaedics and Related Research* **120**:76–82, 1976.

18 Sledge CB, Ewald FC: Total knee arthroplasty. Experience at the Robert Breck Brigham Hospital. *Clinical Orthopaedics and Related Research* **145**:78–84, 1979.

19 Clayton M, Thirupathi R: Patellar complications after total condylar arthroplasty. *Clinical Orthopaedics and Related Research* **170**:152–156, 1982.

20 Eftekhar NS: Adjustable intramedullary replacement of the knee joint. *Journal of Bone and Joint Surgery* [Am] **65**:293–309, 1983.

21 Evanski PM, Waugh TR, Orofino CF, Anzel SH: UCI knee replacement. *Clinical Orthopaedics and Related Research* **120**:33–38, 1976.

22 Freeman MAR, Todd RC, Bambert P, Day WH: ICLH arthroplasty of the knee. *Journal of Bone and Joint Surgery* [Br] **60**:339–344, 1978.

23 Insall J, Lachiewics P, Burnstein A: The posterior stabilised condylar prosthesis—a modification of the total condylar design: two and four year clinical experience. *Journal of Bone and Joint Surgery* [Am] **64**:1317–1323, 1982.

24 Kettlekamp DB, Pryor P, Brady TA: A selective use of the variable axis knee. *Orthopaedic Transactions* **3**:301–302, 1979.

25 Murray DG, Webster DA: Variable axis knee prosthesis. *Journal of Bone and Joint Surgery* [Am] **63**:687–694, 1981.

26 Sheehan J: Arthroplasty of the knee. *Clinical Orthopaedics and Related Research* **145** 101–109, 1979.

27 Soudry M, Mestriner LA, Binazzi R, Insall J: Total knee arthroplasty without patellar resurfacing. *Clinical Orthopaedics and Related Research* **205**:166–170, 1986.

28 Enis JE, Gardener R, Robledo MA *et al.*: Comparison of patellar resurfacing versus non-resurfacing in bilateral total knee arthroplasty. *Clinical Orthopaedics and Related Research* **260**:38–42, 1990.

29 Laskin RS, Bucknell A: The use of metal backed patellar prostheses in total knee arthroplasty. *Clinical Orthopaedics and Related Research* **260**:52–55, 1990.

30 Bayley JC, Scott RD, Ewald FC, Holmes GB: Failure of the metal backed patellar component after total knee replacement. *Journal of Bone and Joint Surgery* [Am] **70**:668–674, 1988.

31 Lombardi AV, Engh GA, Volz RG *et al.*: Fracture/dislocation of the polyethylene in metal-backed patellar components in total knee arthroplasty. *Journal of Bone and Joint Surgery* [Am] **70**:675–679, 1988.

32 Stulberg SD, Stulberg BN, Hamati Y, Tsao A: Failure mechanisms of metal-backed patellar components. *Clinical Orthopaedics and Related Research* **236**:88–105, 1988.

33 Rosenberg AG, Andriacchi TP, Barden R, Galante JO: Patellar component failure in cementless total knee arthroplasty. *Clinical Orthopaedics and Related Research* **236**:106–114, 1988.

34 Insall J, Kelly M: The total condylar prosthesis. *Clinical Orthopaedics and Related Research* **205**:43–48, 1986.

35 Petrie RS, Hanssen AD, Osmon DR, Ilstrup D: Metal-backed patellar component failure in total knee arthroplasty: a possible risk for late infection. *American Journal of Orthopaedics* **27**:172–176, 1998.

36 Marton SD, McManus JL, Scott RD, Thornhill TS: Press-fit condylar total knee arthroplasty, five to nine year follow-up evaluation. *Journal of Arthroplasty* **12**:603–614, 1997.

37 Morgan CG, Pinder IM, Lees TA, Midwinter MJ: Survivorship analysis of the uncemented porous-coated anatomic knee replacement. *Journal of Bone and Joint Surgery* [Am] **73**:848–857, 1991.

38 Smith SR, Stuart P, Pinder IM: Non-resurfaced patella in total knee arthroplasty. *Journal of Arthroplasty* Suppl:581–586, 1989.

39 Picetti GD, McGann WA, Welch RB: The patello-femoral joint after total knee arthroplasty without patellar resurfacing. *Journal of Bone and Joint Surgery* [Am] **72**:1379–1382, 1990.

40 Boyd AD, Ewald FC, Thomas WH *et al.*: Long-term complications after total knee arthroplasty with or without resurfacing of the patella. *Journal of Bone and Joint Surgery* [Am] **75**:674–681, 1993.

41 Steinberg J, Sledge CB, Noble J, Stirratt CR: A tissue culture model of cartilage breakdown in rheumatoid arthritis. *Biochemical Journal* **180**:403–408, 1979.

42 Read L, Alexander KL, Noble J, Collins RF: The action of diseased synovium on cartilage substrate. *Journal of Bone and Joint Surgery* [Br] **64**:383, 1982.

43 Schai PA, Thornhill TS, Scott RD: Total knee arthroplasty with the PFC system. Results at a minimum of 10 years and survivorship analysis. *Journal of Bone and Joint Surgery* [Br] **80**:850–858, 1998.

44 Brick GW, Scott RD: The patello-femoral component of total knee arthroplasty. *Clinical Orthopaedics and Related Research* **231**:163–178, 1988.

45 Scott RD: Prosthetic replacement of the patello-femoral joint. *Orthopaedic Clinics of North America* **10**:129–137, 1979.

46 Deshmuck R, Noble J: Repair of a ruptured patellar ligament in total knee replacement. Submitted for publication, 2000.

47 Deshmuck R, Noble J: Patellar disintegration without resurfacing in total knee replacement. *Journal of Arthroplasty* in press, 1999.

48 Webster DA, Murray DG: Complications of variable axis total knee arthroplasty. *Clinical Orthopaedics and Related Research* **193**:160–167, 1985.

49 Ranawat CS, Rose HA, Bryan WJ: Technique and results of replacement of the patello-femoral joint with total condylar knee replacement. *Orthopaedic Transactions* **5**:414, 1981.

50 Ranawat CS, Rose HA, Bryan WJ: Replacement of the patello-femoral joint with total condylar knee arthroplasty. *International Orthopaedics* **8**:61–65, 1984.

51 Ranawat CS: The patello-femoral joint in total condylar knee arthroplasty. *Clinical Orthopaedics and Related Research* **205**:93–99, 1986.

52 Ritter MA, Campbell ED: Post-operative patellar complications with or without release during total knee arthroplasty. *Clinical Orthopaedics* **219**:163–169, 1987.

53 Haines JF, Noble J: Revision arthroplasty of the knee. Two problem knees. *Journal of the Royal College of Surgeons of Edinburgh* **31**:255–259, 1986.

54 Matsuda S, Ishinishi T, White SE, Whiteside LA: Patello-femoral joint after total knee arthroplasty. Effect on contact area and contact stress. *Journal of Arthroplasty* **12**:790–797, 1997.

55 Monsall F, Noble J, Obeid EM: Eight to thirteen year follow-up of total condylar knee replacements. Presentation to joint meeting of the British Association for Rheumatoid Surgery and the British Orthopaedic Association. Westminster Conference Centre, 1993.

56 Mirza H, Noble J, Jayem M: Ten to nineteen year follow-up of total condylar knee replacements. Presented to British Orthopaedic Association, Glasgow. September, 1999.

57 Levai JP, McLeod HC, Freeman MAR: Why not resurface the patella. *Journal of Bone and Joint Surgery* [Br] **65**:448–451, 1983.

58  Mochizuki RM, Schurmann DJ: Patellar complications following total knee arthroplasty. *Journal of Bone and Joint Surgery* [Am] **61,**879–883, 1979.

59  Gerber BE, Maenza F: Shift and tilt of the bony patella in total knee replacement. *Orthopaedics* **27**:629–636, 1998.

60  Bindelglass DF, Cohen JL and Dorr DL: Patellar tilt and subluxation in total knee arthroplasty. Relationship to pain, fixation and design. *Clinical Orthopaedics and Related Research* **286**:103–109, 1993.

61  Wright J, Ewald FC, Poss R *et al.*: Patello-femoral joint in symmetrical total knee arthroplasty. Presentation to the Combined Meeting of British and Irish Orthopaedic Associations, Dublin, 1998.

62  Bugbee WD, Ammeen DJ, Parks NL, Engh GA: Four to ten year results with the anatomic modular knee. *Clinical Orthopaedics and Related Research* **348**:158–165, 1998.

63  Griffin FM, Scuderi GR, Insall JN, Colizza W: Total knee arthroplasty in patients who were obese with ten years follow-up. *Clinical Orthopaedics and Related Research* **356**:28–33, 1998.

64  Robertson O, Knutson K, Lewold S *et al.*: Knee arthroplasty in rheumatoid arthritis. A report from the Swedish Knee Arthroplasty Register on 4381 primary operations 1985–1995. *Acta Orthopaedica Scandanavica* **68**:545–553, 1997.

65  Kajino A, Yoshino S, Kameyama S *et al.*: Comparison of the results of bilateral total knee arthroplasty with and without patella replacement for rheumatoid arthritis. *Journal of Bone and Joint Surgery* [Am] **79**:570–574, 1997.

66  Keblish PA, Varma AK, Greenwald AS: 1994 Patellar resurfacing or retention in total knee arthroplasty. *Journal of Bone and Joint Surgery* [Br] **76**:930–937.

67  Bourne RB, Rorabeck CH, Vaz M *et al.*: Resurfacing versus not resurfacing the patella during total knee replacement. *Clinical Orthopaedics and Related Research* **321**:156–161, 1995.

68  Barrack RL, Wolfe MW, Waldman DA *et al.*: Resurfacing of the patella in total knee arthroplasty. *Journal of Bone and Joint Surgery* [Am] **79**:1121–1131, 1997.

69  Rorabeck CH: 1999 Personal communication.

70  Newman JH, Ackroyd CE, Shah NA, Karachalios T: Should the patella be resurfaced during total knee replacement. Accepted for publication (2000).

## Questions and answers

*Moderator:* Mr. Noble, is there any situation in which you would not resurface the patella? Could you show us an radiograph of such a situation?

*Mr. Noble:* I have only one absolute contra-indication to PR (apart from patellectomy!), and this is insufficient bone stock. A relative contra-indication in my more recent practice is where the patellar articular cartilage looks in good order. Firstly, I think there are few such cases, certainly in my practice. Secondly, the literature bears out the point that those cases where the patella has not be resurfaced give rise to quite a few cases where that then needs to be done as a second procedure. The literature bears out that that can arise in

208

cases where the articular cartilage looked quite good at the original primary surgery. It is here that the paper by Obeid and the Bristol Group, which I quoted, is probably so important.

You have asked for an radiograph of a patella that I would not replace. I know exactly what you are driving at, but my own practical answer to that question is very simple. To illustrate the point in that way would be extremely misleading, and would convey an impression that I would wish to dispel. Treat the patient, not the radiograph! I have seen lots of rheumatoid cases where the skyline view, in particular, was not encouraging and yet where there was sufficient bone stock to admit a patella button, and the subsequent clinical result was excellent.

*Moderator:* Professor Hagena, several surgeons, including the group from Japan, were initially quite enthusiastic to not resurface the patella but as time and follow-up increased, changed their minds and now recommend PR. Does this concern you?

*Professor Hagena:* I must say that this trend is equated by those colleagues who are going in the opposite direction. Many surgeons have had bad experiences with PR and have stopped doing it routinely. It seems more appropriate to perform selective PR with a reduced rate of revision. Why is it so difficult to perform a well-designed multicenter study to show the significance of patellar resurfacing? My literature review did not show that the outcome of PR, in general, is favorable. This is a fact. I accept that quite a few studies show no revision after PR, but I doubt that this is true for the majority of less experienced surgeons.

*Moderator:* Are you saying that the decision whether or not to resurface the patella should be based on the surgeon's experience performing knee replacement? Is a surgeon suddenly after some number of knee replacements "qualified" to perform the next one with or without a patella replacement?

*Professor Hagena:* Do you think that this is a serious question? I strongly believe that most of the surgeons have normal to excellent surgical skills, but the results of TKA significantly depend on the frequency the operation is performed. Questionnaires at international knee meetings show that the majority of participants perform less than 30 TKAs per year. If that is correct, the authors of very sophisticated prospective studies are representatives of those colleagues who have more experience than the majority. Consequently I speculate that the failure rate of PR in general is much higher than it is reported in the literature. If you think about it, most instrumentations to perform an accurate resection of the femoral condyles and of the tibial surfaces do not offer an instrument for an exact and reproducible resection of the patella. Even more, there is no evident approach to achieve an optimal positioning of the patella implants. Review PR skyline views from various hospitals and in some reports we are often faced with an incorrect or inadequate resection and malposition of the implants. Great efforts are needed to improve the surgical technique and the design of the femoropatellar implant.

*Moderator:* Since you resurface essentially all your patellae, Mr. Noble, let's talk a bit about your technique. The resected patellar surface is normally oval, and yet most patellar prostheses are round. Are you concerned with the unresurfaced portion of the patella? Do you medialize your implant? If so, do you remove the remaining lateral patellar bone, since some have said that this may impinge on the femoral component?

*Mr. Noble:* This is a good series of questions. At present, I think that the patellar prosthesis should probably be oval, and that it should cover as much available bone surface as possible. This makes sense in terms of the simple physics of stress. The practicality of the matter is, as you say, that the vast majority of patellar buttons I put in have been round as opposed to oval. I seem to have had very few problems with them. Generally speaking, if the surface is to be left naked, I leave it naked laterally, rather than medially, which in your terms, I think, means that I do medialize the implant. I make no particular effort to excise or trim back the lateral patellar bone.

*Moderator:* To follow up on that what are your thoughts about using a resurfacing or an inset patellar polyethylene button?

*Mr. Noble:* One of the basic principles of knee replacement, indeed of joint replacement in general, is to be as conservative of bone stock as possible. Providing it is done well, many of us have shown that the results of onlay polyethylene buttons are so good that if really would be difficult to justify inset. I will put this even more strongly. If one were to set up a trial of 100 onlay versus 100 insets, and find that at 5 years the results were the same, then the case would have been overwhelmingly made in favor of onlay, in that a certain number will fail later on and it will be much easier to revise an onlay than an inset. I do not think that there is argument here, but I suspect that you may!

*Moderator:* Actually that study was been done and inset came out slightly better than onlay. Furthermore we obviously differ in which is easier to revise. Since I am the moderator, however, I am bound not to engage in colloquy with my experts. Maybe you and I can debate this in a book by someone else.

Professor Hagena, you have alluded to the fact that the femoral prosthetic trochlear surface has to be "friendly" to the unresurfaced patella. How can the surgeon assure that this is true?

*Professor Hagena:* The choice of the implant is a decision demanding a high degree of experience and responsibility. There are some very important criteria concerning the patellofemoral joint. Some of the available models show a significant increase in retropatellar force during flexion. During flexion of the normal knee more than 70–90°, the retropatellar force is reduced. This decrease in force is induced by the diving of the patella into the intercondylar groove. This changes the moment arm of the extensor mechanism. At the same time the quadriceps tendon starts wrapping over the femoral trochlear, increasing the vector power of the quadriceps muscle. This important interplay of the condyles, the patella, and the quadriceps tendon is not considered in many models. Without this positive effect on the femoropatellar joint we are faced, in fact, with a higher rate of subluxations, delaminations, and fracture of the patella—whether resurfaced or not. Furthermore we are looking for low contact stresses and for a large contact area. If this can be introduced by the retention of the natural patella with a high degree of congruence, the load transfer per unit area may be decreased, and this would be a biomechanical optimum. There is no prosthetic patella implant available which exactly reproduces the size and shape of the normal patella.

A very significant pathological sign of femoropatellar incongruency is peripatellar meniscoid soft tissue formation. This growing abnormal soft tissue may completely cover the patellar implant in some cases. A high incidence of revision surgery may be due to this pathologic soft tissue alteration. Also, point contact of the polyethylene patellar implant during flexion of the knee leads to excessive wear and synovitis. This may be one of the causes and a correlate to anterior knee pain occurring after total knee replacement.

*Moderator:* Actually we have looked at the patella meniscus and found it to be aneural and avascular, so that, in our hands, we do not consider it a cause of anterior knee pain. To change the topic, however, there have been several studies that appear to indicate that merely looking at a patella will not tell you much about whether or not the patient will won't have pain if you don't resurface it. Do you have any guidelines?

*Professor Hagena:* I am glad you asked that, since it gives me the chance to present my very personal recommendations for a selective PR. The patient's history and physical should be performed with attention to discovering the presence of retropatellar or peripatellar pain. Radiographic evaluation of the patellofemoral joint is mandatory. I feel that congruency of the patellar gliding surface within the condylar implant is the most important factor in whether to resurface or not. This congruency can be achieved easily in most cases by shaping the patella, resecting the osteophytes and part of the altered cartilage. Very thin patellae or those with weak bone stock should be trimmed but not resurfaced. This is also true for rheumatoid patients. The cartilage should be removed to reduce the immunological potential. Using a well-designed prosthesis and performing a selective resurfacing of the patella, the incidence of PR in my practice is about 30%.

*Moderator:* Mr. Noble, you have stated in your contribution that the HSS and Knee Society rating systems are not useful in evaluating patellar problems. Could you elaborate on the other systems that you mentioned for evaluating the patella?

*Mr. Noble:* I am slightly on thin ice here, in that I am really quoting the Bristol Group's use of a patellar scoring system. I, personally, have never used that myself, although the way in which I originally assessed the patellofemoral joint, in the old Total Condylar series that we did, is set out in the paper with Paul Rae, which I quoted liberally throughout my contribution.

*Moderator:* This questions may be a bit off base, but what do you do in the patient who does not have a patella? There has been some mention of implanting an implant in a pouch in the quadriceps. Do you have any thoughts (or better yet, any personal experience) with this technique?

*Mr. Noble:* In the absence of a patella, I would not do any fancy procedure, such as putting an implant in a pouch. I think the only utterly unoriginal contribution I would have to make here is that over two decades, I have been an even more wanton destroyer of posterior cruciate ligaments than you own colleagues at Special Surgery. These circumstance, however, are my one exception, and in the post-patellectomy knee I am always very meticulous to preserve and protect the PCL.

*Moderator:* You mentioned, Professor Hagena, that there are economic factors involved in not routinely resurfacing the patella. Are there not also economic factors in having to go back and reiterate on the small percentage of patients who require a patellar implant as a secondary procedure?

*Professor Hagena:* It was shown by the Swedish registry group at the 1999 meeting of the American Academy of Orthopaedic Surgeons that the incidence of reoperation in knees with and without PR is about the same, maybe very slightly higher in the resurfacing group. Resurfacing the patella does not give 100% certainty of preventing anterior knee pain. Even more, aseptic loosening, delamination of the insert, wear of the polyethylene, and septic loosening require revisional surgery. The revision of the resurfaced patella is much more demanding. Also, septic loosening or fractures of the reduced bone stock of the patella may result in a patellectomy. My credo, therefore, would be in general to save the patella for revisional surgery!

*Moderator:* Finally, what percentage of surgeons do you think resurface or don't resurface the patella?

*Professor Hagena:* First of all, I think that there is no strong evidence that can be based on percentages. In Germany I think that PR is performed routinely about a third of the time. Up to now it has been very difficult to get valid information about it. The closest thing we have comes from the Swedish registry paper by Robertsson that I mentioned before. In their registry the ratio of nonPR to PR knee replacements was about 3 to 2 in both OA and RA patients. Their figures did not support the hypothesis that all RA patients should be resurfaced during TKA.

*Moderator:* For completeness, I would like to quote the unofficial figures for knee replacement in the USA: about 90% of all knee replacements are performed with resurfacing of the patella. This ratio is even high in rheumatoid patients, based primarily on the studies of Dr. Bourne and the group from Japan. Furthermore, the ratio of onlay to inset patellar implants in the USA is about 4 to 1.

## 9

*Soft tissue balance is as important as proper bony resections in determining whether or not a total knee replacement arthroplasty will be successful. Our present methods of preparing the tibia articular surface at right angles to the long axis of the tibia, results in a flexion space which is trapezoidal in shape. For proper functioning of the knee the flexion space must be balanced and adequately filled with the prosthetic device. Two ways of achieving this balance are externally rotating the femoral anterior–posterior (AP) resections and using a femoral component with equal thicknesses posteriorly, or not externally rotating the femoral ap resections and using a component with asymmetrical posterior femoral condyles.*

# The optimal way to balance the flexion space is to externally rotate the femoral component

## Pro: Giles Scuderi

Axial alignment in total knee arthroplasty (TKA) has been recognized as an important function in outcome and survivorship. This is achieved by appropriate ligament releases and bone resection. Properly performed these factors achieve balanced and symmetrical flexion and extension spaces. The extension space imparts the intended valgus alignment of the knee; a symmetrical flexion space implies parallelism between the resected tibia and the resected posterior femoral condyles. This is influenced by the method of bone resection and subsequent adjustments.

The anatomic alignment method of bone resection was popularized by Hungerford in 1978 and has been associated with measured resection.[1] This method attempts to preserve the anatomic orientation of the joint line by resecting the tibia in 3° of varus and the distal femur in 9° of valgus. In addition, the amount of bone resected from the distal and posterior femur equals the thickness of the component to be implanted. Since the tibia is cut in varus, the femoral component is oriented parallel to the surface. For this reason the amount of posterior femoral resection is equal and no attempt is made to deliberately externally rotate the femur.

The classic alignment method was introduced by Insall and has become the popular method of bone resection.[2] This technique involves cutting the femur and tibia perpendicular to the mechanical axis. Therefore, the tibia is resected at 90° and the distal femur is cut at 6° valgus. This places the joint line perpendicular to the mechanical axis. Although it may be easy to appreciate the alignment in

215

extension, it is important to realize that in flexion it will be necessary to externally rotate the femoral component relative to the posterior condyles in order to balance the flexion space.

In the normal knee, perpendicular resection of the proximal tibia removes more bone from the lateral plateau than from the medial surface, because the normal tibia has a 3° varus slope. To obtain a rectangular flexion space, a larger amount of bone should be resected off the posteriomedial femoral condyle than off the posterolateral condyle.

The issue of femoral component rotation is coupled with an understanding of knee kinematics, which have been described as two simultaneous rotations occurring about bony fixed axes.[3,4] This implies that the fundamental components of knee motion correspond to flexion–extension and internal–external rotation. The optimal flexion axis passes through the posterior condyles and is closely approximated by the transepicondylar axis. The longitudinal rotation axis is fixed in the tibia and is approximately parallel to the long axis of the tibia and is the true axis of internal and external rotation. Therefore, at the time of surgery, proper positioning of the components along these axes is critical.

At least four ways have been proposed to determine the proper rotational alignment of the femoral component during TKA:

- the transepicondylar axis
- the AP trochlear line
- 3° of external rotation based off the posterior condyles
- the amount of external rotation necessary to form a symmetrical flexion space after ligament balance is complete.

Femoral rotation dictated by ligamentous balancing is potentially imprecise. When rotational alignment is based on ligament balancing, it makes an assumption that the ligament releases are equal and symmetrical. This is technically possible with the use of a tensor and sequential releases of the contracted supporting ligament and capsule, but in practice it does not occur. Soft tissue releases to correct axial malalignment do not reproducibly create equal and symmetrical flexion and extension spaces. Our own experience, with meticulous attempts at soft tissue balancing, revealed that the flexion space was within 1 mm of being rectangular in 89% of knees, and there were some knees that were 3 mm from being perfectly rectangular. The tendency was to over-release the contracted side. Therefore, relying on the soft tissues to dictate bone resection and femoral rotational alignment is imprecise and potentially erroneous. This is especially obvious with a complete release of the lateral supporting structures to correct a fixed valgus deformity. Over-release will result in asymmetry of the flexion space with the resultant trapezoidal space larger on the lateral side than the medial side.

The posterior condyles are inconsistent landmarks for femoral component rotation because they are usually involved with the arthritic process. Erosions of the articular cartilage along with bony deficits will lead to rotational malalignment of the femoral component if the posterior condyles are used as the only rotational landmark. The relationship between the posterior condyles and the transepicondylar axis has been defined as the posterior condylar axis.[5] This angle has been measured in both cadaveric and surgical specimen. Griffin measured the *in vivo* posterior condylar angle during TKA and compared the results between varus, valgus, and nondeformed knees.[6] There was no difference between males and females; the posterior condylar angle averaged $3.3° + 1.9°$ for varus knees (range 0–8°); $3.3° + 2.3°$ for knees with no deformity (range 0–7°); and $5.4° + 2.3°$ for valgus knees (range 3–10°). Griffin and coworkers have shown that 3° of rotation may be appropriate for the majority of varus knees; it may not be the case all the time and may not be sufficient for valgus knees. One explanation is that the valgus knee may have excessive posterolateral femoral wear leading to an increased posterior condylar angle. The other hypothesis is that habitual femoral valgus may result in lateral femoral hypoplasia. This could lead to apparent variation in femoral rotation. If the traditional 3° of external rotation is used in valgus knees, an average 2° of internal rotation relative to the transepicondylar axis results. The posterior condylar angle is variable and the posterior condyles are inconsistent landmarks for femoral rotation. Overall, the standard deviation was over 2° and therefore a significant number of patients will be expected to have more than 2° of malrotation if the posterior condyles are used. Posterior condylar angles of greater than 5° or less than 1° were found in 29% of knees with no deformity, 31.6% with a valgus deformity and 21.9% with a varus deformity. The variability of the posterior condylar angle confirms the point that the posterior condyles are potentially unreliable landmarks for femoral component rotation.

Arima *et al.* proposed a technique for using the AP axis of the distal femur to establish rotational alignment of the femoral component in the valgus knee (Fig. 9.1).[7] These investigators stated that a line perpendicular to the AP axis was approximately in 4° of external rotation relative to the posterior condyles. Poilvache found a similar measurement and determined that the AP axis was perpendicular to the transepicondylar axis.[8] However, these investigators believe that the AP axis is sometimes difficult to identify because of trochlear wear or intercondylar osteophytes. In cases of severe trochlear dysplasia, relying exclusively on the AP axis could induce malrotation of the femoral component. The range of the angle between the AP and the transepicondylar axes was 14°.

Use of the transepicondylar axis for femoral component rotation is logical because, as mentioned above, it approximates the optimal or true flexion axis of the knee and is not defined by the articular

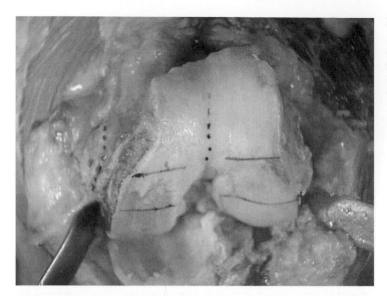

**Fig. 9.1**

Fixed femoral landmarks for determining femoral rotation include the AP axis and the epicondylar axis. See also colour plate section.

surface which may be involved in the arthritic process. When the tibia is resected at right angles to the mechanical axis and the soft tissues are balanced, the transepicondylar axis parallels the resected tibial surface.[9] Yoshioka et al.,[10] in an anatomic study, found that the transepicondylar line was a right angle to the mechanical axis of the femur in the frontal plane, as well as with the knee flexed to 90°. The transepicondylar axis also made a right angle to the long axis of the tibia. Therefore, the transepicondylar axis is a sound landmark when performing the classic method of bone resection.

Familiarity with the anatomy of the distal femur assists the surgeon with identifying the epicondyles since they provide repro-

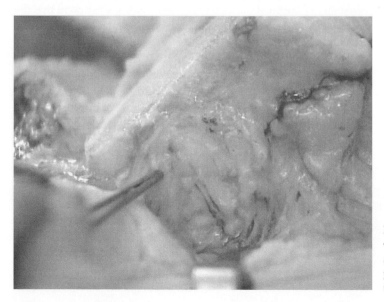

**Fig. 9.2**

The center of the lateral epicondyle is the most prominent point. See also colour plate section.

**Fig. 9.3**

The sulcus is the center of the medial epicondyle. See also colour plate section.

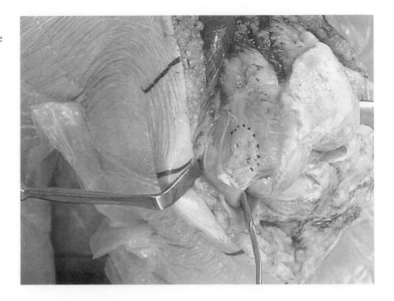

ducible landmarks in both the primary and revision setting. The lateral epicondyle is seen following division of the patellofemoral ligament and elevation of the overlying synovium. It serves as the attachment of the lateral collateral ligament and is the most prominent structure on the lateral side (Fig. 9.2). The medial epicondyle is a crescent-shaped prominence. Whereas the superficial medial collateral ligament attaches to the ridge, the deep fibers of the medial collateral ligament take origin in the sulcus (Fig. 9.3). Since the crescentic ridge is a variable landmark, the center of the medial epicondyle is defined by the base of the sulcus. The transepicondylar axis is defined as the line connecting the medial and lateral epi-

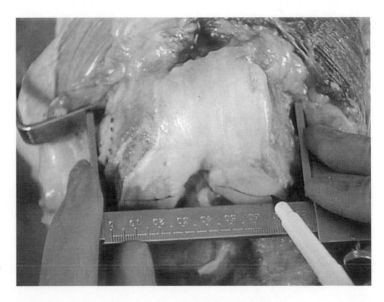

**Fig. 9.4**

The epicondylar axis is determined by a line connecting the medial and lateral epicondyles. See also colour plate section.

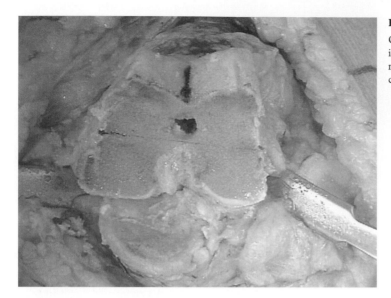

**Fig. 9.5**

Once the epicondylar axis is identified, the femoral component rotation is set. See also colour plate section.

condyles (Fig. 9.4). Once this axis is identified, the femoral component rotation is set (Fig. 9.5).

Malrotation of the femoral component may lead to patellofemoral instability, wear or loosening of the femoral component, or patellar fracture.[11] Internal rotation of the femoral component may also increase stresses on the tibial component leading to wear or loosening. Therefore, internal rotation of the femoral component should be avoided.

Alignment is important to the clinical success of TKA. Along with the axial alignment, femoral component rotation influences knee function. Previous investigators have reported that small amounts of external rotation, relative to the neutral position, significantly improves patellar tracking and reduces patellofemoral complications.[12,13] When the classic method of bone resection is employed, it is necessary to externally rotate the femoral component in order to create a symmetrical flexion space. The transepicondylar axis provides a reproducible method of setting femoral rotation and allows precise positioning of the femoral component.

## References

1   Hungerford DS, Krackow KA, Kenna RV: Alignment in total knee arthroplasty. In *The Knee: Papers of the First Scientific Meeting of the Knee Society*, ed. L Dorr, pp. 9–21. University Park Press, Baltimore, MD, 1985.

2   Insall JN (ed.): *Surgery of the Knee*. Churchill Livingston, New York, 1984.

3   Churchill DL, Incavo SJ, Johnson CC, Beynnon BD: The transepicondylar axis approximates the optimal flexion axis of the knee. *Clinical Orthopedics* **356**:111–118, 1998.

4 Hollister AM, Jatana A, Singh AK *et al.*: The axes of rotation of the knee. *Clinical Orthopedics* **290**:259–268, 1993.

5 Berger RA, Rubash HE, Seel MJ *et al.*: Determining the rotational alignment of the femoral component in total knee arthroplasty using the epicondylar axis. *Clinical Orthopedics* **286**:40, 1993.

6 Griffin FM, Insall JN, Scuderi GR: The posterior condylar angle in osteoathritic knees. *Journal of Arthoplasty* **13**(7):812–815, 1998.

7 Arima J, Whiteside LA, McCarthy DS, White ES: Femoral rotational alignment, based on the anteroposterior axis in total knee arthroplasty in a valgus knee. *Journal of Bone and Joint Surgery* [Am] **77**:1331–1334, 1995.

8 Poilvache PL, Insall JN, Scuderi GR, Font-Rodriguez DE: Rotational landmarks and sizing of the distal femur in total knee arthroplasty. *Clinical Orthopedics* **331**:35–46, 1996.

9 Stiehl JB, Abbott BD: Femoral component rotational alignment using the extramedullary tibial shaft axis: a technical note. *Journal of Orthopaedic Rheumatology* **8**:93, 1995.

10 Yoshioka Y, Siu D, Cooke, TDV: The anatomy and functional axis of the femur. *Journal of Bone and Joint Surgery* [Am] **69**:873–880, 1987.

11 Berger RA, Crossett LS, Jacobs JJ, Rubash HE: Malrotation causing patellofemoral complications after total knee arthroplasty. *Clinical Orthopedics* **356**:144 –153, 1998.

12 Figgie HE, Goldberg VM, Hieple KG *et al.*: The influence of tibial patellofemoral location on the function of the knee in patients with the posterior stabilized prosthesis. *Journal of Bone and Joint Surgery* [Am] **68**:1035, 1986.

13 Rhoads DD, Noble PC, Reuben JD *et al.*: The effect of femoral component position on patellar tracking after total knee arthroplasty. *Clinical Orthopedics* **260**:43, 1990.

# Con: Michael Ries

Placement of the femoral component in appropriate rotational orientation is necessary during TKA to achieve balanced medial and lateral soft tissue tension during flexion. The femoral sulcus of the normal and osteoarthritic knee is located lateral to the midline.[1] External rotation of the femoral component also displaces the proximal end of the trochlear groove laterally, which may facilitate patellar tracking during early flexion.

Rotational orientation of the femoral component can be determined from bony landmarks on the distal femur. The posterior condylar line, epicondylar line, and AP line of the distal femur are often used as reference lines to orient the component position (Fig. 9 .6).[2–11] After the implant position is determined, release of the contracted medial or lateral soft tissues may be necessary. Alternatively, rotational orientation of the femoral component can be determined based on the tension is the soft tissues and ligament balance is achieved by differences in condylar bone resections rather than soft tissue releases.[12,13]

In the normal knee, the femorotibial joint line is oriented at approximately 3° of varus (Fig. 9.7).[14,15] Placement of tibial component in varus, however, is associated with late loosening.[15] Resection

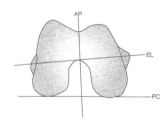

**Fig. 9.6**

Distal femur with the knee flexed. The posterior condylar line (PC) is formed by a line along the posterior aspects of the medial and lateral femoral condyles. The epicondylar line (EL) is formed by a line through the medial and lateral epicondyles. The anteroposterior line (AP) is formed by a line from the trochlear groove to the intercondylar notch.

of the tibial surface perpendicular to the mechanical axis of the tibia results in more bone removal from the lateral compared to the medial plateau. Resection of the distal femoral bone surface perpendicular to the mechanical axis of the femur results in more bone removal from the medial compared to the lateral distal femoral condyle (Fig. 9.7). Resection of the tibial and femoral bone surfaces perpendicular to the mechanical axis of the limb produces a rectangular extension space (Fig. 9.8). When a TKA having equal medial and lateral femoral condylar thicknesses and equal medial and lateral tibial plateau heights is implanted, the joint line is converted from a varus position to one which is perpendicular to the mechanical axis of the limb (Fig. 9.9). Since the overall amount of bone resection equals the height of the prosthetic components, medial and lateral collateral ligament tension remains balanced.

When the knee is flexed to 90°, the normal joint line is also oriented in varus (Fig. 9.10). A tibial resection perpendicular to the mechanical axis results in more bone removal from the lateral compared to the medial tibial plateau. If the posterior femoral condyles are resected in neutral rotation, or parallel to the posterior condylar line, equal amounts of bone are removed from the posteromedial and posterolateral femoral condyles. The symmetric resections of bone produce a trapezoidal flexion space (Fig. 9.9.11). When a TKA with equal posterior femoral condylar thicknesses and equal tibial plateau heights is implanted, the medial collateral soft tissue tension will be greater then the lateral collateral soft tissue tension (Fig. 9.12). This creates imbalance in the soft tissues during knee flexion.

Alternatively, the AP femoral cutting block can be externally rotated relative to the posterior condyle line (Fig. 9.13). This results in more bone removal from posteromedial compared to the posterolateral femoral condyle. The asymmetric bone resections produce a rectangular flexion space (Fig. 9.14). When a total knee arthroplasty having symmetric posterior femoral condylar thicknesses and tibial plateau heights is implanted, collateral ligament tension remains balanced in flexion.

Rotational orientation of the femoral AP cutting block can be based on the position of the posterior condylar line, epicondylar line, or AP line. The AP line and epicondylar line are generally perpendicular to one another and externally rotated approximately 3° relative to the posterior condylar line.[3,5,7,9] External rotation of the femoral AP cutting block 3° from the posterior condylar line will generally result in placement of the transverse axis of the femoral component parallel to the epicondylar line and perpendicular to the AP line.

There may be some anatomic variability in the orientation of the three lines (AP, epicondylar, and posterior condylar) relative to one another. Berger et al.[5] observed an average angle of 3.5° between the epicondylar and posterior condylar lines. Mantas et al.[7] reported an average value for this angle of 5°. Poilvache et al.[9] found the

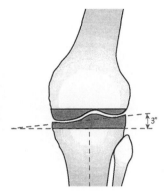

**Fig. 9.7**

Knee in extension. The anatomic joint line is oriented at 3° of varus relative to a line perpendicular to the mechanical axis of the limb. Resection of the tibial surface perpendicular to the mechanical axis causes more bone to be removed from the lateral compared to the medial tibial plateau. Resection of the femoral surface perpendicular to the mechanical axis causes more bone to be removed from the medial compared to the lateral femoral condyle.

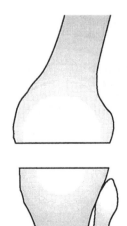

**Fig. 9.8**

After resection of the femoral and tibial surfaces perpendicular to the mechanical axis, a rectangular flexion space is produced.

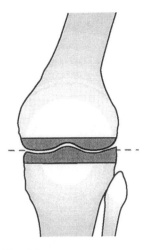

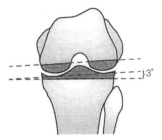

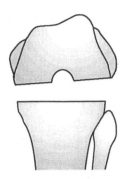

**Fig. 9.9**

After placement of a TKA having equal medial and lateral femoral condylar thicknesses and equal medial and lateral tibial plateau heights, medial and lateral soft tissue tension remains symmetric. The orientation of the joint line (dashed line) has been changed from 3° of varus to perpendicular to the mechanical axis.

**Fig. 9.10**

Knee at 90° of flexion. The anatomic joint line is oriented at 3° of varus relative to a line perpendicular to the mechanical axis of the tibia. Resection of the tibial surface perpendicular to the mechanical axis causes more bone to be removed from the lateral compared to the medial tibial plateau. Resection of the posterior femoral condyles in neutral rotation or parallel to the posterior condylar line causes equal thicknesses of bone to be removed from the posteromedial and posterolateral femoral condyles.

**Fig. 9.11**

After resection of the tibial surface perpendicular to the mechanical axis and resection of the posterior femoral condyles parallel to the posterior condylar line, a trapezoidal flexion space is produced.

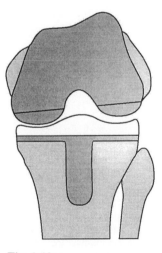

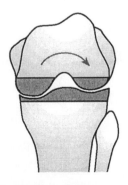

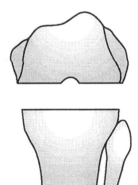

**Fig. 9.12**

After placement of a TKA having equal medial and lateral femoral condylar thicknesses and equal medial and lateral tibial plateau heights, the medial soft tissues will be tighter than the lateral soft tissues.

**Fig. 9.13**

External rotation of the AP femoral cutting block (arrow) causes more bone to be removed from the posteromedial compared to the posterolateral femoral condyle.

**Fig. 9.14**

The asymmetric bone resections produce a rectangular flexion space.

epicondylar line more consistent then the AP line in arthritic knees. The epicondylar line was oriented at $3.51 \pm 2.03°$ relative to the posterior condylar line in neutral or varus knees and $4.41 \pm 1.83°$ in valgus knees. This finding is consistent with the relative hypoplasia of the posterior lateral femoral condyle that can occur in the valgus knee.

Arima *et al.* observed the AP line to be oriented at 4° relative to the epicondylar line but the epicondylar line was difficult to define and not as accurate.[3] The posterior condylar line is easily identified during surgery but may be affected by loss of condylar height from arthrosis. Use of more than one of the three reference lines may be necessary, particularly in severely deformed knees to properly orient the position of the femoral component in TKA (Fig. 9.15).

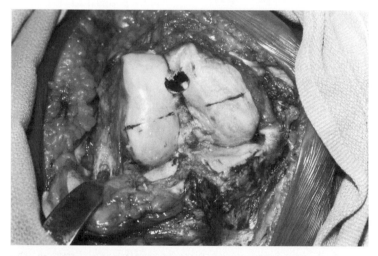

a

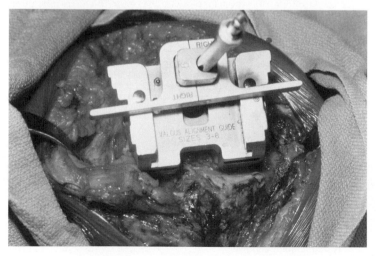

b

**Fig. 9.15**

(a) The AP line and epicondylar line (marked with electrocautery) are approximately perpendicular to each other and rotated 3° relative to the posterior condylar line. (b) Instrumentation to orient the rotational position of the femoral bone cuts (Genesis II, Smith and Nephew, Memphis, TN). Skids which are positioned along the posterior condylar line are oriented at 3° relative to the epicondylar line and 93° relative to the AP line.

In the valgus knee, the lateral femoral condyle is often hypoplastic so if the posterior condylar line is used to reference the rotational position of the femoral component, relative internal rotation of the femoral component could occur. Internal rotation of the femoral component can lead to significant patellar problems. Berger *et al.*[4] found that combined femoral and tibial component internal rotation of 1–4° correlates with lateral patellar tracking and tilt, combined internal rotation of 3–8° correlates with patellar subluxation, and combined internal rotation of 7–17° is associated with patellar dislocation. To avoid internal rotation of the femoral component, use of more than one reference line, particularly in valgus knees is helpful. External rotation of the femoral component in the valgus knee often requires release of the contracted lateral soft tissues. However, this approach provides a balanced flexion space and avoids the problem of femoral component internal rotation.[3]

Rotational orientation of the femoral component may also be determined from the position of resected tibial surface and collateral ligament soft tissue tension rather than with the bony landmarks and reference lines located in the distal femur. Insall described this method of resecting the tibial surface perpendicular to the mechanical axis of the tibia and distracting the knee in flexion with a tensioner.[12] The posterior femoral resection is made parallel to the tibial resection. The thicknesses of the resected posterior medial and lateral femoral condyles as well as rotational orientation of the implant are dependent upon the medial and lateral soft tissue tension. A wide range of femoral component rotation can be achieved with this technique. If one of the collateral ligaments is contracted and not adequately released, excessive internal or external femoral component rotation may occur with this method.

With either the method of cutting the tibia first and distracting the knee to determine rotation or determining rotation from the three reference lines in the distal femur, asymmetric posterior condylar resections are necessary to produce a rectangular flexion space. This positions the femoral component in external rotation relative to the posterior condylar line.

## Adverse effects of femoral component external rotation

There are some potentially undesirable consequences of femoral component external rotation. External rotation of the femoral AP cutting block causes a deeper resection of the anterior lateral femoral surface than the anterior medial surface (Fig. 9.16). This may result in a anterior lateral notch which could predispose to supracondylar femur fracture. If a larger femoral component is used to avoid lateral notching by displacing the externally rotated anterior cut further anterior, the extensor mechanism will be displaced anteriorly which could limit flexion and there may be less contact between the anterior medial distal femoral surface and implant.

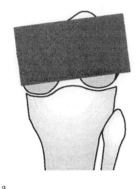

a

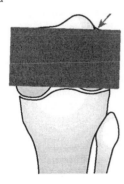

b

**Fig. 9.16**

(a) Neutral rotation of the AP femoral cutting block (parallel to the posterior condylar line) produces an anterior cut roughly parallel to the anterior femoral cortex. (b) External rotation of the AP femoral cutting block causes a deeper anterolateral resection which may create a notch in the distal femur (arrow).

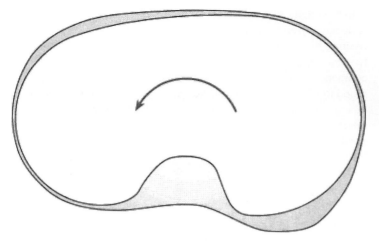

**Fig. 9.17**

Illustration of the tibial surface. If the tibial component is externally rotated, an undersized component may be needed to avoid overhang. This produces areas of incomplete bone coverage posteromedially and anterolaterally. (Reproduced with permission.)

When the femoral component is externally rotated to produce a rectangular flexion space, the component will remain externally rotated when the knee is extended. In order to orient the tibial component with the externally rotated femoral component, external rotation of the tibial component is necessary. This also translates the tibial tubercle medial to the femoral component trochlear groove with the knee in extension which may help prevent patellar subluxation. However, external rotation of the tibial component can cause overhang of the tibial base plate anteromedially and posterolaterally or an undersized component may be required to avoid overhang (Fig. 9.17). In addition rotational incongruity between the femoral and tibial components can occur as the knee is flexed.[17]

If both the femoral and tibial components are externally rotated, the medial femorotibial contact point is moved posteriorly and the lateral femorotibial contact point is moved anteriorly causing rotational malalignment between the femoral and tibial articular surfaces in flexion (Fig. 9.18). External rotation of the tibial surface also moves the medial femoral contact area posteriorly on the tibia. This may contribute to the posteromedial polyethylene wear which is a common failure mechanism in TKA.[18]

**Fig. 9.18**

(a) During knee extension, when both the femoral and tibial components are externally rotated, the contact areas (shown in black) which are parallel to the transverse axis of the femoral component, are aligned with the transverse axis of the tibial component. (b) During knee flexion, when both the femoral and tibial components are externally rotated, the contact areas (shown in black) which are parallel to the transverse axis of the femoral component, are externally rotated relative to the transverse axis of the tibial component. This produces relational incongruity between the femoral and tibial articular surfaces in flexion. (Reproduced with permission.)

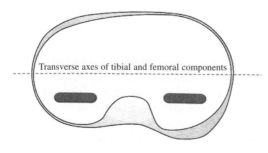

Transverse axes of tibial and femoral components

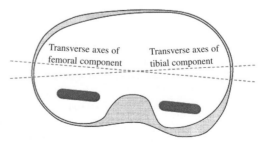

Transverse axes of femoral component

Transverse axes of tibial component

a

b

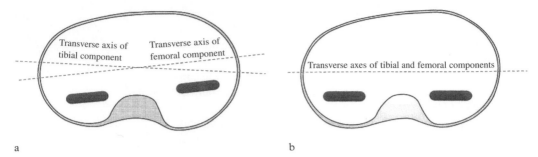

a

b

**Fig. 9.19**

(a) During knee extension, when the femoral component is externally rotated and the tibial component is neutrally rotated, the contact areas (shown in black) which are parallel to the transverse axis of the femoral component are externally rotated relative to the transverse axis of the tibial component. (b) During knee flexion, when the femoral component is externally rotated and the tibial component is neutrally rotated, the contact areas (shown in black) which are parallel to the transverse axis of the femoral component are parallel to the transverse axis of the tibial component. (Reproduced with permission.)

Although most implants permit some rotational incongruity, rotational malalignment in highly conforming knee designs can contribute to failure from polyethylene wear.[19] However, if the femoral component is externally rotated and the tibial component is neutrally rotated, the two articular surfaces will be rotationally malaligned in extension (Fig. 9.19). This implies that when the femoral component is externally rotated, there will be rotational malalignment in flexion if the tibial component is externally rotated and in extension if the tibial component is not externally rotated.[17]

The position of the femoral component trochlear groove is also affected by femoral component rotation. The plane through which the femoral component is rotated is at the level of the distal femoral bone cut. The proximal end of the trochlear groove will be displaced laterally as a result of femoral component external rotation (Fig. 9.20). This may contribute favorably to patellar tracking during extension and early flexion. However, external rotation of the femoral component can cause relative medialization of the trochlear groove which articulates with the patella during flexion (Fig. 9.21). At flexion angles past 90°, external rotation of the femoral component causes significant medial displacement of the patella and at 120° of knee flexion, 10° of femoral component external rotation can cause 10 mm of the medial patellar displacement.[10] Medialization of the trochlear groove during flexion, when patellofemoral compressive forces are maximal, may contribute to lateral patellar wear, loosening, and fracture.

If the tibial cut is posteriorly sloped, external rotation of the cutting block can also influence axial alignment. For a 10° posteriorly sloped cut, rotation of 6° results in a change in limb alignment of 1°.[20]

In the normal knee, the axis of knee flexion can be represented by a line through the epicondyles.[21] It has been suggested that after TKA, the axis of knee flexion can also be represented by a line through the epicondyles. However, there are marked structural differences between the normal and replaced knee. Therefore it is not surprising that the kinematics of the normal knee are quite different than the kinematics of the replaced knee.[22-27]

In the normal knee, the joint line is oriented at 3° of varus, both cruciate ligaments and menisci are present, and the extensor mechanism is preserved. In the replaced knee, the joint line is changed to an orientation perpendicular to the mechanical axis, one or both cruciate ligaments are removed, both menisci are removed, the conformity of the articular surfaces is changed, the joint line may be raised, collateral ligaments may be released, limb alignment may not be restored perfectly, and the extensor mechanism is altered. This can lead to a pattern of AP motion after TKA which is the opposite of the normal knee.

During normal knee flexion, the femur rolls back or moves posteriorly on the tibia (Fig. 9.22). However, after knee replacement the femur moves anteriorly on the tibia during knee flexion.[22–24,27] This "paradoxical" movement may be related primarily to the loss of anterior cruciate ligament function (Fig. 9.23). It occurs with both posterior cruciate ligament retaining and substituting total knee replacements (Fig. 9.24). The axis of knee flexion is quite variable also and not constant during motion. Results of numerous fluoroscopic studies of kinematics after TKA indicate that the axis of knee flexion is not represented by a single line through the epicondyles.[22–24,27]

Total knee replacements, however, function quite well when balanced flexion and extension spaces or gaps are obtained during surgery. The resultant effect, which may be called "gap kinematics," does not produce normal knee kinematics. However, it does produce very satisfactory knee function. Because of the excellent function achieved after total knee replacement, but kinematics which are markedly different from those of the normal knee, the question is raised whether or not restoration of "normal" knee kinematics is desirable or realistic after TKA. If restoration of "normal" knee kinematics after TKA can be achieved by modifications in design or surgical technique, then it would seem desirable and appropriate provided that the changes necessary to achieve the "normal" knee kinematics do not compromise the excellent longevity and function of total knee replacements that have "abnormal" kinematics.

The issue of how to achieve good gap kinematics or balanced flexion and extension spaces can be addressed by external rotation of the femoral component relative to the posterior condylar line. However, external rotation of the femoral component can also lead to notching the anterolateral femoral cortex, medialization of the trochlear groove during flexion, rotational incongruity between the femoral and tibial articular surfaces, and decreased tibial bone coverage.

## Neutral rotation of a femoral component with asymmetric posterior condyles

Balanced flexion and extension spaces can also be achieved by neutral femoral resections (parallel to the posterior condylar line)

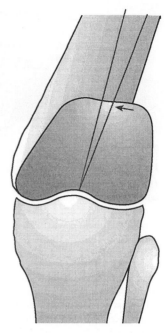

**Fig. 9.20**

Knee in extension. External rotation of the femoral component causes relative lateralization of the proximal end of the trochlear groove (arrow).

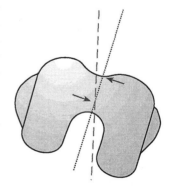

**Fig. 9.21**

Knee in flexion. External rotation of the femoral component (orientation shown by dotted line) causes relative lateralization of the proximal trochlear groove (upper arrow). However, the distal trochlear groove (lower arrow) is medialized relative to a position of the trochlear groove in neutral rotation (dashed line).

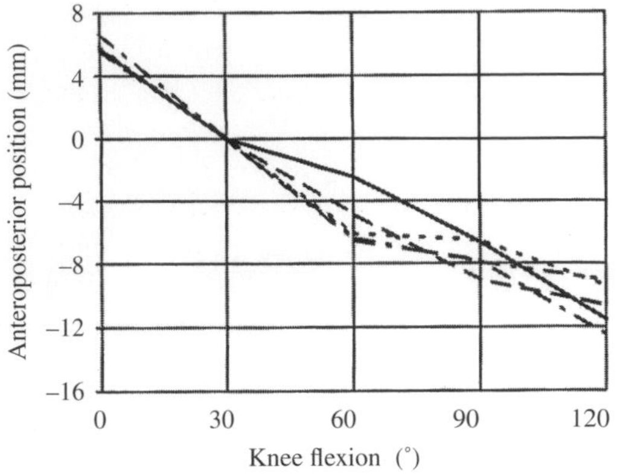

**Fig. 9.22**

*In vivo* fluoroscopic analysis of five patients with normal knees. During knee flexion, the femur moves posteriorly or rolls back on the tibia (Reproduced with permission from Dennis *et al.*[24]).

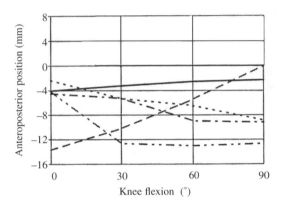

**Fig. 9.23**

*In vivo* fluoroscopic analysis of five patients with ACL-deficient knees. Normal femoral rollback no longer occurs (Reproduced with permission from Dennis *et al.*[24]).

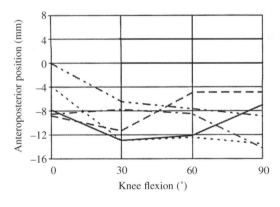

**Fig. 9.24**

*In vivo* fluoroscopic analysis of patients with PCL-retaining TKAs. AP motion is quite variable (Reproduced with permission from Dennis *et al.*[24]).

and modification of the femoral component with posterior condyles having different thicknesses. In order to avoid the adverse effects of femoral component external rotation, the distal femoral bone cuts may be made in neutral rotation and the posterior lateral condyle of the implant is made thicker than the posterior medial

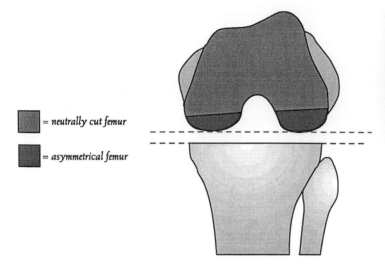

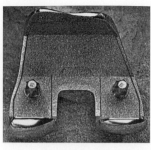

b

= *neutrally cut femur*

= *asymmetrical femur*

a

**Fig. 9.25**

(a) Flexed knee after a tibial resection perpendicular to the mechanical axis. The posterior femoral condyles are resected in neutral rotation (parallel to the posterior condylar line) producing a trapezoidal flexion space. A modified femoral component having thicker posterolateral than posteromedial femoral condyles maintains the joint line perpendicular to the mechanical axis of the tibia and collateral ligament tension is balanced during flexion. Note the boundary between the neutrally cut femur (lighter gray shading) and the asymmetrical femur (darker gray). (b) Genesis II (Smith and Nephew, Memphis, TN) femoral component with asymmetric posterior condyles.

condyle (Fig. 9.25). Equal thicknesses of bone are removed from the posteromedial and posterolateral condyles producing a trapezoidal flexion space. The unequal thickness of the implant posterior condyles produces a joint line perpendicular to the mechanical axis and balanced collateral ligament tension in flexion. Since the anterior femoral flange is not lateralized by externally rotating the component, modification of the trochlear groove is also necessary (Fig. 9.26). A modified femoral component having both asymmetric posterior condyles and a proximal trochlear groove which is translated laterally can provide more lateral patellar tracking throughout the entire range of motion than an externally rotated conventional symmetrical femoral component. Because the component is not rotated, the trochlear groove is not medialized during flexion.

With use of a femoral component having asymmetric posterior condyles, only 3 of 100 consecutive patients undergoing primary TKA required a lateral retinacular release.[28] Two of 3 patients requiring lateral retinacular release had preoperative valgus deformities of

**Fig. 9.26**

(a) Modified femoral component in extension. The trochlear groove is translated laterally (offset between arrows) so external rotation of the component is not needed to lateralize the proximal trochlear groove. (b) Modified femoral component in flexion. The trochlear groove which articulates with the patella during flexion lies in the midline rather than in a medialized position which would occur if the component was externally rotated.

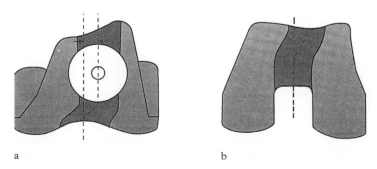

a                                        b

**Fig. 9.27**

*In vivo* fluoroscopic analysis of patients with PCL-retaining and PCL-substituting Genesis II knee replacements implanted in neutral rotation.[23] Consistent AP motion is observed.

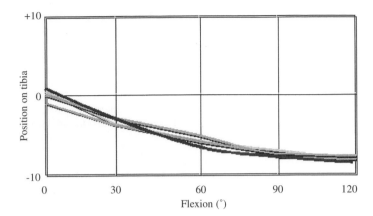

over 15° and preoperative patellar subluxation. Average patellar tilt in this series of patients was 1.3° and average patellar shift was 1.5 mm measured on merchant views one year post operatively. The incidence of anterior knee pain was 2%.[28]

Use of a femoral component having asymmetric posterior condyles implanted in neutral rotation with a tibial component implanted in neutral rotation provides balanced flexion and extension spaces. *In vivo* fluoroscopic analysis of these patients with either posterior cruciate retaining or substituting prostheses demonstrates a consistent kinematic pattern of femoral movement from anterior to posterior during knee flexion (Fig. 9.27).[22]

## References

1  Eckhoff DG, Montgomery WK, Stamm ER, Kilcoyne RF: Location of the femoral sulcus in the osteoarthritic knee. *Journal of Arthroplasty* **11**:163–165, 1996.

2  Anouchi YS, Whiteside LA, Kaiser AD, Milliano MT: The effects of axial rotational alignment of the femoral component on knee stability and patellar tracking in total knee arthroplasty demonstrated on autopsy specimens. *Clinical Orthopedics* **287**:170–177, 1993.

3  Arima J, Whiteside LA, McCarthy DS, White SE: Femoral rotational alignment, based on the anteroposterior axis, in total knee arthroplasty in a valgus knee. A technical note. *Journal of Bone and Joint Surgery* [Am] **77**:1331–1334, 1995.

4  Berger RA, Crossett LS, Jacobs JJ, Rubash HE: Malrotation causing patellofemoral complications after total knee arthroplasty. *Clinical Orthopedics*, **356**:144–153, 1998.

5  Berger RA, Rubash HE, Seel MJ *et al.*: Determining the rotational alignment of the femoral component in total knee arthroplasty using the epicondylar axis. *Clinical Orthopedics* **286**:40–47, 1993.

6  Laskin RS: Flexion space configuration in total knee arthroplasty. *Journal of Arthroplasty* **10**:657–660, 1995.

7  Mantas JP, Bloebaum RD, Skedros JG, Hofmann AA: Implications of reference axes used for rotational alignment of the femoral component in primary and revision knee arthroplasty. *Journal of Arthroplasty* **7**:531–535, 1992.

8   Nagamine R, White SE, McCarthy DS, Whiteside LA: 1995 Effect of rotational malposition of the femoral component on knee stability kinematics after total knee arthroplasty. *Journal of Arthroplasty* **10**:265–270.

9   Poilvache PL, Insall JN, Scuderi GR, Font-Rodriguez DE: Rotational landmarks and sizing of the distal femur in total knee arthroplasty. *Clinical Orthopedics*, **331**:35–46, 1995.

10  Rhoads DD, Noble PC, Reuben JD, Tullos HS: The effect of femoral component position on the kinematics of total knee arthroplasty. *Clinical Orthopedics* **286**:122–129, 1993.

11  Stiehl JB, Abbott BD: Morphology of the transepicondylar axis and its application in primary and revision total knee arthroplasty. *Journal of Arthroplasty* **10**:785–789, 1995.

12  Insall J (ed.): *Surgery of the Knee*. Churchill Livingstone, New York, 1984.

13  Stiehl JB, Cherveny PM: Femoral rotational alignment using the tibial shaft axis in total knee arthroplasty. *Clinical Orthopedics* **331**:47–55, 1996.

14  Yoshioka Y, Siu D, Cooke TD: The anatomy and functional axes of the femur. *Journal of Bone and Joint Surgery* [Am] **69**:873–880, 1987.

15  Yoshioka Y, Siu DW, Scudamore RA, Cooke TD: Tibial anatomy and functional axes. *Journal of Orthopedic Research* **7**:132–137, 1989.

16  Ritter MA, Faris PM, Keating ME, Meding JB: Postoperative alignment of total knee replacement. Its effect on survival. *Clinical Orthopedics* **299**:153–156, 1994.

17  Ries MD, Salehi A, Laskin RS *et al.*: Can rotational congruity be achieved in both flexion and extension when the femoral component is externally rotated in total knee arthroplasty? *Knee* **5**:37–41, 1998.

18  Lewis P, Rorabeck CH, Bourne RB, Devane P: Posteromedial tibial polyethylene failure in total knee replacement. *Clinical Orthopedics* **299**:11–17, 1994.

19  Northmore-Ball MD, Freeman MAR, Barnes KA: Subclinical rotational malposition: A potential cause of catastrophic wear in conforming condylar knee arthroplasty. *Knee* **2**:177–180, 1995.

20  Ries MD: Relationship between posterior tibial slope and rotation on axial alignment in total knee arthroplasty. *Knee* **2**:223–226, 1996.

21  Hollister AM, Jatana S, Singh AK *et al.*: The axes of rotation of the knee. *Clinical Orthopedics* **290**:259–268, 1993.

22  Banks SA, Markovich GD, Hodge WA: In vivo kinematics of cruciate-retaining and -substituting knee arthroplasties. *Journal of Arthroplasty* **12**:297–304, 1997.

23  Banks SA Otis JC, Bakus SL *et al.*: Integrated analysis of knee arthroplasty mechanics using simultaneous flouroscopy, force plates, and motion analysis. *Transactions of the Orthopedics Research Society* **24**:747, 1999.

24  Dennis DA, Komistek RD, Hoff WA, Gabriel SM: In vivo knee kinematics derived using an inverse perspective technique. *Clinical Orthopedics* **331**:107–117, 1996.

25  Nilsson KG, Kärrholm J, Gadegaard P: Abnormal kinematics of the artificial knee. Roentgen stereophotogrammetric analysis of 10 Miller–Galante and five New Jersey LCS knees. *Acta Orthopaedica Scandinavica* **62**:440–446, 1991.

26  Nilsson KG, Kärrholm J, Ekelund L: Knee motion in total knee arthroplasty. A roentgen stereophotogrammetric analysis of the kinematics of the Tricon-M knee prosthesis. *Clinical Orthopedics* **256**:147–161, 1990.

27  Stiehl JB, Komistek RD, Dennis DA *et al.*: Fluoroscopic analysis of
      kinematics after posterior-cruciate-retaining knee arthroplasty.
      *Journal of Bone and Joint Surgery* [Br] **77**:884–889, 1995.
28  Laskin RS: Patellar tracking and flexion space balancing using a
      femoral component with asymmetrical femoral condyles. *Knee*
      **6**:87–93, 1999.

## Questions and answers

*Moderator:* Many people have stated that it isn't easy to find the
epicondyles precisely. Do you do anything special to facilitate this?

*Dr. Scuderi:* Familiarity with the distal femoral anatomy makes it
easy to identify the femoral epicondyles. Although it may be necessary to excise the overlying synovium, careful surgical technique will
avoid damaging the origin of the collateral ligaments.

*Moderator:* If you use the ligament tension technique, of determining the amount of femoral component rotation to balance the
flexion space, you are assuming that you have completely corrected
any deformity. How can you be sure that you have? What I am saying is that if the ligaments are not balanced prior to using them to
determine rotation, the rotation will be inaccurate. Is this premise
correct?

*Dr. Ries:* With the ligament tension technique, soft tissue releases
are performed to balance collateral ligament tension in extension.
The femoral component is then rotated internally or externally to
balance the flexion space. This technique is based on the assumption
that soft tissue releases which balance the knee in extension will also
balance the knee in flexion. However, structures such as the posterior capsule and hamstring tendons contribute to varus–valgus stability in extension but not in flexion. Soft tissue releases in extension
may not correct contracted soft tissues in flexion. With the ligament
tension technique, excessive internal or external rotation of the
femoral component may be necessary to balance the flexion space.
However, malrotation of the femoral component can cause problems with patellar tracking (Berger RA *et al.*, *Clinical Orthopedics*
1998;**356**:144–153). The most appropriate method of balancing contracted soft tissues in both flexion and extension is to balance the
flexion and extension spaces simultaneously. This requires orienting
the rotational position of the femoral bone cuts relative to the bony
anatomy (posterior condylar line, epicondylar line, and AP line) and
balancing the soft tissues using spacer blocks or trial implants.

*Moderator:* Just how accurate, Dr. Scuderi, is using the epicondylar
axis to judge rotation?

*Dr. Scuderi:* The epicondylar axis is a reliable method of determining femoral rotation. Variability does exist between varus and
valgus knees. When measuring the angle between the epicondylar

axis and the posterior condyles, the posterior condylar angle averages $3.3° + 1.9°$ for the varus knee (range 0–8°); $3.3° + 2.3°$ for knees with no deformity; and $5.4° + 2.3°$ for the valgus knee (range 3–10°).

*Moderator:* We have been talking up to this point about femoral component rotation. How about tibial component rotation? How do you determine where to set it?

*Dr. Scuderi:* Tibial component rotation is set in line with the anterior cortex of the tibia and in line with the tibial tubercle. Since the tibial plateau is asymmetrical—with the AP dimension of the medial side being greater than the lateral side—a symmetrical tibial component that covers the entire medial tibia will overhang the posterolateral corner. This has been of little or no clinical significance.

*Moderator:* Actually I have to put my experience in here. I have found that posterolateral overhang can be of clinical significance in that it can impinge on the popliteus tendon, causing anything from an annoying snap, to posterolateral pain and eventually attrition of the tendon. However, as a follow-up question on tibial rotation, Dr. Ries, since every fixed bearing tibial component must be inserted in one position, which do you choose? Should it be congruous in extension, congruous in flexion, or somewhere in the middle and why?

*Dr. Ries:* If both the femoral and tibial components are externally rotated, the articular surfaces will be congruous in extension but incongruous in flexion. If the femoral component is externally rotated and the tibial component is neutrally rotated, the articular surfaces will be congruous in flexion but incongruous in extension. Since most weightbearing activities during gait occur during early flexion (approximately 0–30°), maintaining high congruity in extension may be more important than during deep flexion. If it is necessary to externally rotate the femoral component, then external rotation of the tibial component by the same amount or nearly the same amount as the femoral component would seem appropriate to maintain joint congruity during early flexion. Alternatively, use of a femoral component with asymmetric posterior condyles implanted in a neutral rotation can be combined with a tibial component placed in a neutral rotation which maintains joint congruity throughout the flexion arc (for a more detailed account see Ries MD et al., *Knee* 1998;**5**:37–41).

*Moderator:* In previous chapters we discussed the concept of a medial pivot knee. How does this concept integrate with your use of the epicondylar axis?

*Dr. Scuderi:* Although kinematic studies have shown that the knee will pivot on the medial tibia and slide on the lateral side, the flexion axis of the knee has been shown to be the epicondylar axis. Yoshiokia *et al.* found the epicondylar axis to be at a right angle to the mechanical axis of the femur in extension, as well as at 90° of flexion. This is similar to the observations of Churchill *et al.*

*Moderator:* If you externally rotate the femoral component, you will, on many occasions notch the anterolateral cortex. Doesn't this bother you, Dr. Scuderi?

*Dr. Scuderi:* Notching of the anterior cortex is a consequence of femoral component. I would agree that when the femoral component is externally rotated, the osteotomized anterior femur has the appearance of a "boot" or "grand piano" with the lateral side being cut more proximally than the medial side. This is the result of more bone being resected from the anterolateral condyle than the antero-medial condyle. Remember, this is the opposite of what is happening posteriorly, where more bone is resected from the posteromedial condyle.In cases of extra-articular deformity or post-traumatic arthritis secondary to a femur fracture, the epicondylar axis may not be reliable and the surgeon should be prepared to use alternate methods for determining femoral rotation, such as the tibial shaft or soft tissue tension.

*Moderator:* Dr. Ries, the prosthesis that you describe has an effective external rotation of 3°. Is this always the correct amount and, if not, what do you do?

*Dr. Ries:* The anatomic joint line is oriented at approximately 3° of varus relative to the mechanical axis of the limb and the posterior condylar line in most knees is oriented at 3 and 93° respectively, relative to the epicondylar and AP lines (Yoshioka Y *et al.*, *Journal of Bone and Joint Surgery* 1987;**69A**:873–880; Yoshioka Y *et al.*, *Journal of Orthopedic Research* 1989;7:132–137, Berger RA *et al.*, *Clinical Orthopedics* 1993;**286**:40–47). In the arthritic knee, the articular surfaces of the posterior condyles may be eroded and in the valgus knee, the lateral condyle is often hypoplastic (Arima J *et al.*, *Journal of Bone and Joint Surgery* 1995;**77A**:1131–1134). The prosthetic joint line in flexion therefore may need to be positioned in slightly more or less than 3° of external rotation relative to the posterior condylar line of the arthritic knee. Use of a femoral component having asymmetric posterior condyles oriented at 3° relative to the arthritic posterior condylar line will position the femoral component in neutral rotation in most knees. Slight internal or external rotation of the asymmetric component may be necessary in some knees to orient the prosthetic joint line parallel to the epicondylar line.However, if a component with symmetric condyles is used, 3° of external rotation is necessary in most knees to position the prosthetic joint line in flexion parallel to the epicondylar line. Several degrees more or less of rotation may be necessary in some situations. For example, if additional external rotation of 2° is necessary, the femoral component will be externally rotated 5°. The tibial component would also need to be externally rotated 5° to be rotationally aligned with the femoral component in extension. This can compromise tibial bone coverage and cause rotational malalignment between the two articular surfaces in flexion (Ries MD *et al.*, *Knee* 1998;5:37–41). However, if the asymmetric femoral component is used in this example, it would require only 2° of femoral component external rotation and a corresponding rotation of 2° rather than 5° of the tibial component. With the asymmetric component oriented in neutral rotation, the starting position of the joint line in flexion is relatively parallel to the epicondylar axis, whereas with a symmetric component 3° of external rotation is needed to place the joint line in the same orientation.

*Moderator:* What do you do in a revision situation, Dr. Ries, where there is no trochlear groove, the epicondyles have fractured and the posterior femoral condyles are abnormal secondary to osteolysis?

*Dr. Ries:* In most revisions, the position of the posterior condylar line and AP line cannot be determined. Rotation of the femoral component is determined from either the epicondylar line or by the ligament tension technique. If the epicondyles are fractured, the collateral ligaments are also deficient so the epicondylar line as well as the ligament tension technique are unreliable in determining the femoral component rotation. Because the collateral ligaments are deficient, a constrained prosthesis is indicated. In this situation the distal femoral and tibial bone cuts are made using intramedullary instrumentation referenced from the endosteal canal of the femur and tibia (Ries MD *et al.*, *Knee* 1998;5:37–41). With the knee fully extended and a spacer block placed in the extension space, tension in the posterior capsule and hamstring tendons rotationally aligns the femur and the tibia. A rough approximation of femoral component rotation can be made based on the remaining distal femoral anatomy. Constrained stemmed trial femoral and tibial components are then implanted and the knee fully extended. The tibial base plate trial should be free to rotate on the cut tibial bone surface. Since the femoral and tibial components are constrained relative to one another in rotation, if the femoral component rotation has been correctly determined, the AP axis of the tibial component should align with the medial third of the tibial tubercle. If the tibial component is malrotated, the femoral component should be repositioned in proper rotation by recutting the posterior condyles and using appropriate thicknesses of posterior femoral wedges to augment bone deficiency.

# 10

*Deep venous thrombosis (DVT) is yet another complication which can turn an otherwise successful total knee arthroplasty (TKA) into a problem case. Over the years many pharmacological agents have been suggested to control the problem of DVT.*

# Aspirin is sufficient prophylaxis for deep venous thrombosis for most total knee patients

## Pro: Kim M. Koffler and Paul A. Lotke

Venous thromboembolism is reported to be the most common serious complication following total joint arthroplasty. However, the incidence of symptomatic pulmonary embolism (PE) is approximately 1% and the rate of fatal PE only 0.1–0.3%.[1] Historically, PE was thought to have a much higher incidence and the concern about fatal PE has prompted considerable investigation into the area of thromboembolic disease. However, despite decades of investigation, controversy still persists in regard to some of the most basic concepts, such as the significance of DVT and its relationship to PE following total joint arthroplasty as well as in the appropriate balance between the risks and benefits of regimens for prevention. Indeed, there is a reasonable school of thought that suggests the risks from chemoprophylaxis are not worth the benefits. That is the proposal for our contribution.

It is known that chemical thromboprophylaxis reduces the venographic prevalence of DVT. It is unclear whether this results in a reduction of symptomatic PE. It has been assumed that a reduction in the venographic DVT rate will lead to a similar reduction in the rates of PE and fatal PE. However, several more recent reports indicate that this assumption may not be true and that there may be no difference in the rate of fatal PE with or without routine anticoagulation.[1–5] Thus, rates of asymptomatic DVT may not be the most appropriate marker for the patient at risk for PE, although it may be a satisfactory end-point for comparing the efficacy of various prophylactic regimens. The use of thromboprophylaxis also has side effects and cost considerations. Therefore, if a fall in the DVT rate is not associated with a similar fall in the fatal PE rate, or if prophylaxis increases the risk of hemorrhagic complications or other causes of death, the question to ask may be whether routine anticoagulation is indicated at all after total knee arthroplasty (TKA) rather than which prophylactic regimen is best.

For many reasons, some noted above, there is significant controversy in the orthopaedic literature regarding thromboprophylaxis in TKA. Chemical prophylaxis is known to reduce the relatively common episodes of venographically detected DVT, but whether it reduces symptomatic thrombosis and fatal and nonfatal PE is unclear. It is also unclear whether the clinical complications of fatal and nonfatal PE, DVT, and postphlebitic syndrome are sufficiently common to justify routine thromboprophylaxis. Some authors have suggested that mortality from postoperative venous thrombosis is rare.[1,3,4,6] Although there are no large randomized trials with clinical end-points, the literature contains increasing numbers of consensus and guideline articles on thromboprophylaxis[7] which rely largely on the data from clinical trials, mainly the early International Multicenter Trial of heparin prophylaxis in elective surgical patients[8] and the subsequent meta-analysis of heparin prophylaxis.[9] Some surgeons consider the conclusions of these articles, that anti-coagulant prophylaxis should be given to all moderate- and high-risk patients, are risky and based on insufficient clinical evidence. A recent article in the British literature showed that only about 36% of UK orthopaedic surgeons considered low-dose anticoagulants to be a necessity.[10] A number of those surveyed used thrombophrophylaxis only for fear of medicolegal repercussions rather than from a conviction of benefit to the patient.[11] This gap between recommendation and practice has risen because of doubts about the clinical benefits of thromboprophylaxis compared to the potential risks.

## Significance of DVT

One of the reasons for a lack of firm evidence in favor of thromboprophylaxis is that many of the trials rely on the rates of asymptomatic DVT diagnosed by venography, fibrinogen scanning, plethysmography, ultrasound, or clinical assessment. These techniques have been widely used, yet some are inaccurate in their ability to diagnose and quantify thrombus.[12] As a result, many of the reports in the earlier literature that depend upon these techniques may have inappropriate conclusions. The venogram is generally recognized as the most accurate method of confirming the presence of a clot because it can diagnose, localize, and quantify the thrombosis. Although there are some inaccuracies related to nonfilling veins and some difficulty in diagnosing pelvic thrombi if the femoral vein is not directly cannulated, this technique is currently considered the most accurate method. Because of patient discomfort from its invasive nature, potential of renal toxicity, allergic reactions and dye-inducing thrombus or phlebitis, as well as the inability to cannulate the veins of a swollen foot postoperatively, venography has not been universally used to diagnose DVT. In addition, many studies using venography inconsistently report the size or location of clots and intermix data pertaining to distal and proximal clots to achieve statistical significance.

An interesting observation is the variability among multiple centers in the rates of DVT by surgical site and treatment group. In one multicenter study on the use of low molecular weight heparin (LMWH) for total joint arthroplasty, the interinstitutional incidence of clot formation in one treatment regimen ranged from 28% to 54%.[13] Jorgenson et al.[14] also noted this interobserver variability in venogram interpretations. From a primary individual reading to a consensus decision of a venogram, there was agreement for positive findings in only 70–90% of the cases. This factor of uncertainty was felt important enough to be considered in studies with venographic end-points. Although these differences are difficult to explain, they indicate the variables and potential inaccuracies in establishing a diagnosis of DVT even with the gold standard, and in comparing treatment regimens.

B-mode duplex ultrasonography has become a popular method for diagnosis of DVT.[15] This study has the potential to be very accurate, especially for proximal thrombosis, with sensitivity in symptomatic patients approaching 97%.[16] However, it is less accurate in the popliteal and calf areas, especially when used for routine surveillance in asymptomatic patients, and cannot show pelvic clots or clots anywhere above the inguinal ligament. The technique is highly technician dependent, with accuracy varying from 0% to 90%, and the literature has shown great inconsistency in the reported sensitivity.[16–18] Reports that do not validate their ultrasonography results may have misleading conclusions.

In addition to the inconsistency and potential inaccuracy in reporting DVT, recent data in the literature suggest that asymptomatic DVT may not be an appropriate surrogate measure for the major efficacy end-point of interest, symptomatic DVT and fatal PE.[19] Although the efficacy of various prophylactic agents in decreasing the rate of asymptomatic DVT has been well documented, it is unclear whether these agents alter the symptomatic expression of thromboembolism. Warwick et al., in a study looking at symptomatic DVT after TKA, found that symptomatic, radiologically confirmed venous thromboembolism was common with a rate of 10.6% in a follow-up study of 1000 consecutive primary TKAs in which 33.9% of patients had chemoprophylaxis. Moreover, this rate was unchanged with or without chemoprophylaxis, with rates of 10.1% and 10.5% respectively.[5]

The significance of these asymptomatic clots also has yet to be fully understood.[20,21] DVTs may occur in an array of sizes and locations in the postoperative period. There may be small clots in the calf, moderate sized clots in the popliteal area, small femoral clots around valve cusps, or large iliofemoral thromboses involving a substantial portion of the proximal venous system. It is believed that each of these clots has a different potential risk for the patient. However, because of the inaccuracies in the diagnosis of clots and the inconsistency in the reporting of the size and location, the significance of DVT in a given location and size has not been well defined.

An example of the difficulty in determining the significance of a clot is the observation that calf thrombi are two and a half times more common after TKA than after total hip arthroplasty (THA).[20] Nevertheless, PE is much less common after TKA. In fact, fatal PE after THA may be as much as seven times more common. One study looking at venous thromboembolism in 5024 THA and TKA patients reported a PE rate after THA of 0.35% compared to 0.05% after TKA.[22] If calf thrombi represent significant risks to patients, one would expect an increased incidence of PE after TKA.

In addition to its location, the size of the lower extremity clot is also significant. It appears that a large clot is necessary to create a symptomatic PE.[23,24] Although the exact size of the clot that creates pulmonary symptoms is yet undetermined, in a recent study describing asymptomatic PE, there was a positive correlation between the size of DVT and the probability of developing asymptomatic PE on ventilation perfusion (V/Q) scan. Although most V/Q scan defects were in patients who were completely asymptomatic, the data indicate that small clots embolize regularly but do not cause symptoms nor appear to have clinical significance until they reach a larger size.[20]

The temporal sequence of postoperative DVT and embolic events has also not been well defined and in theory should effect the duration of thromboprophylaxis. It is generally agreed that clots that are adherent to the endothelium begin to organize, mature, and are less likely to detach to become symptomatic emboli. Many clots are formed within the first 24 h of surgery. One must then speculate on which clots are related to PE and when they were formed. One report on 343 fatal PE cases concluded that the clots formed very quickly in large veins and thus did not have the opportunity to adhere firmly. If large enough they caused a fatal PE.[25] This same report noted that only half the patients with fatal PE had thrombus in their lower extremities. In one study looking at LMWH prophylaxis in knee and hip arthroplasty, the authors noted two deaths from PE which were unlikely to have been preventable except possibly by preoperative prophylaxis.[26] These authors concluded that there was little to gain in extending postoperative prophylaxis.[26] One report in 1000 total knee patients noted only a 1.1% incidence of problems after discharge, which was not significantly different in those with or without prophylaxis while hospitalized. These clots were also of dubious significance and the authors concluded that the risk of thromboembolism is too low to justify extended prophylaxis following discharge and there was no evidence that prolonged prophylaxis would even influence late complications.[4,5] As hospital stays shorten and the length of in-hospital prophylaxis decreases, one must ask whether there is any real clinical benefit compared to known hemorrhagic risks with these agents.

Part of the problem in establishing the significance of size, location, and timing of the thromboembolic events is related to the assumption that data from the internal medicine literature is equally valid for postsurgical patients. When nonoperative patients develop clots—for example patients with congestive heart failure, carcinomatosis or those on oral contraceptives—the clot indicates a coagulopathy predisposing to thromboembolic disease.[24] Although the calf clot itself may not be dangerous, it is a marker for the coagulopathy and the patient at risk for potential PE. Many in the medical community have transferred the significance of a calf clot in a medical patient to the postsurgical patient. However, the prognostic significance of a clot following significant local endothelial injury at the time of surgery may be different. Many patients develop clots but it is unclear which of these clots are reliable markers for the patient at increased risk of PE. Considering 50–80% of patients develop DVT after TKA, while the incidence of fatal PE ranges from 0.05% to 0.2%, it is difficult to determine which of the patients are truly at increased risk from the clot.

## Pulmonary embolism

When discussing prophylaxis for DVT or PE, we are really discussing risks versus benefits. To assess this problem intelligently, we have to know the risks. The greatest risk is fatal PE. It has been assumed that a reduction in asymptomatic DVT with chemoprophylaxis can be extrapolated to a reduction in the rate of fatal PE and overall mortality rate following TKA. This may be a false assumption. Formerly, the fatal PE rate without chemoprophylaxis following total joint arthroplasty was thought to be 3–6%.[27] Recently, however, numerous studies have shown the fatal PE rate to be much lower, ranging from 0.05% to 0.2%. In a meta-analysis of 93 000 patients, Murray et al.[3] found the fatal PE rate in patients who had no chemoprophylaxis to be 0.12%. The fatal PE rate with prophylaxis also averaged 0.12%. He also noted a progressive fall in fatal PE over the past few decades, which he presumed to be due to improved surgical technique, anesthesia, and rehabilitation rather than the increased use of thromboprophylaxis.[3] Ansari et al.[2] reviewed 1390 consecutive TKAs without routine prophylactic anticoagulation except in high-risk cases and found a fatal PE rate of 0.22%. Warwick et al.[5] reported a fatal PE rate of 0.1% in 1000 patients who had undergone primary TKA with only one-third of the patients receiving any chemoprophylaxis. Fender et al. recently found an overall fatal PE rate of 0.19% in 2111 primary THAs. The fatal PE rate in patients with anticoagulation was 0.24% and without anticoagulation was 0.15%, which was not significantly different.[1]

Several other studies looking at various chemoprophylactic regimens have noted similar fatal PE rates. Westrich,[28] in a report on the use of hypotensive epidurals, aspirin, stockings, and early mobilization after TKA, found the incidence of fatal PE was 0.04%. Colwell,[29] in a comparison between a LMWH and warfarin, noted a fatal PE fate of 0.2% in the LMWH group and 0.1% in the warfarin group. Another study by Leclerc et al.,[26] looking at venous thromboembolism during prophylaxis with LMWH, found a fatal PE rate of 0.15%. Sarmiento[30] reported a fatal PE rate of 0.13% in 1492 patients using aspirin, exercise and graded elastic stockings or intermittent compression devices as thromboembolic prophylaxis. Another study by Lieberman et al.[31] using low-dose warfarin for prophylaxis found a fatal PE rate of 0.1%. Lotke et al.[32] reported in a controlled study with aspirin and warfarin that the death rate from PE was 0.15%. The Mayo Clinic, reporting on 5024 patients, found that the death rate from PE in TKA was only 0.05% with all combined methods of prophylaxis.[22]

Additionally, the diagnosis of PE should be clearly demonstrated. However, if the methods by which PE is diagnosed and reported are evaluated, it becomes clear that there may be significant inaccuracies in the data. If all patients believed to have PE by clinical history and examination have a full evaluation, including blood gases, V/Q scans, and/or pulmonary angiography, only 5–20% will truly have had a PE.[33] Therefore, studies depending on clinical evaluation alone may have inaccuracies in their database.

V/Q scans have traditionally been the most accurate method of diagnosing PE. Recently, however, they also have been shown to have significant shortcomings.[33] A large, multi-institutional study on PE concluded that a high-probability scan usually indicates a PE, but only a minority of patients with PE have a high-probability scan. A low-probability scan, with a weak clinical impression of PE, makes the possibility of PE remote, whereas an intermediate probability scan is not of help in establishing a diagnosis. Therefore, the V/Q scan has significant limitations. The pulmonary angiogram is probably the best way to determine the diagnosis of PE but in general has not been used as an end-point in the literature, largely because of its invasive nature.

The recognition of fat embolism after total joint arthroplasty has become particularly important.[34] It is now recognized that this is a significant factor in the postoperative period when a patient has reduced oxygenation and fails to thrive. In the past, these patients were felt to have had a PE, but in reality many had fat embolism syndrome. This entity has certainly affected conclusions regarding PE in the literature. Considering that the clinical diagnosis of PE is unreliable, V/Q scans are often inconclusive, pulmonary angiography is rarely performed, and postoperative fat embolism has only recently been recognized and not considered in earlier reports of PE, it is not surprising that PE has not been well defined in many studies.

## Chemoprophylaxis and bleeding complications

Although PE does represent a threat to patients after TKA, it may be significantly less than previously thought, and must be balanced against the potential risks of thromboprophylactic agents. There are two general types of prophylaxis: chemoprophylactic agents such as LMWH, warfarin, and aspirin, and mechanical aids such as calf or plantar compression devices. The studies noted above have shown no decrease in the fatal PE rate with chemoprophylaxis. Prophylaxis to reduce thromboembolic disease is therefore only justified if the agent does not produce a significant alternative morbidity—bleeding. The more effective the chemoprophylaxis is in preventing clots, the greater the risk of developing a bleeding complication. Most studies in the literature looking at bleeding risk divide bleeds into major and minor. A major bleed is variably defined, but generally includes death, intracranial bleeding or bleeding within a critical organ, transfusion of more than two units of blood, and reoperation because of bleeding. All other bleeding, such as wound hematoma not requiring reoperation, is considered minor bleeding. If we look at the bleeding complications with the use of LMWH, most of the studies show higher bleeding rates than with other methods of anticoagulation. Colwell *et al.*[35] reported on the efficacy and safety of LMWH versus unfractionated heparin. They found a major bleed rate of 1.3% for both, with minor bleed rates of 18.9% and 21.8% respectively. Operative site hemorrhage occurred in 3.9% of patients treated with LMWH and 2.2% of patients treated with unfractionated heparin. An earlier study by Colwell[29] comparing two different doses of LMWH and unfractionated heparin showed an even higher bleed rate. The group that received 30 mg of LMWH every 12 h had a major bleed rate of 4% compared to 1% in the group that received 40 mg of LMWH a day and 6% in the unfractionated heparin group. Spiro *et al.*,[36] in a study comparing three different doses of LMWH, found a major bleed rate of 5% and an overall incidence of hemorrhagic episodes of 13% in the group receiving 30 mg of LMWH every 12 h. Most of the major bleeds occurred at the operative site. Leclerc *et al.* reported bleeding complications in 2.9% of patients treated with LMWH after TKA with the most common being wound hematoma.[26]

There are also several studies looking at the bleeding complications of warfarin. Leclerc,[37] in a study comparing warfarin to LMWH after knee arthroplasty, found a major bleed rate of 1.8% in the warfarin group compared to 2.1% in the LMWH group. Francis *et al.*[38] found a major bleed rate of 1% with warfarin and 2% with LMWH. There was a 4% minor bleed rate with warfarin and a 6% minor bleed rate with LMWH. Of note, the authors in this study found a significant increase in the number of blood transfusions, both whole blood and packed red blood cells, in the LMWH group compared to the warfarin group. In the LMWH group 20% of patients received whole blood transfusions and 48% received packed red cells, compared with 14% whole blood transfusions and 31% packed red blood cell transfusions in the warfarin group. Another study on the efficacy of low-dose warfarin found a major bleed rate of 2.9%.[31] Lotke *et al.*[32] found major bleed rates of less than 1% for both warfarin and aspirin. This was consistent with the Antiplatelet Trialists' Collaboration major bleed rate of 0.7% with aspirin therapy.[39]

A meta-analysis published in *JAMA* compared clinically important bleed rates among multiple chemoprophylactic regimens. They found a rate of 0.3% in the control group, 0.4% for aspirin, 2.6% for unfractionated subcutaneous heparin, 1.8% for LMWH, and 1.3% for warfarin.[40] Warfarin is known to predispose to bleeding especially if prothrombin times become higher than anticipated. Lieberman et al.[31] found that an international normalized ratio (INR) of 1.8 was associated with an increased risk of bleeding, especially wound hematoma. A clinical epidemiology study on anticoagulant-related bleeding showed an average frequency of fatal, major, and major and minor bleeding of 1%, 5%, and 17% with warfarin therapy during an average 1.8 years of treatment. The risk for anticoagulant-related bleeding is highest at the start of therapy. During warfarin therapy, the risk for major bleeding during the first month of therapy is approximately 10 times the risk after the first year of therapy.[41] This information is especially significant for total joint arthroplasty patients who undergo warfarin therapy only for a limited period of time, usually 6 weeks or less. This study also noted the average frequency of fatal, major, and major or minor bleeding during heparin therapy to be 0.05%, 0.8%, and 2%; these frequencies are approximately twice those expected without heparin therapy.[41]

Again, these numbers emphasize the very real risks associated with anticoagulation. Murray et al.,[3] in their meta-analysis on thromboprophylaxis and death after total hip replacement, suggested that prophylaxis would not decrease the fatal PE rate by more than 0.05%. If the death rate due to anticoagulant complications is 0.05% or more, then the use of these agents may actually cause harm. We must keep in mind that we are trying to protect our patients from a 0.1% risk of fatal PE with agents that have much higher major bleed rates and some agents that may have higher death rates. We also cannot discount the significant morbidity associated with wound hematoma, whether reoperation is required or not. Warwick quotes a complication rate of up to 45% with full anticoagulation after a joint replacement and notes a patient in that series who required a local flap and eventually an arthrodesis after developing a wound hematoma during therapeutic anticoagulation.[5] The high transfusion rate seen with some chemoprophylactic agents should also be of concern as transfusion is certainly not without risk. There is as yet no good evidence that any pharmacological agent does more good than harm after routine total joint arthroplasty.[3]

## Aspirin for DVT prophylaxis

Although the argument against routine chemoprophylaxis is convincing, the current medicolegal environment is prohibitive, making the choice of no routine prophylaxis imprudent. Because the risks of many chemoprophylactic regimens are so high, there has been an increased interest in the use of aspirin. It is well known that aspirin inhibits platelet function. In doses less than 100 mg per day, the inhibition is dose dependent. However, if more than 100 mg of aspirin is given per day, there is immediate and complete suppression of platelet aggregation that lasts the entire lifespan of the platelet. In assessing the clinical studies which show the efficacy of aspirin, many have divided them into arterial and venous studies. On the arterial side, aspirin has been shown to reduce the mortality related to unstable angina by 60%, reduce the infarction fate for nonfatal MI by 43%, reduce cerebrovascular accidents (CVA) and transient ischemic attacks (TIA) by 25%, and reduce occlusion of the vascular system following vascular surgery by 50%. On the venous side, the Antiplatelet Trialist Group has shown a significant reduction in DVT and PE with the use of aspirin.[39] They also noted a significantly reduced fatal PE rate, from 0.9% in controls to 0.2% in the aspirin group. Aspirin is also relatively safe, with a major bleed rate of 0.7% compared to 0.4% in controls which did not achieve statistical significance.[39] In looking at all-cause mortality, they noted a trend toward a decrease in all deaths with the use of aspirin.

When comparing aspirin to other prophylactic agents, there is no significant difference in fatal PE rates. Lotke et al.[32] found a fatal PE rate of 0.15% with the use of aspirin following TKA, which is comparable to the Antiplatelet Trialist Group's findings. In addition to a lower rate of bleeding compared to warfarin or LMWH, the use of aspirin may avoid other complications such as thrombocytopenia, skin necrosis, and epidural anesthetic risk. Aspirin has other advantages including ease of use for prolonged periods of time. There is a risk of thromboembolic disease after patients leave the hospital, and the duration of prophylaxis is controversial. The length of hospital stay following TKA is dramatically shortening and it is difficult to adequately administer warfarin in that short time. It is also inconvenient and expensive to administer subcutaneous drugs to outpatients. Aspirin can be easily continued after hospitalization, is effective, inexpensive, well tolerated, relatively safe, and requires no monitoring. In today's cost-conscious health care environment, it may be the best and most logical choice.

## High-risk patients

It may be likely, however, that there is a subgroup of patients that would benefit from more aggressive thromboprophylaxis. This subgroup consists of thrombophilics who have some coagulopathy or prothrombin gene mutation that contributes to their increased risk from thromboembolic disease. The risk of venous thrombosis of the lower extremities is increased by factors that cause hypercoagulability or venous stasis, such as the use of oral contraceptives, pregnancy or the postpartum state, surgery, trauma, prolonged immobilization, or the presence of cancer.[42,43] There are also known molecular causes for thrombophilia, including defects in protein S, protein C, antithrombin, plasminogen and fibrinogen, as well as acquired abnormalities such as the presence of antiphospholipid antibodies.[42,43] More recently, resistance to activated protein C, a newly discovered hereditary trait potentially accounting for a far greater proportion of patients with thromboembolic disorders, has been described.[43] This mutation is in the gene for factor V and is called factor V Leiden. Up to 40% of patients with this mutation develop venous thromboembolism.[43] Another inherited abnormality of the coagulation system, this one in the gene for prothrombin called *G20210A*, has been identified. Next to the mutation in the factor V gene, it is the most common genetic determinant of DVT of the lower extremities.[42] This mutation increases the risk of thrombosis by a factor of 10. There currently is no easy way to screen patients for these inheritable mutations or protein defects, although this may be a focus for the future.

Traditionally there are groups of patients that are believed to have risk factors for postoperative thromboembolism. These include prior thromboembolism (possibly a thrombophilic), advanced age, obesity, malignancy, varicose veins, congestive heart failure, extended operative time, estrogen usage, and bilateral procedures.[44] Only a few have been truly validated. It may be that the only patients who require or should receive routine anticoagulation are the thrombophilics who have known clotting disorders or other risk factors.

## Conclusion

The need for thromboprophylaxis following total joint arthroplasty remains controversial. There is no "best" prophylaxis and each physician must make a choice based on the risks and benefits of the chemoprophylactic agent. A prospective, randomized controlled clinical trial is required to answer the question of the most effective yet safe treatment. However, the outcome of interest, namely fatal PE, has such a low incidence that between 20 000 and 50 000 patients would be required in each arm of the study to detect any difference. The extensive studies needed to demonstrate the small reduction in death rate from this cause might not be worthwhile. Several studies noted in this chapter support the idea of no routine chemoprophylaxis since anticoagulation has shown no reduction in the rate of fatal PE but does have significant potential for harm due to bleeding complications. Today's medico-legal environment makes this an unlikely choice. In the absence of other risk factors, aspirin then becomes a very good alternative for prophylaxis against thromboembolic disease. It is safe, effective, inexpensive, well tolerated, and may actually help prevent non-PE deaths.

## References

1   Fender D; Harper WM, Thompson JR, Gregg PJ: Mortality and fatal
    pulmonary embolism after primary total hip replacement. *Journal
    of Bone and Joint Surgery* [Br] **79**:896–899, 1997.

2   Ansari S, Warwick D, Ackroyd CE, Newman JH: Incidence of fatal pulmonary embolism after 1,390 knee arthroplasties without routine prophylactic anticoagulation, except in high-risk cases. *Journal of Arthroplasty* **12**:599–602, 1997.

3   Murray DW, Britton AR, Bulstrode CJK: Thromboprophylaxis and death after total hip replacement. *Journal of Bone and Joint Surgery* [Br] **78**:863–870, 1996.

4   Warwick D, Williams MH, and Bannister GC: Death and thromboembolic disease after total hip replacement: a series of 1162 cases with no routine chemical prophylaxis. *Journal of Bone and Joint Surgery* [Br] **77**:6–10, 1995.

5   Warwick DJ, Whitehouse S: Symptomatic venous thromboembolism after total knee replacement. *Journal of Bone and Joint Surgery* [Br] **79**:780–786, 1997.

6   Wroblewski BM, Siney PD, White R: Fatal pulmonary embolism after total hip arthroplasty. Seasonal variation. *Clinical Orthopaedics and Related Research* **276**:222–224, 1992.

7   Prentice CRM: Thromboprophylaxis in elective orthopaedic surgery—what is the purpose? *Journal of Bone and Joint Surgery* [Br] **79**:889–890, 1997.

8   International Multicentre Trial: Prevention of fatal postoperative pulmonary embolism by low doses of heparin. *Lancet* **2**:45–51, 1975.

9   Collins R, Scrimgeour A, Yusuf S, Peto R: Reduction in fatal pulmonary embolism and venous thrombosis by perioperative administration of subcutaneous heparin: an overview of results of randomized trials in general, orthopaedic and urological surgery. *New England Journal of Medicine* **18**:1162–1173, 1988.

10  Unwin AJ, Jones JR, Harries WJ: Current UK opinion on thromboprophylaxis in orthopaedic surgery: its use in routine total hip and knee arthroplasty. *Annals of the Royal College of Surgeons of England* **77**:351–354, 1995.

11  Parker-Williams J, Vickers R: Major orthopaedic surgery on the leg and thromboembolism. *BMJ* **303**:531–532, 1991.

12  Lieberman JR, Geerts WH: Prevention of venous thromboembolism after total hip and knee arthroplasty: current concepts review. *Journal of Bone and Joint Surgery* [Am] **76**:1239–1250, 1994.

13  Hull R, Raskob G, Pineo G *et al*. A comparison of subcutaneous low molecular weight heparin with warfarin sodium for prophylaxis against deep venous thrombosis after hip or knee implantation. *New England Journal of Medicine* **329**:1370–1376, 1993.

14  Wille-Jorgenson P, Borris L, Jorgensen LN *et al*. Phlebography as the gold standard in thromboprophylactic studies? A multicenter interobserver variation study. *Acta Radiologica* **33**:24–28, 1992.

15  Grady-Benson JC, Oishi CS, Hanssen PB, *et al*. Postoperative surveillance for deep venous thrombosis for duplex ultrasonography after total knee arthroplasty. *Journal of Bone and Joint Surgery* [Am] **76**:1649–1657, 1994.

16  Ciccone WJ, Fox PS, Neumyer M *et al.*: Ultrasound surveillance for asymptomatic deep venous thrombosis after total joint replacement. *Journal of Bone and Joint Surgery* [Am] **80**:1167–1174, 1998.

17  Davidson BL, Elliot CG, Lensing AWA: RD-heparin arthroplasty group. Low accuracy of color doppler ultrasound in teh detection of proximal leg vein thrombosis in asymptomatic high risk patients. *Annals of Internal Medicine* **117**:735–738, 1992.

18  Garino JP, Lotke PA, Kitziger K, Steinberg MD Deep venous thrombosis after total joint arthroplasty. the role of compression ultrasonography and the importance of the experience of the

technician. *Journal of Bone and Joint Surgery* [Am] **78**:1359–1365, 1996.

19  Clagett GP, Anderson FA Jr., Geerts W *et al.*: Prevention of venous thromboembolism. *Chest* **114**:531S–560S, 1998.

20  Lotke PA, Steinberg MD, Ecker ML Significance of deep venous thrombosis in the lower extremity after total joint arthroplasty. *Clinical Orthopaedics and Related Research* **299**:25–30, 1994.

21  Haas SB, Tribus CB, Insall JN *et al.* The significance of calf thrombi after total knee arthroplasty. *Journal of Bone and Joint Surgery* [Br] **74**:799–802, 1992.

22  Mohr DN, Silverstein MC, Ilstrup DM *et al.*: Venous thromboembolism associated with hip and knee arthroplasty: current prophylactic practices and outcomes. *Mayo Clinic Proceedings* **67**:861–870, 1992.

23  Foley M, Maslack MM, Rothman RH *et al.*: Course of pulmonary embolism. *Radiology* **172**:481–485, 1989.

24  Carson J, Kelley MA, Duff A *et al.*: The clinical course of pulmonary embolism. *New England Journal of Medicine* **326**:1240–1245, 1992.

25  Priestly JT, Barker NW: Postoperative thrombosis and embolism. *Surgical Gynecology and Obstetrics* **75**:193–201, 1942.

26  Leclerc JR, Gent M, Hirsh J *et al.*: The incidence of symptomatic venous thromboembolism during and after prophylaxis with enoxaparin: a multi-institutional cohort study of patients who underwent hip or knee arthroplasty. *Archives of Internal Medicine* **158**:873–878, 1998.

27  Clagett GP, Anderson FA Jr., Heit J *et al.*: Prevention of vvenous thromboembolism. *Chest* 108S:312S–334S, 1995.

28  Westrich GH, Sculco TP: Prophylaxis against deep venous thrombosis after total knee arthroplasty. Pneumatic plantar compression and aspirin compared with aspirin alone. *Journal of Bone and Joint Surgery* [Am] **78**:826–834, 1996.

29  Colwell CW Jr., Spiro TE, Trowbridge AA *et al.* Use of enoxaparin, a low-molecular-weight heparin, and unfractionated heparin for the prevention of deep venous thrombosis after elective hip replacement. *Journal of Bone and Joint Surgery* [Am] **76**:3–14, 1994.

30  Sarmiento A, Goswami ADK. Thromboembolic prophylaxis with use of aspirin, exercise, and graded elastic stockings or intermittent compression devices in patients managed with total hip arthroplasty. *Journal of Bone and Joint Surgery* [Am] **81**:339–346, 1999.

31  Lieberman JR, Wollaeger J, Dorey F *et al.*: The efficacy of prophylaxis with low-dose warfarin for prevention of pulmonary embolism following total hip arthroplasty. *Journal of Bone and Joint Surgery* [Am] **79**:319–325, 1997.

32  Lotke PA, Rees HW, Beck TD *et al.*: Incidence of fatal pulmonary embolism after total knee arthroplasty with aspirin prophylaxis. Scientific presentation, American Academy of Orthopaedic Surgeons Annual Meeting, Anaheim, 1998.

33  PIOPED Investigators. Value of the ventilation/perfusion scan in acute pulmonary embolism: results of the prospective investigation of pulmonary embolism diagnosis. *JAMA* **263**:2753–2795, 1990.

34  Johnson JM, Lucas GL: Fat embolism syndrome. Review. *Orthopaedics* **19**:41–49, 1996.

35  Colwell CW Jr., Spiro TE, Trowbridge AA *et al.*: Efficacy and safety of enoxaparin versus unfractionated heparin for prevention of deep venous thrombosis after elective knee arthroplasty. *Clinical Orthopaedics and Related Research* **321**:19–27, 1995.

36  Spiro TE, Johnson GJ, Christie MJ *et al.*: Efficacy and safety of enoxaparin to prevent deep venous thrombosis after hip replacement surgery. *Annals of Internal Medicine* **121**:81–89, 1994.

37  Leclerc JR, Geerts WH, Desjardins L *et al.*: Prevention of venous thromboembolism after knee arthroplasty: a randomized, double-blind trial comparing enoxaparin with warfarin. *Annals of Internal Medicine* **124**:619–626, 1996.

38  Francis CW, Pellegrini VD Jr., Totterman S *et al.*: Prevention of deep-vein thrombosis after total hip arthroplasty: comparison of warfarin and dalteparin. *Journal of Bone and Joint Surgery* [Am] **79**:1365–1372, 1997.

39  Antiplatelet Trialists' Collaboration. Collaborative review of randomised trials of antiplatelet therapy–III: reduction in venous thrombosis and pulmonary embolism by antiplatelet prophylaxis among surgical and medical patients. *BMJ* **308**:235–246, 1994.

40  Imperiale TF, Speroff T A meta-analysis of methods to prevent venous thromboembolism following total hip replacement. *JAMA* **271**:1780–1785, 1994.

41  Landefeld CS, Beyth RJ: Anticoagulant-related bleeding: clinical epidemiology, prediction, and prevention. *American Journal of Medicine* **95**:315–328, 1993.

42  Martinelli I, Sacchi E, Landi G *et al.*: High risk of cerebral-vein thrombosis in carriers of a prothrombin-gene mutation and in users of oral contraceptives. *New England Journal of Medicine* **338**:1793–1797, 1998.

43  Simioni P, Prandoni P, Lensing AWA *et al.*: The risk of recurrent venous thromboembolism in patients with an arg506 to gln mutation in the gene for factor V (factor V Leiden). *New England Journal of Medicine* **336**:399–403, 1997.

44  Della Valle CJ, Steiger DJ, Di Cesara PE: Thromboembolism after hip and knee arthroplasty: diagnosis and treatment. *Journal of the American Academy of Orthopaedic Surgeons* **6**:327–336, 1998.

# Con: Geoffrey H. Westrich

Patients who undergo elective TKA are at a high risk for the development of a DVT, which can potentially lead to a fatal PE. The incidence of DVT after TKA has been reported to be 50–88%.[1-3] DVT following TKA occurs commonly in the calf, and is observed more often after bilateral than unilateral TKA. Isolated proximal DVT is infrequent after TKA, unlike THA. Propagation of thrombosis in the veins of the calf proximally into the popliteal and femoral venous system is well documented, and is the causative factor for the majority of fatal PE after TKA. Although the majority of DVTs occur in the calf veins and resolve without symptoms, up to 24% may propagate to the proximal veins.[2]

In addition, there is a known association between DVT and PE. In TKA, Haas *et al.*[4] reported a 1.9% incidence of asymptomatic PE in patients with a negative venogram and 6.4% incidence of asymptomatic PE in patients with a positive venogram. Symptomatic PE was noted in 0.2% of patients with a negative venogram and 1.6% of patients with a positive venogram. Similarly, Lotke[5] (see Chapter 10, "Pro") noted an association between the location of a DVT diagnosed by venography and the incidence of PE diagnosed by V/Q scan. Lotke found that the incidence of asymptomatic PE was 9% with a negative venogram, 19% with a small DVT, 42% with a large DVT, and 50% with a proximal DVT. Lotke noted a direct correlation with the location of a DVT and the development of a PE.

In spite of the above, the occurrence of clinically significant PE is relatively uncommon and the symptoms are easily confused with other cardiac or pulmonary conditions found in an older population. The incidence of PE detected by routine lung scans has been reported to be 7–17%.[1,2] The reported incidence of symptomatic PE is generally reported to be 1–3%,[4,6] but this is probably an underestimation since many PE do not occur until several weeks or even months after surgery.

Clearly, prevention is the best solution for thromboembolic disease. This is especially true if one considers the potential hemorrhagic risks involved in the treatment of early proximal deep vein thrombosis and PE. Paterson et al.[7] reported that intravenous heparin therapy used within the first 5 days following total joint replacement surgery was associated with a 51% complication rate. However, the morbidity and mortality associated with untreated symptomatic PE and proximal DVT is also high.[8]

## Prophylactic regimens

The ultimate goal of any prophylactic regimen is to prevent not only the formation of a DVT, but also the occurrence of symptomatic or fatal PE. However, the incidence of symptomatic and fatal PE is low, and as a result, a definitive evaluation of the various prophylaxis regimens would require many thousands of patients. Therefore, most studies have focused on the prevention of DVT. Although there are limitations in this methodology, studies have shown that DVT places a patient at risk for PE.[9,10] Numerous prophylactic regimens have been studied in orthopedic surgery and include pharmacological agents such as warfarin, LMWH and aspirin as well as mechanical devices such as compression stockings and foot pumps.

### Warfarin

Warfarin has become a popular form of prophylaxis following orthopedic surgery. It is an oral anticoagulant that inhibits the blood coagulation cascade by affecting the synthesis of active Vitamin K-dependent coagulation factors (factors 2,7,9 and 10 as well as protein C). Since warfarin inhibits synthesis of active coagulation factors, it has no effect on existing circulating coagulation factors. Therapeutic anticoagulation is reached 24–72 h after the initial dose of warfarin. Most commonly 5 or 10 mg of warfarin is started the night before or the night of surgery and then dosing is adjusted to maintain an INR of 2.0–2.5.

Risks of using warfarin include bleeding and less frequently, warfarin-induced skin necrosis. Bleeding complications have been reported in 0–4% of patients receiving warfarin prophylaxis.[11–13] Another pitfall associated with the use of warfarin is the need to monitor the prothrombin time. The advantages of warfarin prophylaxis are that warfarin is administered orally and that it can be continued as treatment if DVT is detected.

As with most prophylactic regimens, the incidence of DVT using low-dose warfarin depends considerably on the patient population at risk. Although warfarin appears to be an effective agent in reducing the incidence of DVT after THA, its efficacy in knee replacement surgery is not clear. Warfarin may limit propagation and embolization of a thrombus after TKA, but it has not clearly been shown to decrease the occurrence of DVT.

## Low molecular weight heparin

LMWHs are a relatively new form of prophylaxis that has been popularized in Europe and is currently being evaluated in the USA. They were was developed in the 1970s and has been shown to have very good antithrombotic activity. When compared to standard heparin, the LMWHs have less bleeding per unit of equivalent antithrombotic effect. LMWHs are fractionated forms of heparin, with a molecular weight of 4000–6000 Da. There are several LMWH compounds produced by various pharmaceutical companies, each differing in its fractionation technique and dosing schedule. However, all LMWHs contain a specific tetrasaccharide that binds antithrombin III. Because of their smaller size they can bind antithrombin III and this complex can inactivate coagulation factor Xa, and to a lesser extent, factor IIa. Their small size also inhibits their combining with heparin cofactor II, a specific mediator that inactivates factor IIa. These compounds have a high bioavailability at low doses, unlike standard heparin, since they only bind to one circulating protein. LMWHs are administered in a fixed dose without daily monitoring of partial thromboplastin time.

Currently only Enoxaparin (Rhone Poulenc Rorer) is approved by the FDA for DVT prophylaxis in patients undergoing orthopedic surgery or trauma. Dalteparin (Upjohn) is approved by the FDA for general surgical use, but has not yet been approved for orthopedic surgery at this time. The advantages of a LMWH is that it is easily administered in the hospital by subcutaneous injection, and does not require monitoring with partial thromboplastin times. Risks associated with LMWH use include bleeding and heparin-induced thrombocytopenia. Major bleeding complications have been reported in 0–2.8% of patients. Other disadvantages are that it is relatively expensive, requires self-injection or help with injection if administered following discharge, and has a known associated risk of bleeding.

## Aspirin

Aspirin (acetylsalicylic acid) is a nonsteroidal anti-inflammatory agent that irreversibly inhibits the cyclo-oxygenase of platelets, thereby inhibiting the synthesis of thromboxane $A_2$.[14] Thromboxane $A_2$ causes platelet aggregation and vasoconstriction. Aspirin has been reported to be an effective antithrombotic agent in patients with ischemic heart disease and cerebrovascular disease. It gained much popularity as a prophylactic modality in orthopedic patients after early reports of success in THA.[14] Follow-up reports and further evaluation, however, revealed that aspirin is not an effective agent in preventing DVT in patients who had total joint replacement surgery or trauma.

Some authors have recommended the continued use of aspirin after hospital discharge as a secondary prophylactic agent.[5] These authors note that aspirin is safe and associated with a low rate of PE, and most thrombi that occur with the use of aspirin are found in the calf veins. Risks of using aspirin include gastritis, gastric erosions, and gastric ulcers. These side-effects appear to be dose related. Most regimens employ aspirin by mouth, 325–650 mg twice daily.

We do not routinely use aspirin as a single prophylactic agent after major knee surgery; however, we have noted that when aspirin is combined with mechanical compression, routine venographic screening, and treatment of detected thrombi, it is associated with a low rate of symptomatic and fatal pulmonary emboli.

## Mechanical devices

Mechanical devices and physical agents have been used for the prophylaxis of DVT after a variety of surgical procedures or trauma. Devices currently on the market incorporate different parameters such as foot pumps, foot–calf pumps, calf pumps, and calf–thigh pumps; some are single chamber, but others have a number sequential chambers. Although the optimal characteristics of these pumps to reduce DVT and PE are not yet known, it has been proposed that pneumatic compression devices act by two mechanisms: decreased stasis (accelerated venous emptying) and increased fibrinolysis.[15–36] Newer devices that produce impulse pumping, as opposed to a slow rise in venous return, have recently been introduced, and although some of these devices are thought to produce an increased peak venous velocity, it is unclear what is the optimal contribution of increased venous velocity or increased venous volume necessary to provide adequate DVT prophylaxis in the leg.[15,17,18,20–25,27,30,33,35,37,38]

Intermittent pneumatic devices include polyvinyl boots or leggings, stockings with inflatable bladders, multi-compartment vinyl leggings, and more recently foot pumps.[39,40] Generally pressures reach 35–55 mm Hg and inflate in cycles of 60–90 s. The devices are intended to decrease stasis by augmenting venous flow in the legs. In addition, studies have shown stimulation of the fibrinolytic system with the intermittent compression.[12]

The boot or stockings can be applied to the nonoperative leg preoperatively and postoperatively begun on the operative leg. The pneumatic devices are continued until the patient is walking independently. The pneumatic devices can also be used in conjunction with continuous passive motion. The incidence of DVT with the use of calf- and thigh-length devices has been reported to be 7.5–33% after unilateral TKA.[23,41–46] Haas et al.[47] evaluated the efficacy of a multi-chamber thigh-length pneumatic compression stockings compared to aspirin in a randomized prospective study and found that the incidence of DVT was reduced to 22% with pneumatic stockings compared to 47% with aspirin. The greatest reduction was seen in large thrombi (greater than 6 cm) which were reduced from 31% with aspirin to 6% with the pneumatic stockings. Patients undergoing simultaneous bilateral TKA are at even higher risk for development of DVT: despite the use of pneumatic compression stockings, 48% of these patients developed a DVT.

Woolson et al.[48] conducted a prospective study of the prevalence of proximal DVT in TKA patients who had prophylaxis for thrombosis with a combination of low-dose warfarin and intermittent pneumatic compression. They studied 297 who underwent 377 consecutive TKAs. All patients were treated with low-dose warfarin and intermittent pneumatic compression using thigh-high sleeves. Surveillance for proximal thrombosis was done by duplex ultrasonography. Proximal thrombosis was detected in 19 patients, for a prevalence of 5%. There were 3 patients who had a major bleeding complication, giving a prevalence of 0.9% for the 337 procedures performed. Although there was no concurrent control group of patients treated with another means of prophylaxis to compare with these patients, the low prevalence of proximal thrombosis and the low risk of major bleeding complications that was found indicates the safety and efficacy of intermittent pneumatic compression with low-dose warfarin.

Grady-Benson et al.[25] studied 100 patients who had had a TKA and had been managed with pneumatic compression stockings and aspirin for prophylaxis against DVT. These patients had screening of both legs with duplex ultrasonography on the 4th postoperative day. Duplex ultrasonography demonstrated proximal DVT in 7 patients (7%) and distal DVT in 22 patients (22%); all 29 patients were asymptomatic. The patients who had distal DVT had surveillance with serial duplex ultrasonography on the 7th and 14th postoperative days; 5 of these patients were found to have had propagation of the thrombosis to the proximal deep veins.

In 1959, Lovgren and Rastgeldi first evaluated intermittent pneumatic pedal compression. Henry and Winsor continued the research in the 1960s. In the 1970s, Gaskell and Parrott used a pneumatic foot pump to increase blood flow to the foot in patients with compromised vasculature. In 1983, Gardner and Fox described a physiologic venous foot pump in the sole of the foot involving the venae comitans of the lateral plantar artery.[49] This "pump" has a 20 ml stroke volume that empties only through the deep venous system, and is activated solely on weight bearing.[49]

Pneumatic compression devices that compress the plantar plexus are starting to gain appeal because the range of applicability is increased and is not influenced by any postoperative dressing or external immobilization. The compliance from both nurses and patients has seemingly improved, owing to the simplicity and comfort of the devices. The stroke volume of these devices is relatively small, approximately 30 ml, and the increase in peak venous velocity in the common femoral vein is considerably less than devices that pump the calf, specifically the soleal sinus. However, the foot pumps are capable of generating a 250% increase in peak venous velocity in the popliteal vein, and this may explain their efficacy.

Studies have shown that these devices can lead to a significant increase in venous flow in the leg.[21] Two studies have evaluated foot pumps in knee replacement. Westrich and Sculco evaluated the efficacy of the PlexiPulse (NuTech, San Antonio, TX) device combined with aspirin compared to aspirin alone.[50] The authors found a significant reduction in DVT with the use of a PlexiPulse; 27% of patients using the PlexiPulse developed a DVT compared to 59% with aspirin alone. No patient using the PlexiPulse developed proximal thrombi, but 14% of the patients using aspirin alone were found to have proximal thrombi. Westrich also evaluated compliance and found a relationship between DVT and the duration for which the device was used. Wilson et al.[40] evaluated the efficacy of foot compression after TKA. They found a significant reduction in proximal thrombi; 19% in the control group compared to 0% with foot pumps. The foot pump devices appear to be well tolerated and we are now using them routinely on our knee replacement patients at Hospital for Special Surgery.

## Meta-analysis data

A meta-analysis was performed at Hospital for Special Surgery to assess the efficacy of four common modalities of thromboembolic prophylaxis after TKA: intermittent pneumatic compression, warfarin, aspirin, and LMWH.[51] All published studies in the English literature in which TKA was performed on patients who were postoperatively assessed for DVT were reviewed. Only papers that used routine venography to assess DVT and perfusion lung scan, V/Q lung scan, or angiography to assess PE were included. The study identified and reviewed 136 articles and abstracts, and a total of 23 studies (6001 patients) were included in the analysis.

The incidence of DVT was 53% in the aspirin group, 45% in the warfarin group, 29% in the LMWH group, and 17% in the pneumatic compression device group. Intermittent pneumatic compression devices and LMWH were significantly better than warfarin ($p < 0.0001$) or aspirin ($p < 0.0001$) in preventing deep vein thrombosis. Warfarin was significantly better than aspirin ($p < 0.0001$) in preventing DVT. There was no statistically significant difference

**Table 10.1** Meta-analysis results (figures are percentages)

| Type of prophylaxis | DVT | Asymptomatic PE | Symptomatic PE |
| --- | --- | --- | --- |
| Aspirin | 53 | 11.7 | 1.3 |
| Warfarin | 45 | 8.2 | 0.4 |
| LMWH | 29 | not available | 0.5 |
| IPCD | 17 | 6.3 | 0 |

IPCD, intermittent pneumatic compression device; LMWH, low molecular weight heparin.

between LMWH and intermittent pneumatic compression prophylaxis (Table 10.1).

In assessing asymptomatic pulmonary emboli, the incidence with aspirin was 11.7%, warfarin 8.2%, and pneumatic compression 6.3%. No studies with LMWH used routine lung scans, so the rate of symptomatic PE was not evaluated. Warfarin and pneumatic compression were significantly better than aspirin in preventing asymptomatic PE ($p < 0.05$). No statistically significant difference was noted between warfarin and pneumatic compression (Table 10.1).

In assessing symptomatic pulmonary emboli, the incidence with aspirin was 1.3%, warfarin 0.4%, LMWH 0.5%, and a pneumatic compression device 0%. No statistically significant difference was noted between the above prophylaxis modalities due to the very small incidence of symptomatic PE in each group (Table 10.1).

## Conclusion

Aspirin alone for the prophylaxis of DVT after TKA is clearly not appropriate. Numerous studies have documented a very high incidence of DVT with aspirin alone, and a direct correlation between DVT and PE is well documented. Mechanical prophylaxis offers several advantages over pharmacological prophylaxis in that it is safe, efficacious, and maybe more cost-effective. According to the current literature, intermittent pneumatic compression devices are the most effective modality in preventing the occurrence of DVT after TKA. Both intermittent pneumatic compression devices and warfarin may also be better than aspirin in reducing the incidence of PE. Large, prospective randomized trials are needed to identify the benefit of combining prophylactic regimens.

## References

1    Lotke PA, Ecker ML, Alavi A, Berkowitz H: Indications for the treatment of deep venous thrombosis following total knee replacement. *Journal of Bone and Joint Surgery* [Am] **66**:202–208, 1984.

2    McKenna R, Bachmann F, Kaushal SP, Galante JO: Thromboembolic disease in patients undergoing total knee replacement. *Journal of Bone and Joint Surgery* [Am] **58**:928–932, 1976.

3   Stulberg BN, Insall JN, Williams GW, Ghelman B: Deep-vein throm-
    bosis following total knee replacement. An analysis of six hundred
    and thirty-eight arthroplasties. *Journal of Bone and Joint Surgery*
    **66**:194–201, 1984.

4   Haas SB, Tribus CB, Insall JN *et al.*: The significance of calf thrombi
    after total knee arthroplasty. *Journal of Bone and Joint Surgery* [Br]
    **74**:799–802, 1992.

5   Lotke PA: *Aspirin prophylaxis for thromboembolic disease*. CV Mosby, St.
    Louis, 1995.

6   Lieberman JR, Huo M, Hanaway J *et al.*: The prevalence of deep
    venous thrombosis after total hip arthroplasty with hypotensive
    epidural anesthesia. *Journal of Bone and Joint Surgery* [Am]
    **76**:341–348, 1994.

7   Patterson BM, Marchand R, Ranawat C: Complications of heparin
    therapy after total joint arthroplasty. *Journal of Bone and Joint
    Surgery* [Am] **71**:1130–1134, 1989.

8   Barritt DW, Jordan SC, Brist MB: Anticoagulant drugs in the treat-
    ment of pulmonary embolism: A controlled trial. *Lancet*
    **18**:1309–1312, 1960.

9   Clagett GP, Reisch JS: Prevention of venous thrombosis in general sur-
    gical patients. Results of meta-analysis. *Annals of Surgery* 208–227,
    1988.

10  Paiement GD, Bell D, Wessinger SJ: New advances in prevention, diag-
    nosis, and cost effectiveness of venous thromboembolic disease in
    patients with total hip replacement. In *The hip*, Proceedings of the
    Fourteenth Open Scientific Meeting of the Hip Society,
    pp. 94–119. CV Mosby, St. Louis, 1987.

11  Bern MM, Lokich JJ, Wallach SR: Very low doses of warfarin can
    prevent thrombosis in central venous catheters. A randomized
    prospective trial. *Annals of Internal Medicine* **112**:423–428,
    1990.

12  Knight MTN, Dawson R: Effect of intermittent compression of the
    arms on deep venous thrombosis in the legs. *Lancet* **ii**:1265–1267,
    1976.

13  Wells PS, Lensing AWA, Hirsch J: Graduated compression stockings in
    the prevention of postoperative venous thromboembolism. *Archives
    of Internal Medicine* **154**:67–71, 1994.

14  Hirsh J, Salzman EW, Harker L: Aspirin and other platelet active
    drugs: Relationship among dose, effectiveness and side effects.
    *Chest* **95**:12s–16s, 1989.

15  Agnelli G: Anticoagulation in the prevention and treatment of pul-
    monary embolism. *Chest* **107**:39S–44S, 1995.

16  Cade JF: High risk of the critically ill for venous thromboembolism.
    *Critical Care Medicine* **10**:448–450, 1982.

17  Carter CA, Skoutakis VA, Spiro TE: Enoxaparin: The low-molecular-
    weight heparin for prevention of postoperative thromboembolic
    complications. *Annals of Pharmacotherapy* **27**:1223–1230, 1993.

18  Collignon F, Frydman A, Caplain H: Comparison of the pharmacoki-
    netic profiles of three low molecular mass heparins: dalteparin,
    enoxaparin, and nadroparin administered subcutaneously in
    healthy volunteers (doses for prevention of thromboembolism).
    *Thrombosis and Haemostasis* **73**:630–640, 1995.

19  Donaldson GA, Williams C, Scannel JG: A reappraisal of the applica-
    tion of the Trendelenburg operation to massive fatal embolism:
    Report of a successful pulmonary-artery thrombectomy using a
    cardiopulmonary bypass. *New England Journal of Medicine*
    **268**:171–174, 1963.

20 Frampton JE, Faulds D: Pamaparin: a review of its pharmacology, and clinical application in the prevention and treatment of thromboembolic and other vascular disorders. *Drugs* **47**:652–676, 1994.

21 Friedel HA, Balfour JA: Tinzaparin: a review of its pharmacology and clinical potential in the prevention and treatment of thromboembolic disorders. *Drugs* **48**:638–660, 1994.

22 Garlund B: Randomised, controlled trial of low-dose heparin for prevention of fatal pulmonary embolism in patients with infectious diseases. *Lancet* **347**:1357–1361, 1996.

23 Geerts WH, Code KI, Jay RM *et al.*: A prospective study of venous thromboembolism after major trauma. *New England Journal of Medicine* **331**:1601–1606, 1994.

24 Geerts WH, Jay RM, Code KI: A comparison of low-dose heparin with low-molecular-weight heparin as prophylaxis against venous thromboembolism after major trauma. *New England Journal of Medicine* **335**:701–707, 1996.

25 Grady-Benson JC, Oishi CS, Hannson PB *et al.*: Postoperative surveillance for deep venous thrombosis with duplex ultrasound after total knee arthroplasty. *Journal of Bone and Joint Surgery* [Am] **76**:1649–1657, 1994.

26 Green D, Chen D, Chmiel JS: Prevention of thromboembolism in spinal cord injury: role of low-molecular weight heparin. *Archives of Physical Medicine and Rehabilitation* **75**:290–292, 1995.

27 Halkin H, Goldberg J, Modan M: Reduction of mortality in general medical inpatients by low-dose heparin prophylaxis. *Annals of Internal Medicine* **96**:561–565, 1982.

28 Hamilton MD, Hull RD, Pineo GF: Prophylaxis of venous thromboembolism in brain tumor patients. *Journal of Neurooncology* **22**:111–1289, 1994.

29 Howell R, Fidler J, Letsky E: The risks of antenatal subcutaneous heparin prophylaxis: a controlled trial. *British Journal of Obstetrics and Gynaecology* **90**:1124–1128, 1983.

30 Janku GV, Paiement GD, Green HD: Prevention of venous thromboembolism in orthopaedics in the United States. *Clinical Orthopaedics* **325**:313–321, 1996.

31 Jorgensen LN, Willie-Jörgensen P, Hauch O: Prophylaxis of postoperative thromboebolism with low molecular weight heparins. *British Journal of Surgery* **80**:689–704, 1993.

32 Kakkar VV, Cohen AT, Edmonson RA: Low molecular weight versus standard heparin for prevention of venous thromboembolism after major abdominal surgery. *Lancet* **341**:259–265, 1993.

33 Keane MG, Ingenito FP, Goldhaber SZ: Utilization of venous prophylaxis in the medical intensive care unit. *Chest* **106**:13–14, 1994.

34 Keith SL, McLaughlin DJ, Anderson FA: Do graduated compression stocking and pneumatic boots have additive effect on the peak velocity of venous blood flow? *Archives of Surgery* **127**:727–730, 1992.

35 Noble S, Peters DH, Goa KL: Enoxaparin: a reappraisal of its pharmacology and clinical applications in the prevention and treatment of thromboembolic disease. *Drugs* **49**:388–410, 1995.

36 Ziomek S, Read RC, Tobler HG: Thromboembolism in patients undergoing thoracotomy. Annals of Thoracic Surgery **56**:223–227, 1993.

37 Barbour LA, Pickard J: Controversies in thromboembolic disease during pregnancy: a critical review. *Obstetrics and Gynecology* **86**:621–633, 1995.

38  Westrich GH, Specht LM, Sharrock NE, Windsor RE: Venous haemo-
    dynamics after total knee arthroplasty. *Journal of Bone and Joint
    Surgery* [Br] **80**:1057–1066, 1998.

39  Tarnay TJ, Rohr PR, Davidson AG *et al.* Pneumatic calf compression,
    fibrinolysis, and the prevention of deep venous thrombosis. *Surgery*
    **88**:489–496, 1980.

40  Wilson NV, Das SK, Kakkar VV *et al.* Thrombo-embolic prophylaxis in
    total knee replacement. Evaluation of the A-V impulse system.
    *Journal of Bone and Joint Surgery* [Br] **74**:1992.

41  Graor RA, Davis AW, Borden LS, Young J: Comparative evaluation of
    deep vein thrombosis prophylaxis in total joint replacement
    patients. Presented at AAOS, Las Vegas, 1989.

42  Hodge WA: Warfarin and sequential calf compression in the prevention
    of deep vein thrombi following total knee replacement. Presented
    at the Knee Society, Las Vegas, 1989.

43  Hood RW, Flawn LB, Insall JN: The use of pulsatile compression
    stockings in total knee replacement for prevention of venous
    thromboembolism: A prospective study. Presented at the ORS,
    New Orleans, 1982.

44  Hull R, Delmore TJ, Hirsh J, Gent M *et al.*: Effectiveness of intermit-
    tent pulsatile elastic stockings for the prevention of calf and thigh
    vein thrombosis in patients undergoing elective knee surgery.
    *Thrombosis Research* **16**:37–45, 1979.

45  Kaempffe FA, Lifeso RM, Meinding C: Intermittent pneumatic com-
    pression versus coumadin: Prevention of deep vein thrombosis in
    lower-extremity total joint arthroplasty. *Clinical Orthopedics*
    **269**:79–89, 1991.

46  Lynch JA, Baker PL, Polly RE: Mechanical measures in the propylaxis
    of post-operative thromboembolism in total knee arthroplasty.
    *Clinical Orthopedics* **260**:24–29, 1990.

47  Haas SB, Insall JN, Scuderi GR *et al.*: Pneumatic sequential-compres-
    sion boots compared with aspirin prophylaxis of deep-vein throm-
    bosis after total knee arthroplasty. *Journal of Bone and Joint Surgery*
    [Am] **72**:27–31, 1990.

48  Woolson ST, Robinson RK, Khan NQ *et al.*: Deep venous thrombosis
    prophylaxis for knee replacement: Warfarin and pneumatic com-
    pression. *American Journal of Orthopedics* **27**:299–304, 1998.

49  Gardner AM, Fox RH: The venous pump of the human foot-prelimi-
    nary report. *Bristol Medical-Chirurgical Journal* **98**:109–112, 1983.

50  Westrich GH, Sculco TP: Prophylaxis against deep vein thrombosis
    after total knee arthroplasty. Pneumatic plantar compression and
    aspirin compared to aspirin alone. *Journal of Bone and Joint Surgery*
    [Am] **78**:826, 1996.

51  Westrich GH, Haas SB, Mosca P, Peterson M: Meta-analysis of throm-
    boembolic prophylaxis after total knee arthroplasty. *Journal of Bone
    and Joint Surgery* [Br] **82**:795–8000, 2000.

## Questions and answers

*Moderator:* Dr. Westrich, if a relative of yours were having a TKA,
what would you like to have as the thromboembolic prophylaxis?
We will assume that he is 72 years old and has no prior history of
thromboembolic disease.

*Dr. Westrich:* First and foremost I would recommend a pneumatic
compression device. At Hospital for Special Surgery we have had

great success with pneumatic foot compression with PlexiPulse. This device would be applied immediately after surgery and begun in the recovery room. I would also use an additional prophylaxis agent for an additive or synergistic effect. If screening with Doppler ultrasound were to be utilized in the postoperative period, then I would feel comfortable with a pneumatic compression device with aspirin. Should the Doppler test be negative, then I would continue aspirin for approximately 4 weeks after surgery. However, if the Doppler revealed a DVT, then I would discontinue the aspirin and use warfarin. Due to cost containment issues in many centers, routine postoperative screening is not utilized, and therefore, I would recommend a pneumatic compression device such as the PlexiPulse foot pump in conjunction with warfarin as an anticoagulant. In this scenario warfarin would be started the night of surgery and continued for 4 weeks postoperatively.

*Moderator:* Let's expand on that, Dr. Westrich. Do you think that there is sufficient data to suggest using mechanical means alone as a prophylaxis method?

*Dr. Westrich:* Although I do think that there is significant data to warrant pneumatic compression alone during the patient's hospitalization, I am always concerned with the very few patients that may develop a DVT after hospital discharge. At this point most people are ambulatory and would not be using a pneumatic compression device. The oral anticoagulants are utilized after hospital discharge, but I do not feel they are very effective while the patient is in the hospital, since these medications take several days to approach therapeutic levels.

*Moderator:* What is your response to that question, Dr. Lotke?

*Dr. Lotke:* I really think that chemoprophylaxis does reduce the incidence of DVT in the calf, but this comes at the risk of increasing bleeding. Since there is no evidence to show that DVT is an accurate marker for the patient at risk for PE, it does not seem reasonable to expose all the patients to increased bleeding in order to reduce the incidence of DVT without evidence that this also will reduce the risk of PE. The incidence of symptomatic and fatal PE appears to be the same whether the patients are on chemoprophylaxis or not. Therefore, the ability to reduce clots in the leg may not be worth the risk of the increased morbidity from increased bleeding complications.

The mechanical methods, on the other hand are an interesting way to reduce the incidence of DVT without the risk of bleeding. Unfortunately they have never been shown to reduce the incidence of PE. There are several problems with mechanical boots which should be addressed. These problems include the compliance of the patient and the duration of their use during hospitalization. Furthermore, it is unknown whether these devices actually reduce the incidence of PE that occur 3–4 weeks after surgery. Although there is no data to show that the boots offer any protection against

PE, they are relatively inexpensive, and have no complications associated with them. Therefore, they may offer some protection in the medicolegal environment in which we currently live.

*Moderator:* Dr. Lotke, you have mentioned the possibility of renal toxicity or allergic reactions to the dyes used in venography. Don't the nonanionic dyes obviate this problem?

*Dr. Lotke:* Yes, the nonanionic dyes reduce the problems with the venogram, but this question really relates to the best methods to establish a diagnosis of DVT with minimal patient discomfort. At first response, the answer appears simple, i.e., diagnosing DVT should be done with the least toxic and minimally evasive technique available. However, two considerations are very important when ordering a study to establish the diagnosis of a DVT. First, what is the accuracy of the study that is being used to determine the presence of a DVT, and secondly, what is the response of the surgeon to the results of the study. Venography is used infrequently at present because of the patient inconvenience, the potential for toxicity, even with nonanionic dyes, and the cost. It still remains the gold standard, however because a DVT can be well visualized and quantified. In actual practice, however, Doppler ultrasonography is replacing contrast venography. Ultrasonography is a very attractive testing method, because of patient acceptance and absence of toxicity. The surgeon should be aware, however, that the accuracy of ultrasonography can vary broadly from 0–90%. The surgeon should therefore know the reliability of the technician who is performing the study. It has been demonstrated that for scientific purposes the unpredictable accuracy in ultrasonography makes it a rather unreliable tool; for clinical problems, however, it may be acceptable.

The second question, which is probably more important, is how do we respond to the results of whatever study we are obtaining. It is generally believed that DVTs are not accurate surrogate markers for the patients at risk for thromboembolic disease. Therefore, when you obtain the study, the surgeon should have a clear idea how to respond if this study shows small calf clots, large calf clots, popliteal clots, small thigh clots, or large thigh clots. Currently, there is no clear answer and the response to this questions varies from surgeon to surgeon. My own practice is to continue routine prophylactic measures (i.e., not change my normal prophylactic regimen) for all but the largest of clots.

*Moderator:* Let's continue with discussing diagnostic tests, Dr. Lotke. If you say that only a minority of patients with a true PE have a high-probability scan, are you not underestimating your number of PE patients?

*Dr. Lotke:* There are many small, silent, and clinically insignificant PEs. However, the precise incidence of PE is difficult to assess because the symptoms are frequently confused with other problems such as fat embolism syndrome, as well as the tools that are available to assess PE (such as the V/Q scan) are basically inaccurate. The PIPOPED study showed that in the presence of classic symptoms for PE the accuracy of the V/Q scan might be as high as 96%. However, without a high clinical suspicion for a PE, the accuracy of V/Q scans was as low as 46%. Therefore, we do not have clear statistics on the incidence of PE because of the confounding variables, fat embolism syndrome, lack of accuracy of the V/Q scan, lack of clinical findings, and apparent lack of significance for small asymptomatic clots.

*Moderator:* Many surgeons do not start their anticoagulation regimen until after surgery in order not to have bleeding problems with their epidural anesthetic catheter. Is this really accomplishing anything in the crucial first few days after surgery other than making surgeons feel that they "did something"?

*Dr. Westrich:* Here in lies the advantage of a pneumatic compression device for prophylaxis of thromboembolic disease after TKA. There is a real concern in combining epidural anesthesia or postoperative epidural analgesia with anticoagulation. Certainly many case reports have noted epidural hematomas when using epidural anesthesia/analgesia in conjunction with Lovenox, a LMWH. The FDA has actually mandated now that Lovenox not be used with epidural anesthesia or analgesia due to this risk, as the package insert from Lovenox now states. Therefore, if epidural anesthesia is utilized, the epidural catheter must be removed before beginning Lovenox. If postoperative epidural analgesia is utilized, the same protocol is followed. Clearly, postoperative paralysis from an epidural hematoma would negate any and all benefit of DVT prophylaxis with this regimen. As far as anticoagulation with warfarin, this takes approximately 3 days on average to reach a therapeutic range and it is not felt that epidural catheter use is problematic with respect to this.

*Moderator:* Dr. Lotke, some have said that advanced age is a factor in your choice of a chemoprophylactic agent to help prevent DVT. How old is advanced age; let me warn you that it must be at least 20 years older then I am.

*Dr. Lotke:* There really is no data suggesting that age should be a factor in the decision to use a chemoprophylactic agent. Age may be a risk factor for the development of DVT, but at present it has not been proven as a risk factor for PE. There is some data that patients over 70 have a slightly higher incidence of distal DVT and have a greater risk of mortality after TKA, but since the incidence of symptomatic PE is so low, it is impossible to make statements regarding age factors and recommendations for chemoprophylaxis.

*Moderator:* How about "extended operative time" as a risk factor for the development of DVT?

*Dr. Lotke:* I do not believe that we can define "extended operating time," but we can compare the risks of DVT for primary versus revision surgery. To date, there is no evidence to show that there is an increased incidence of thromboembolic disease in revisions. Therefore, we may assume that the time of surgery does not significantly appear to be a major factor in the development of DVT or PE. This response, however, could change with appropriate scientific study.

*Moderator:* There have been reported problems using LMWH in knee replacement patients as related to bleeding. Would you please comment on this?

*Dr. Westrich:* Many authors have noted that the use of LMWH is associated with postoperative bleeding after TKA. The greatest risk of postoperative bleeding is within the first several hours after surgery and the dosing for LMWH has therefore been adjusted. It is now recommended that surgeons wait 18–24 h to begin the first dose of Lovenox after TKA. It is noted that the hemorrhagic complications are a true risk and that the longer one waits to dose the anticoagulant the less risk of postoperative bleeding. Hematoma after TKA is problematic in that not only can it cause pain, swelling and decreased range of motion, but it also places the patient at greater risk for infection.

*Moderator:* Do you think that at some critical weight, one should use some other form of prophylaxis other than aspirin, Dr. Lotke?

*Dr. Lotke:* TKA is very common in the obese patients. Fortunately, there does not appear to be any studies that show obesity as a risk factor for DVT and clearly none have shown for the incidence of PE. Therefore, obesity should not affect your choice of chemo-prophylaxis.

*Moderator:* Are there any studies, Dr. Lotke, to show that the presence of superficial varicosities in the absence of deep venous incompetence really increases the risk of DVT?

*Dr. Lotke:* Several studies have looked at whether varicosities are correlated with the presence of DVT. To date, none have been able to show any correlation with superficial venous incompetence and the risk of DVT or PE.

*Moderator:* Dr. Westrich, a basic philosophical difference between you and Dr. Lotke relates to the importance or otherwise of calf clots. He says that they rarely cause lethal PE and therefore their mere presence is not, if I may paraphrase him, a catastrophic event. What are your thoughts on this?

*Dr. Westrich:* Although minor calf clots and major calf clots in themselves may not cause a lethal PE, they are at risk for propagation to a more proximal clot. Colwell *et al.* noted a 24% propagation rate from a calf clot to a proximal clot after TKA using serial Doppler examination. Therefore, there is a 1 in 4 chance that a calf clot can become a more proximal clot. The more proximal clot is obviously a concern for a lethal PE, and therefore, I do feel that prophylaxis is indicated for calf clots. The other issue is that we tend to downplay the detrimental effects of postphlebitic syndrome. This is a real entity that produces pain and chronic swelling of the limb. Vascular surgeons have a much greater appreciation for postphlebitic syndrome than orthopedic surgeons; however, there should be a greater state of awareness among orthopedic surgeons as to the deleterious effects of a postphlebitic syndrome. This is another reason to treat calf clots with anticoagulation.

*Moderator:* I would like to end this debate with several questions regarding the use of aspirin. First, you mentioned doses of aspirin lower than 100 mg per day. How much aspirin should a patient take? Secondly, can you give aspirin to patients who are having an epidural anesthetic. Doesn't the antiplatelet effect of aspirin incrase the risk of epidural bleeding?

**Dr. Lotke:** Aspirin is available in "baby" sizes of 80 mg. It is a unique drug in that in relatively low doses (100 mg), it completely suppresses platelet functions and reduces adhesiveness for the entire life of that particular platelet. With doses less than 100 mg, this inhibitory effect is dose dependent. Our colleagues in cardiology routinely may recommend the use of one baby aspirin a day to prevent thrombotic cardiac disease and protect patients from transient ischemic attacks.

As for your second question, the problem of anticoagulation and epidural anesthesia has recently come into question primarily as related to the use of LMWHs. Their use definitely increases the risk of epidural bleeding complications. However, aspirin has been used for a long period of time without this problem. The anticoagulant effect from aspirin is probably not as intense, and therefore less likely to cause bleeding than is the anticoagulant effects of heparin. However, since the anesthesiologists have been sensitized to the potential risk of epidural bleeds, some have generalized this to all agents that reduce coagulation. At present, there is great diversity among anesthesiologists as to whether the use of aspirin contraindicates the use of an epidural catheter. From our own experience, which is anecdotal, we do not hesitate to use epidural catheters with aspirin prophylaxis.

*Moderator:* Equally as anecdotal, our anesthesia group here at the Hospital for Special Surgery does indeed have problems using epidural cathethers in patients who are taking aspirin.

263

# 11

*Unicompartmental osteoarthritis has, in the past, been treated by a variety of methods, including bracing, tibia osteotomy, unicompartmental replacement, and total joint replacement. This problem can occur both in the young patient (especially after knee injuries such as rupture of the anterior cruciate ligament or meniscal tear) and in the older patient (without prior history of trauma). What is the optimal treatment, and is it the same for both groups?*

# Unicompartmental osteoarthritis of the knee is best treated by an osteotomy rather than unicompartmental arthroplasty

## Pro: John A. L. Hart

Degenerative joint disease (DJD) is the most common form of arthritis and the knee joint is most commonly affected,[1] with this condition occurring in approximately 1% of men and women under the age of 65 and in 2% of men and 6.6% of women over the age of 65.[2]

DJD may be primary or secondary to a variety of causes including direct trauma, malalignment and malunion,[3,4] inflammatory joint disease, osteochondritis dissecans. and sepsis. Meniscectomy[4-9] and recurrent patellar subluxation[10] can also lead to DJD. The severity of the disease and the number of compartments involved significantly affect management. Statistically it is the medial compartment that is most commonly involved.[11]

## Treatment options

### Nonoperative treatment

Weight reduction is important. The resultant axis, which represents the load on the knee during standing, passes through the center of the knee.[12] Increased body weight displaces the axis medially and overloads the medial compartment, as does loss of the medial meniscus. This leads to the vicious cycle of the varus knee, resulting in increased medial compartment stress, destruction of articular cartilage, joint space narrowing and worsening of the varus deformity.[1,13] Other measures such as soft-soled shoes to decrease impact loading, physiotherapy (particularly hydrotherapy) and walking aids, may be beneficial.

Uniaxial unloading knee braces[14] are useful in younger patients to maintain activity and in older patients who are unfit for surgery. These are, however, cumbersome and difficult to fit, which limits their use in many patients. The important concept to convey to patients is that they should maintain an active exercise program, but avoid impact loading.

Nonsteroidal anti-inflammatory drugs have a useful role.[15] Articular cartilage debris induces a synovitis which leads to further degeneration of articular cartilage.[16] Articular cartilage fragments themselves may induce cartilage degeneration. There has been considerable research to determine the role of chondroprotective agents in the treatment of joint disease.[17,18] Chondroprotective agents such as pentosan polysulfate[19] and hyaluran[20] have produced symptomatic relief in some patients, but there is little evidence to suggest that they can reverse the disease process and improve long-term outcomes. Odenbring and his colleagues[21] in an elegant study, demonstrated that unicompartmental osteoarthrosis of the knee is progressive. Their conclusions are summarized in Fig. 11.1. If conservative measures fail, surgery should be considered.

**Fig. 11.1**

Flow chart for unicompartmental osteoarthritis.[21]

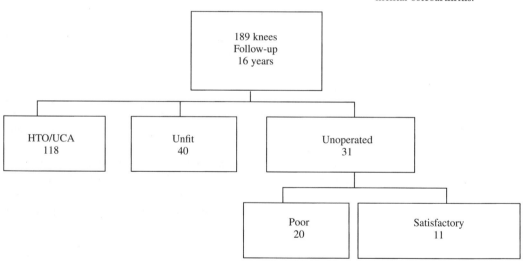

Table 11.1 Roles of arthroscopy

| Diagnostic role | Therapeutic role |
| --- | --- |
| Confirms extent of lesion | Manipulation |
| • within compartment | Treatment of mechanical derangement |
| • other compartments | Removal of loose bodies |
| Excludes other diseases | Removal of debris |
| • meniscal tears | Trimming of flaps |
| • synovitis | Resurfacing procedures |
| • chondrocalcinosis | Removal of osteophytes |

## Surgical options

Arthroscopic surgery has both a diagnostic and a therapeutic role in the management of DJD. (Table 11.1). The results of arthroscopic debridement have varied, with some authors reporting up to 79% good results[22-24] whereas others, such as Rand,[25] have reported good results in only 39%. Patient selection is important.[26] In my experience, patients with greater than 1° of flexion, minimal deformity, and identifiable internal derangements do best. Excision of the anterior tibial osteophyte may improve knee extension. Abrasion arthroplasty has given disappointing results.[27,28]

If conservative treatment including arthroscopic debridement fails for established unicompartmental DJD, the choice lies between osteotomy, unicompartmental arthroplasty (UCA), and total knee arthroplasty (TKA).

Osteotomy as a treatment for DJD of the knee has had a dubious reputation because of unreliable results and complications. Often, these opinions are based on procedures carried out in the 1970s and 1980s. These problems can be overcome by:

- careful patient selection
- preoperative planning
- precise operative technique
- rigid fixation
- active rehabilitation.

## Indications and contra-indications

Osteotomy is ideally suited to the young patient (less than 65 years of age) with normal weight, high activity levels, and a high pain threshold with early progressive disease.[7]

Concomitant PFD can be treated by advancement of the tibial tuberosity. Contra-indications may be absolute or relative (Table 11.2). The results of tibial osteotomy may be compromised by ligamentous instability, but modification of techniques and associated ligamentous reconstruction have produced good results. Medial opening wedge osteotomy[38,39] and simultaneous ligament advancement[40] can correct genu varum with medial laxity. Good results have

**Table 11.2** Contraindications for osteotomy

| Absolute | Relative |
| --- | --- |
| Inflammatory joint disease[1,29,30] | Osteoporosis |
| Metabolic joint disease[1,31] | Patellofemoral disease (PDF) |
| Contralateral compartment disease | Obesity[7,29] |
| FFD >15° | Cast intolerance[7] |
| ROM <100°[7] | Instability (ACL) |
| Instability with shift[32,33] | |
| Bone loss[1,7] | |

been reported by the simultaneous correction of genu varum and anterior cruciate ligament (ACL) instability by combined tibial osteotomy and intra-articular reconstruction of the ACL.[41–43] Latterman and Jakob recommended simultaneous procedures in the young, but staged procedures in the older patient.[44] Fowler[45] recently reported the use of an opening wedge flexion osteotomy to correct posterior instability.

## Preoperative planning

A general assessment is essential and should include some estimate as to the patient's activity, goals and co-morbidities. Other joints should be carefully assessed. Local disorders, such as vascular impairment, may require specialist referral. The clinical assessment of the knee should evaluate pain and function according to a knee scoring system and should be documented. Gait evaluation is particularly important to assess the degree of deformity and the presence of a varus thrust.[7,32,33]

## Radiography

Standard anterior–posterior (AP) and lateral views and a Merchant view[46] should be taken to evaluate the patellofemoral joint. The Rosenberg view (standing PA film with the knee flexed at 45°) is useful for detecting early joint space narrowing.[47] A three-joint standing view to include the hip, knee, and ankle allows measurement of the mechanical axis, represented by a line drawn from the center of the femoral head to the center of the talus. This axis should pass through or just medial to the center of the knee.[48,49] (Fig. 11.2)° of varus or valgus angulation are measured as the angle between the mechanical axis and a second line drawn from the center of the knee to the center of the talus.[50]

This method of assessment has been criticized by some,[51,52] but practical alternative methods of assessment have not been forthcoming.[2] The angulation of the joint line to the femoral and tibial axes may influence the type of osteotomy to be performed. Miniaci[53] described a technique using the three-joint film to estimate the angle of correction for genu varum (Fig. 11.3).

The predicted mechanical axis is drawn from the center of the femoral head through a point, 30–40% of the width of the lateral tibial plateau and is extrapolated to the intended center of the ankle. A second line from the center of the knee is drawn from the center of the ankle to the pivotal point of the osteotomy on the medial cortex and a third line from the pivotal point to the projected center of the ankle. The angle between the second and third lines is the desired amount of correction. The technique is designed to place the weight-bearing axis correctly in the lateral compartment and to overcome anatomical variables. Whether this technique gives better long-term results is not yet determined. We have compared a series of three-joint standing radiographs using the two techniques. Miniaci's angle

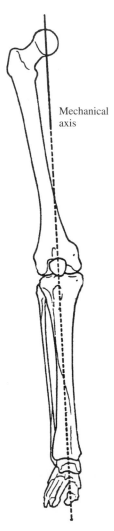

Mechanical axis

**Fig. 11.2**

Mechanical axis.

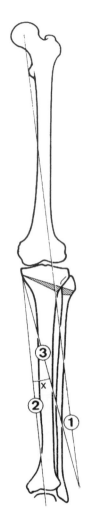

**Fig. 11.3**
Miniaci's axis.

**Table 11.3** Advantages and disadvantages of computer analysis

| Advantages | Disadvantages |
| --- | --- |
| Elimination of magnification errors | Cost (up to $US50 000) |
| Easier cross comparison | Learning curve |
| Accurate integration of measurement | Time consuming |
| Implants can be superimposed | |
| Data transmission | |
| Clinical studies | |

was equivalent to 5° of overcorrection with a narrow range of 4–6°. Stress views may be useful to confirm joint space loss and collateral ligament laxity. Unrecognized intra-articular shift due to lax collateral ligaments can result in overcorrection.[54] Where instability and shift is suspected, gait analysis may be useful. It can be used to determine adduction moment in genu varum, since a high adduction moment gives poor results.[32,33]

Computer analysis gives more precise information.[55,56] The advantages and disadvantages of computer analysis are presented in Table 11.3. Computer analysis certainly gives very accurate estimates, but because of the disadvantages, it is best reserved for complex cases.

## Genu varum

The aim of valgus tibial osteotomy is to transfer the weightbearing axis from the medial compartment to 30–40% of the distance across the lateral compartment.[57] Valgus tibial osteotomy is absolutely contra-indicated in some situations in genu varum (Table 11.4).

### Osteotomy site

Jackson and Waugh[58] performed a domed osteotomy distal to the tibial tuberosity. This osteotomy was remote from the deformity, had a high nonunion rate, produced less precise correction, and required greater dissection and plaster immobilization postoperatively. Schwartsman[59] improved the results with domed osteotomy by using external fixation. This eliminated the need for a cast, produced a higher union rate and more precise correction which could be adjusted, and allowed full weightbearing.[59] Complex deformities

**Table 11.4** Absolute contra-indications to valgus tibial osteotomy

| Problem | Solution |
| --- | --- |
| Femoral deformity | Opening medial wedge femoral osteotomy |
| Marked medial laxity with shift | Opening medial wedge with ligament tensioning or TKA |
| Tibial bone loss with ligamentous laxity (Pagoda knee) | TKA |

can be more readily corrected using this method.[40] However, the technique is time-consuming, knee motion is limited and non-acceptability to patients is significant. Pin tract infection can create a difficult situation for a subsequent total knee arthroplasty (TKA), being close to the knee. Coventry popularized the high tibial valgus closing wedge osteotomy (HTO).[60] This procedure had the advantage of a low nonunion rate[61-63] and producesa correction close to the deformity,[2;63] although a number of disadvantages[2;7] have been described:

- limited bone stock for internal fixation
- decreased distance between the tibial tuberosity and tibial plateau
- laxity of the lateral collateral ligaments[40]
- patella baja[64]
- intra-articular fracture
- osteonecrosis
- correction limited to less than $15°$[60]
- increased Q angle.[2]

**Fig. 11.4**
Hofmann technique.

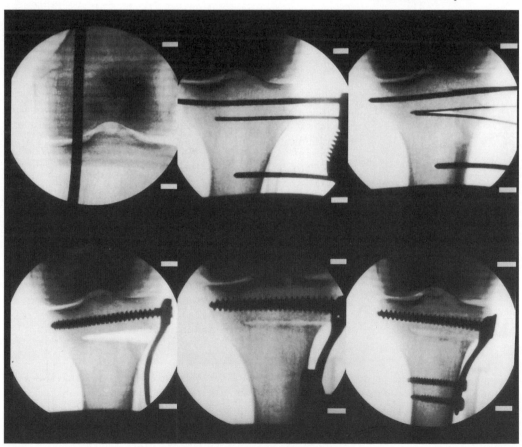

Coventry[60] excised a complete wedge extending to the medial cortex and used staples for fixation which sometimes led to translation and rotational deformity at the osteotomy. Hofmann et al.[65] described an incomplete valgus closing wedge osteotomy. They used a slotted jig to cut the required angle precisely and progressively closed the osteotomy with a compression clamp applied to an L-shaped titanium plate. The incomplete osteotomy eliminated the problems of translation and rotation. The slotted osteotomy jig enables a very precise wedge to be removed, rather than relying on techniques where 1 mm of wedge is excised for each 1° of correction required (Fig. 11.4). Hofmann and his colleagues compared the results using this technique with osteotomies which were fixed with staples and casts or by cast alone (Fig 11.5). They reduced their complication rate from 42% in the latter group to 5% in those where the compression plate was used. They also considered that their correction was much more precise and that their patients were able to mobilize earlier, which resulted in a better range of movement at 6 months.

Deformities greater than 15° are best treated by a domed osteotomy stabilized by external fixation.[40,59] Although the closing wedge osteotomy is used most often, there are alternatives. A medial opening wedge osteotomy is indicated where there is leg shortening or laxity of the medial collateral ligament.[38] This procedure requires a bone graft usually taken from the iliac crest, thus creating donor site morbidity. Puddu[39] has designed a toothed plate and a jigging system, which makes opening wedge osteotomies much more precise and more stable, but bone grafting is still required. Combined closing and opening wedges can be used for large deformities to preserve leg length.[2,7]

Jakob and Murphy[54] described a retrotubercular osteotomy and claimed they had a high union rate and a greater correction range. This procedure allegedly preserves more proximal bone stock and avoids raising the tibial tuberosity; however, it increases the Q angle. Patients with mild patellofemoral disease have not been worsened by HTO.[66,67] For those with severe patellofemoral disease, elevation of the tibial tuberosity can be performed simultaneously.[68–70] Combined procedures are technically more difficult and may have a high complication rate and poorer outcomes.[36,37]

## Fixation

Cast immobilization in isolation[58] or in combination with staple fixation[60] immobilizes the knee, causing knee stiffness and patella baja, and increases the risk of thromboembolic disease.[65] External fixation[40,59] allows early movement but does not allow full excursion of the knee. Rigid fixation with blade plates[54] or compression plates[65] overcomes these disadvantages. Despite this, some authors[72–74] have reported no advantage in buttress plate fixation compared to staple fixation and have stated that buttress plating is associated with a higher infection rate owing to the increased exposure.[75]

Fibular mobilization is required to allow correction with a closing wedge valgus osteotomy. The fibular osteotomy may be carried out in a variety of ways and at different levels, but it is important to avoid damage to the common peroneal nerve.[2]

## Personal preference

I prefer to carry out an incomplete closing wedge valgus osteotomy above the tibial tuberosity using the oblique jigging system and malleable titanium L plate described by Hofmann *et al.*[65] The operation can be considerably simplified by the use of an image intensifier, which allows placement of the first drill parallel and at an exact distance from the joint line, thus avoiding intra-articular fracture. The use of an image intensifier is also necessary to determine the line of the mechanical axis once the osteotomy has been performed. I perform a fibular neck osteotomy with a hand drill and osteotome following mobilization of the common peroneal nerve at the fibular neck. This procedure is performed through the universal lateral incision of Muller,[76] which can easily be utilized for a subsequent TKA. This technique can be readily combined with anteriorization of the extensor mechanism (AEM) for PFD. The accuracy of correction using this technique is shown in Fig. 11.5. The zero on the horizontal scale represents 5° of mechanical valgus. There appears to be a tendency to undercorrect, but in patients where osteotomies were combined with resurfacing procedures, 5° of mechanical axis valgus was not always attempted.

## Results

Grelsamer[7] reviewed the results of high valgus closing wedge osteotomy (Table 11.5) concluded that the best results were

**Fig. 11.5**

Accuracy of correction for genu varum using Hofmann technique. 21 cases in 1995–96 (gray bars); 16 cases in 1997–98 (white bars); total 37 (black bars).

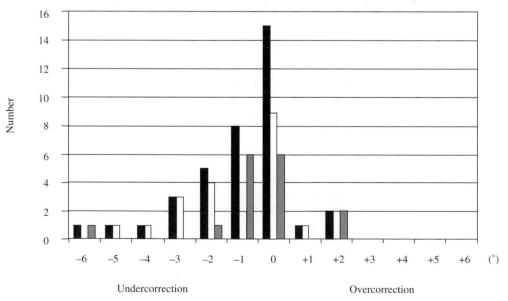

**Table 11.5** Results of HTO[7]

| Author | Year | No. | Follow-up (years) | Good/Excellent | Deterioration |
|---|---|---|---|---|---|
| Tjornstrand[63] | 1981 | 89 | 7 | 53% | – |
| Aglietti[78] | 1983 | 139 | | 76% | No |
| Insall[30] | 1984 | 95 | 5 | 85% | Yes (63%) |
| Sundaram[79] | 1986 | 105 | 5 | 75% | – |
| Hernigou[38] | 1987 | 93 | 10 | 45% | – |
| Matthews[80] | 1988 | 40 | 1 | 85% | Yes (28%) |
| Morrey[81] | 1989 | 33 | 7.5 | 73% | – |
| Berman[82] | 1991 | 39 | 8.5 | 87% | Yes (59%) |

achieved in patients with a low adduction moment, metaphyseal bowing, and early disease, who were younger with low body weight and were overcorrected into valgus (3–8° beyond neutral).

### Degree of correction (see Table 11.6)

There has been an increasing awareness that overcorrection is required to obtain a good or excellent result. Coventry recommended correction to −1° in 1973,[79] 1° degree in 1987[86] and greater than 2° in 1993.[87] Yasuda and his colleagues[88] found that 88% of patients had satisfactory results at 15 years follow-up, where the mechanical axis was corrected to between 6–10° of valgus. I aim to correct to 5° beyond the neutral mechanical axis, i.e., 11° of femorotibial valgus. Overcorrection of this magnitude may have a significant cosmetic effect, particularly in angular women, and this does need to be explained to the patient before the operation. In those patients who undergo a corrective osteotomy to unload an affected compartment in conjunction with a resurfacing procedure and where there is little or no pre-existing varus deformity, this amount of overcorrection may not be required.

### Complications

Complications following valgus HTO are well documented with the use of staples and a cast or a cast alone for fixation.[1,30,38,65,77,89,90] Dearbon et al.[1] classified complications as early and late.

**Table 11.6** Recommended correction

| Author | Degrees of mechanical axis |
|---|---|
| Bauer et al.[83] | −4–9° |
| Insall[30] | −1–6° |
| Torgerson et al.[68] | 1–2° |
| Kettlecamp et al.[84] | 2–5° |
| Engel and Lippett[85] | −1–9° |
| Vainionpää et al.[86] | −1–9° |
| Aglietti et al.[78] | 1–4° |

EARLY COMPLICATIONS

Undercorrection of deformity is a consequence of either inadequate preoperative planning or inadequate correction at the time of surgery. Loss of correction is due to inadequate fixation.[1] Intra-articular fracture can be avoided by creating an adequate bone bridge using an image intensifier. Common peroneal nerve (CPN) injury has been frequently reported[1,2] but is especially high with mid-shaft fibular osteotomy.[91] Neurolysis of the CPN at the time of fibular neck osteotomy is recommended; no postoperative palsies have occurred in a consecutive series of 37 osteotomies.[35] Compartment syndrome has been reported[1] and may require early fasciotomy. Direct vascular injury is a potential complication of high tibial osteotomy which Coventry considered was due to the increased exposure required for plate fixation.[81] A series of 207 HTOs internally fixed by a blade plate resulted in only one vascular complication.[93] Performing the osteotomy with the knee fully extended is safer than when the knee is flexed, as this results in more posterior displacement of the neurovascular bundle. Deep vein thrombosis and pulmonary embolism are reduced with early mobilization, but antithrombotic prophylaxis is recommended.

Nonunion and delayed union are uncommon with this osteotomy[94] and are related to inadequate fixation[65] or instability due to loss of the medial hinge when the medial cortex and periosteum are disrupted.

Joint stiffness impairs function and has deleterious effects on articular cartilage.[66,95,96] Early mobilization with a continuous passive motion (CPM) machine and early weightbearing overcomes these problems and rigid fixation allows these techniques to be safely used.[65] Infection may be related to exposure.[65] Hsu et al.[75] reported a 9.3% infection rate with buttress plate fixation compared to 0.8% with staple fixation. Pin tract infection is a potential risk with external fixators.[97] Prophylactic antibiotic administration with a preoperative dose and two doses in the first 12 h postoperatively is advisable and does not produce drug resistance.[98]

## Late complications

Progression of medial DJD following HTO may be due to inadequate correction or loss of correction.[30,79,81] Progression of DJD in the lateral compartment is due to overcorrection[1] or to unrecognized lateral compartment disease. Patella baja may occur in up to 89% of patients owing to shortening of the patellar tendon,[1] but its significance is unclear.[99] Patella baja is not common after HTO if patellar height is related to the femur.[100]

In a personal series of 37 HTOs using the Hofmann technique with image intensifier control and CPM and early partial weightbearing immediately postoperatively, there were no nonunions, peroneal palsies, or infections. No patients have required conversion to TKA.

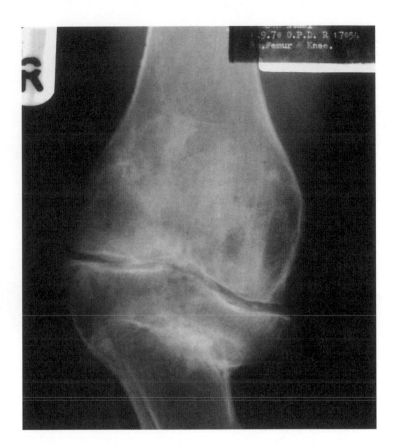

**Fig. 11.6**

Oblique joint line following varus osteotomy for genu valgum.

Although it has been frequently stated that the outcome of TKA following HTO is not as good as primary TKA,[101,102] recent studies[103–106] have shown that outcome after HTO is no worse than after a primary TKA.

## Genu valgum

Corrective osteotomies for genu valgum may be performed in the tibia,[86] but correction of larger deformities leads to obliquity of the joint line and lateral subluxation of the tibia[107–109] as seen in Fig. 11.6. It may occasionally be indicated for primary deformity of the tibia after a depressed tibial plateau fracture. Correction is generally preferred in the femur for these reasons.[108,109]

### Technique

A medial closing wedge is generally preferred because of a high union rate and because it avoids the need for bone grafting. A lateral opening wedge is indicated where the lateral femoral condyle is deficient or where there is shortening of the extremity. A lateral approach is used for an opening wedge osteotomy. A closing wedge osteotomy may be performed through a lateral incision, but the osteotomy is more easily performed through a medial approach reflecting the vastus medialis forward. Fixation with staples, plates,

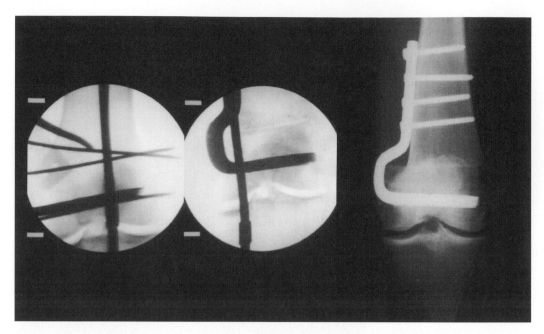

and screws is ineffective;[109] a blade plate is required (Fig. 11.7). For the lateral approach a condylar blade plate or Association Osteosynthesis dynamic condylar screw can be used, but for the medial side, a 95° condylar blade plate is required to accommodate the prominence of the medial femoral condyle. Puddu[39] has used his tooth plate laterally in combination with an oblique opening edge osteotomy and has reported good early results. Grafting, with bone or bone substitute, is still required (Fig. 11. 8).

## Degree of correction

Terry and Comino[110] recommended correction to a zero mechanical axis, which restores the normal femorotibial valgus angle of 6°. Maquet[107] suggested that the deformity be overcorrected to a zero anatomical axis (6–7° of mechanical varus) or beyond, and other authors have supported this concept (Table 11.7).[105,109,111] The best results were obtained by McDermott *et al.*[108] who corrected to a zero anatomical axis or more. Healy's group also achieved good results, but Terry and Comino[110] had the worst results, where they only corrected to a zero mechanical axis. The results from the Mayo Clinic[109] were very varied; there was a high complication rate owing to inadequate fixation in many of the cases.

I prefer to use a medial closed wedge performed through a medial incision using a 95° condylar blade plate for fixation under image intensifier control. A variance of correction analysis demonstrated there was a tendency to undercorrect. I therefore use the following formula to determine the amount of correction obtained from the three-joint standing views:

**Fig. 11.7**

Closing wedge supracondylar osteotomy using medial blade plate.

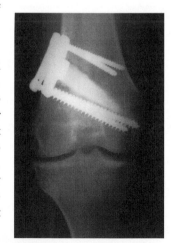

**Fig. 11.8**

Opening wedge lateral supracondylar osteotomy using a Puddu tooth plate and hydroxyapatite bone substitute.

**Table 11.7** Supracondylar varus osteotomy

| Author | Healey *et al.* | McDermott *et al.* | Edgerton *et al.* | Terry & Camino |
|---|---|---|---|---|
| Year | 1988 | 1988 | 1993 | 1992 |
| No. Rev | 23/23 | 24/24 | 24/101 | 35/36 |
| F/U | 4 years | 4 years | 8.3 years | 5.4 years 5.5 |
| AIM | Mech. axis + 4 deg | Anat. axis | Anat. axis | Mech. axis |
| METHOD | Medial wedge blade plate | Medial wedge blade plate | Varied | Medial wedge lateral wedge blade plate |
| CORR. | Anat. axis −2 deg | All knees to 0 deg or more | 14/24 0 or varus. 10/24 valgus | 3.8 deg. valgus |
| RES G/E | 83% | 92% | 71% overall 77% corrected to 0 deg. 60% undercorrected | 67% |
| COMP | 13% | 4% | 63% | 8% |

valgus deformity + 6° + 2° of overcorrection.

A varus overcorrection is more cosmetically acceptable than a valgus overcorrection.

## Conclusion

Osteotomy is an effective method of treating unicompartmental DJD. The result can be considerably improved by preoperative planning, image intensifier control, more precise techniques, and improved fixation allowing earlier mobilization and weightbearing. Krackow[112] defined the role of osteotomy according to age. In patients under the age of 50 years he strongly recommended osteotomy and in patients over the age of 65, TKA. In the middle age group he calculated that there was a 90% probable satisfactory outcome for a TKA and a subsequent revision compared to an 80% probably satisfactory outcome for an osteotomy. He felt that the latter scenario was preferable, and I agree.

### Osteotomy versus unicompartmental arthroplasty

The obvious surgical alternative for unicompartmental DJD is the unicompartmental arthroplasty (UCA). This concept was first introduced by McKeever[113] as a resurfacing disk placed on the tibia.

A variety of prostheses have been introduced since then, including the design of Marmor, which was specifically a resurfacing procedure rather than a full arthroplasty.[114] Goodfellow and O'Connor[115] introduced the concept of a meniscal bearing knee. Other designs have incorporated the features developed from TKAs. The indications for UCA and HTO are similar, but the contra-indications differ (Table 11.8).

**Table 11.8** Contra-indications

|                 | Osteotomy | UCA |
|-----------------|-----------|-----|
| FFD >15         | Yes       | Yes |
| Absent ACL      | No        | Yes |
| PFD             | No        | Yes |
| Inflammatory JD | Yes       | Yes |
| Chondrocalcinosis | ?       | Yes |
| Lateral DJD     | Yes       | Yes |
| Instability     | No        | Yes |

Osteotomy is a more flexible procedure, which can be performed with larger deformities and in the presence of patellofemoral disease and instability. The comparative disadvantages of osteotomy and UCA are presented in Table 11.9. Given equivalent outcomes, the potential disadvantages of a UCA outweigh those of an osteotomy.

Stenstrom et al.[116] presented the results from the Swedish Knee Arthroplasty Register for the years 1986–95. The 9 year survival rate was 91% for 75 404 TKAs and 85% for 11 046 UCAs. TKAs had a steady decline in revision at 5 years to 4% whereas the UCA revision rate has remained high at 8%. Some prostheses fare better than others. The revision rates were 6% for the Marmor and the St George UCAs at 5 years, but 15% for the PCA. Scott in 1997[117] described his experience with three designs used between 1974 and 1997. The unicondylar UCA used between 1974 and 1981 had a survival rate of 82% at 11 years, the Brigham used in 1987–90 was good at 5 years but failed rapidly between 6 and 10 years owing to polyethylene wear. The PFC UCA used since 1990 had 9% good or excellent results at 5 years in 29 younger patients, but 2 of these had developed femoral loosening. Attempts to thicken the polyethylene have resulted in more bone loss, and attempts to reduce wear by increasing congruity, have caused femoral loosening.

**Table 11.9** Disadvantages

|                         | Osteotomy    | UCA           |
|-------------------------|--------------|---------------|
| Wear                    | No           | Yes           |
| Loosening               | No           | Yes           |
| Non-union               | Yes          | No            |
| Technical difficulty    | Decreasing   | Yes           |
| ROM                     | Good         | Good          |
| Consequence of infection | Moderate    | Severe        |
| Deformity               | <15°         | <6°           |
| Revision problems       | Patella baja | Bone loss     |
|                         | Bone stock   | Infection     |
| Results                 | Improving    | Not improving |
| COST                    | AUD $5,000   | AUD $11,000   |

The Oxford meniscal knee[115] may provide solutions to some of these problems. Although good results have been reported for the medial compartment with this prothesis, there has been a 12.9% failure rate at 3.5 years for the lateral compartment.[118] Figures from the Swedish Knee Arthroplasty Register[119] have shown a revision rate of 12% for the Oxford knee at 6 years. A 1996 study by Gill and his colleagues[120] demonstrated that UCAs are more difficult to revise than osteotomised knees because of bone loss, and have less favorable outcomes.

## Summary

Osteotomy is a valuable option for the treatment of unicompartmental DJD of the knee where conservative methods have failed. It is the treatment of choice in patients under the age of 65. Careful selection of patients, adequate preoperative planning, more precise surgery, and improved fixation allowing early mobilization and weightbearing will reduce complications and improve outcomes. The procedure is a low-cost alternative and is preferred to UCA. Over the age of 65, TKA is generally the treatment of choice although the UCA may have a limited place in some older, lighter patients with unicompartmental DJD and a good range of movement. The role of osteotomy has expanded beyond treatment for established DJD. It has important roles to unload the affected compartment in resurfacing procedures, and as a combined procedure in patients with PFD and specific ligamentous instability.

## References

1  Dearbon J, Eakin C, Skinner H: Medial compartment arthrosis of the knee. *American Journal of Orthopaedics* **25**(1):18–26, 1996.

2  Phillips M, Krackow K: High tibial osteotomy and distal femoral osteotomy for valgus or varus deformity around the knee. *Instructional Course Lectures* **47**, 1998.

3  Reimann I: Experimental osteoarthritis of the knee in rabbits induced by alteration of the load-bearing. *Acta Orthopaedica Scandinavica* **44**:496–504, 1973.

4  Tetsworth K, Paley D: Malalignment and degenerative arthroscopy. *Orthopedic Clinics of North America* **25**:367–377, 1994.

5  King D: The function of semlunar cartilages. *Journal of Bone and Joint Surgery* **18**:1069–1076, 1936.

6  Fairbank TJ: Knee joint changes after meniscectomy. *Journal of Bone and Joint Surgery* [Br] **30**:664–670, 1948.

7  Grelsamer RP: Unicompartmental osteoarthritis of the knee. *Journal of Bone and Joint Surgery* [Am] **77**:278–292, 1995.

8  Simon WH, Friedenberg S, Richardson S: Joint congruence: a correlation of joint congruence and thickness of articular cartilage in dogs. *Journal of Bone and Joint Surgery* [Am] **55**:1614–1620, 1973.

9  Walker PS, Erkman MJ: The role of the menisci in force transmission across the knee. *Clinical Orthopedics and Related Research* 109–184, 1975.

10   Fulkerson JP, Hungerford DS: *Disorders of the patello-femoral joint,* 2nd edn. Williams and Wilkins, Baltimore, 1990.

11   Hernborg JS, Nilsson BE: The natural course of untreated osteoarthritis of the knee. *Clinical Orthopedics and Related Research* **123**:130–137, 1977.

12   Maquet P: *Biomechanics of the knee,* 2nd edn. Springer-Verlag, New York, 1984.

13   Thornhill TS: Unicompartmental knee arthroplasty. *Clinical Orthopedics and Related Research* **205**:121–131, 1986.

14   Hewett TE, Noyes FR, Barber-Wilson, Heckmann TP: Decrease in joint pain and increase in joint function in patients with medial compartment arthrosis: a prospective analysis of valgus bracing. *Orthopaedics* **21**:131–138, 1998.

15   Oddis CV: New perspectives on osteoarthritis. *American Journal of Medicine* **100**:10S–15S, 1996.

16   Grande DA, Pitman MI, Peterson L *et al.*: *Orthopaedics Research* **7**:208–218, 1989.

17   Howell DS, Altman RD: Cartilage repair and conservation in osteoarthritis. *Rheumatic Diseases Clinics of North America* **19**:713–724, 1993.

18   Burchardt D, Ghosh P: Laboratory evaluation of anti-arthritic drugs as potential chondroprotective agents. *Seminars on Arthritis and Rheumatism* **17**:3–24, 1987.

19   Edelman J, Smith MM, March L, Ghosh P: A double-blind placebo-controlled clinical study of a pleiotropic osteoarthritis drug (entosan Polysulphate, Cartrophin) in 105 patients with osteoarthritis (OA) of the knee and hip joints. *Osteoarthritis Cartilage* **2**(Suppl.1):60, 1994.

20   Wobig M, Dickhut A, Maier R, Vetter G: Viscosupplementation with hylan G-F 20: A 26-week controlled trial of efficacy and safety in the osteoarthritic knee. *Clinical Therapeutics* **20**:410–423, 1988.

21   Odenbring S, Lindstrand A, Egund N *et al.*: Prognosis for patients with medial gonarthrosis. *Clinical Orthopedics* **266**:152–155, 1991.

22   Ewing JW: Uni-compartmental gonarthrosis of the knee managed by arthroscopic surgical techniques. Eighth International Seminar on Operative Arthroscopy, Maui, Hawaii. 18–25 October, 1986.

23   Jennings JE: Arthroscopic debridement as an alternative to total knee replacement. *Arthroscopy* **2**:123, 1986.

24   Merchan EC, Galindo E: Arthroscope-guided surgery versus non-operative treatment for limited degenerative osteoarthritis of the femoro-tibial joint in patients over 50 years of age. A prospective comparative study. *Arthroscopy* **9**:663–667, 1993.

25   Rand JA: Role of arthroscopy in osteoarthritis of the knee. *Arthroscopy* **7**:358–363, 1991.

26   Baumgaertner MR, Cannon WD, Jr.; Vittori, S *et al.*: Arthroscopic debridement of the arthritic knee. *Clinical Orthopedics* **253**:197–202, 1990.

27   Rand JA, Ritts GD: Abrasion arthroplasty as a salvage for failed upper tibial osteotomy. Journal of Arthroplasty **4**(suppl):S45–S48, 1989.

28   Singh S, Lee CC, Tay BK: Results of arthroscopic abrasion arthro-plasty in osteoarthritis of the knee joint. *Singapore Medical Journal* **32**:34–37, 1991.

29   Coventry MB: Osteotomy of the upper portion of the tibia for degen-erative arthritis of the knee. A preliminary report. *Journal of Bone and Joint Surgery* [Am] **47**:984–990, 1965.

30  Insall JN, Joseph DM, Msika C: High tibial osteotomy for varus
    gonarthrosis. A long-term follow-up study. *Journal of Bone and Joint
    Surgery* [Am] **66**:1040–1048, 1984.

31  Kozinn SC, and Scott R: Current concepts review. Unicondylar knee
    arthoplasty. *Journal of Bone and Joint Surgery* **71A**:145–150, 1989.

32  Prodromos CC, Andriacchi TP, Galante JO: A relationship between
    gait and clinical changes following high tibial osteotomy. *Journal of
    Bone and Joint Surgery* [Am] **67**:1188, 1985.

33  Goh JC H, Bose K, Khoo BCC: Gait analysis study on patients with
    varus osteoarthritis of the knee. *Clinical Orthopedics* **294**:223–231,
    1993.

35  Hart JAL: Surgical treatment of patello-femoral disease. Patello-
    femoral Disease Symposium, SICOT, 21st World Congress,
    Sydney, Australia 18–23 April, 1999.

36  Insall JN: Patella pain syndromes and chondromalacia patellae.
    *Instructional Course Lectures* **30**:342–356, 1981.

37  Hofman AA, Wyatt RW, Jones RE: Combined Coventry–Marquet pro-
    cedure for two- compartment degenerative arthritis. *Clinical
    Orthopedics* **190**:186–191, 1984.

38  Hernigou P, Medevielle D, Debeyre J, Goutallier D: Proximal tibial
    osteotomy for osteo-arthritis with varus deformity. A ten to thir-
    teen year follow-up study. *Journal of Bone and Joint Surgery* [Am]
    **69**:332–354, 1987.

39  Puddu G: A plate for open wedge tibial and femoral osteotomies.
    ISAKOS Congress, Washington DC, 29 May–2 June, 1999.

40  Paley D, Bhatnagar J, Herzenberg JE *et al.*: New proceedings for tight-
    ening knee collateral ligaments in conjunction with knee realign-
    ment osteotomy. *Orthopedic Clinics of North America.* **25**:533–555,
    1994.

41  O'Neill DF, James SL: Valgus osteotomy with anterior cruciate liga-
    ment laxity. *Clinical Orthopedics* **278**:153–159, 1992.

42  Noyes FR, Barber SD, Simon R: High tibial osteotomy and ligament
    reconstruction in varus angulated, anterior cruciate ligament-
    deficient knees: A two-to-seven-year follow-up study. *American
    Journal of Sports Medicine* **21**:2–12, 1993.

43  Neuschwander DC, Drez D Jr., Paine RM: Simultaneous high tibial
    osteotomy and ACL reconstruction for combined genu varum and
    symptomatic ACL tear. *Orthopaedics* **16**:679–684, 1983.

44  Lattermann C, Jakob RP: High tibial osteotomy alone or combined
    with ligament reconstruction in anterior cruciate-deficient knees.
    *Knee Surgery, Sports Traumatology, Arthroscopy* **4**:32–38, 1996.

45  Fowler PJ: Osteotomies about the knee. Instructional Course Lecture,
    ISAKOS Congress, Washington DC, 29 May–2 June, 1999.

46  Merchant AC, Mercer AL, Jacobsen RH, Cool CR: Roentgenographic
    analysis of patello-femoral congruence. *Journal of Bone and Joint
    Surgery* [Am] **56**:1391–1396, 1974.

47  Rosenberg TD, Paulos LE, Parker RD *et al.*: The forty-five-degree
    postero anterior flexion weight-bearing radiograph of the knee.
    *Journal of Bone and Joint Surgery* [Am] **70**:1479–1483, 1988.

48  Chao EY, Neluheni EV, Hsu, RW, Paley D: Biomechanics of malalign-
    ment. *Orthopedic Clinics of North America* **25**:379–386, 1994.

49  Moreland JR, Bassett LW, Hanker GJ: Radiographic analysis of the
    axial alignment of the lower extremity. *Journal of Bone and Joint
    Surgery* [Am] **69**:745–749, 1987.

50  Cooke TD V, Scudamore RA, Bryant JT *et al.*: A quantitative
    approach to radiography of the lower limb. Principles and applica-
    tions. Journal of Bone and Joint Surgery [Br] **73**(5):715–720, 1991.

51  Andriacchi TP: Dynamics of knee malalignment. *Orthopedic Clinics of North America* **25**:395–403, 1994.

52  Shaw JA, Moulton MJ: High tibial osteotomy. an operation based on a spurious mechanical concept. A theoretic treatise. *American Journal of Orthopedics* **25**:429–436, 1996.

53  Miniaci A, Ballmer FT, Ballmer PM, Jakob RP: Proximal tibial osteotomy a new fixation device. *Clinical Orthopedics* **246**:250–259, 1989.

54  Jakob RP, Murphy SB: Tibial osteotomy for varus gonarthrosis: Indication, planning and operative technique. *Instructional Course Lectures* **41**;87–93, 1992.

55  Chao EY, Sim PH: Computer-aided pre-operative planning in knee osteotomy. *Iowa Orthopedic Journal* **15**:4–18, 1995.

56  Santore RF: Computers for surgical planning of orthopaedic procedures. *Instructional Course Lectures* 199?

57  Fujisawa Y, Masuhara K, and Shiomi S: The effect of high tibial osteotomy on arthritis of the knee. An arthroscopic study of 54 knee joints. *Orthopedic Clinics of North America* **10**:585–608, 1979.

58  Jackson JP, Waugh W: Tibial osteotomy for osteoarthritis of the knee. Journal of Bone and Joint Surgery [Br] **43**:746–751, 1961.

59  Schwartsman V: Circular external fixation in high tibial osteotomy. *Instructional Course Lectures* **44**:469–474, 1995.

60  Coventry MB: Osteotomy of the upper portion of the tibia for degenerative arthritis of the knee: A preliminary report. *Journal of Bone and Joint Surgery* [Am] **47**:984–990, 1965.

61  Myrnerts R: High tibial osteotomy with over-correction of varus malalignment in medial gonarthrosis. *Acta Orthopaedica Scandinavica* **51**:557–560, 1980.

62  Bauer GC, Insall J, Koshine T: Tibial osteotomy in gonarthrosis (osteoarthritis of the knee). *Journal of Bone and Joint Surgery* **51**:1545–1563, 1969.

63  Tjornstrand B, Hagstedt B, Persson BM: Results of surgical treatment for non-union after high tibial osteotomy in osteoarthritis of the knee. *Journal of Bone and Joint Surgery* [Am] **60**:973–977, 1978.

64  Katz MM, Hungerford DS, Krackow KA *et al.*: Results of total knee arthroplasty after failed proximal tibial osteotomy for osteoarthritis. *Journal of Bone and Joint Surgery* [Am] **69**:225–233, 1987.

65  Hofmann AA, Wyatt RW B, Beck SW: High tibial osteotomy: Use of an osteotomy jig, rigid fixation and early motion versus conventional surgical technique and cast immobilisation. *Clinical Orthopedics and Related Research* **271**:212–217, 1991.

66  Tjornstrand BAE, Egund N, Hagstedt BV: High tibial osteotomy. A seven-year clinical and radiographic follow-up. *Clinical Orthopedics* **160**:124–136, 1981.

67  Torgerson WR, Kettelkamp DP, Igou RA Jr., Leach RE: Tibial osteotomy for the treatment of degenerative arthritis of the knee. *Clinical Orthopedics* **101**:46–52, 1974.

68  Bourguigon RL: Combined Coventry–Maquet tibial osteotomy. Preliminary report of two cases. *Clinical Orthopedics* **160**:144–148, 1981.

69  Maquet P: Valgus osteotomy for osteoarthritis of the knee. *Clinical Orthopedics* **120**:143–148, 1976.

70  Putnam MD, Mears DC, Fu FH: Combined Maquet and proximal tibial valgus osteotomy. *Clinical Orthopedics* **197**:217–223, 1985.

71  Insall JN: Patella pain syndromes and chondromalacia patellae. *Instructional Course Lectures* **30**:342–356, 1981.

72    Coventry MB: Stepped staple for upper tibial osteotomy. *Journal of Bone and Joint Surgery* [Am] **51**:1011, 1969.

73    Ebel R: High tibial osteotomy for gonarthrosis. Zeitschrift für Orthopädie **116**:716–724, 1978.

74    Wildner M, Peters A, Heilich J *et al.*: Complications of high tibial osteotomy and internal fixation with staples. *Archives of Orthopaedics and Trauma Surgery* **111**:210–212, 1992.

75    Hsu RW, Himeno S, Coventry MB *et al.*: Normal axial alignment of the lower extremity and load-bearing distribution at the knee. *Clinical Orthopedics* **255**:215–227, 1990.

76    Muller W: *The knee*, p. 166. Springer-Verlag, Berlin, 1983.

77    Aglietti P, Rinonapoli E, Stringa G, Taviani A: Tibial osteotomy for the varus osteoarthritic knee. *Clinical Orthopedics* **176**:239–251, 1983.

78.   Sundaram NA, Hallet JP, Sullivan MF: Dome osteotomy of the tibia for osteoarthritis of the knee. *Journal of Bone and Joint Surgery* [Br] **68**(5):782–786, 1986.

79    Matthews LS, Goldstein SA, Malvitz TA *et al.*: Proximal tibial osteotomy. Factors that influence the duration of satisfactory function. *Clinical Orthopedics* **229**:193–200, 1988.

80    Morrey BF: Upper tibial osteotomy for secondary osteoarthritis of the knee. *Journal of Bone and Joint Surgery* [Br] **71**(4):554–559, 1989.

81    Berman AT, Bosacco SJ, Kirshner S, Avolio A Jr.: Factors influencing long-term results in high tibial osteotomy. *Clinical Orthopedics* **272**:192–198, 1991.

82    Bauer GCH, Insall J, Koshino T: Tibial osteotomy in gonarthrosis (osteo-arthritis of the knee). *Journal of Bone and Joint Surgery* [Am] **51**:1545–1563, 1969.

83    Kettelkamp DB, Wenger DR, Chao EYS, Thompson C: Results of proximal tibial osteotomy. The effects of tibiofemoral angle, stance-phase flexion-extension, and medial-plateau force. *Journal of Bone and Joint Surgery* [Am] **58**:9520–9960, 1976.

84    Engel GM, Lippert FG III: Valgus tibial osteotomy: avoiding the pitfalls. *Clinical Orthopedics* **160**:137–143, 1981.

85    Vainionpää S, Läike E, Kirves P, Tiusanen P: Tibial osteotomy for osteoarthritis of the knee. A five to ten-year follow-up study. *Journal of Bone and Joint Surgery* [Am] **63**:938–946, 1981.

86    Coventry MB: Proximal tibial varus osteotomy for osteoarthritis of the lateral compartment of the knee. *Journal of Bone and Joint Surgery* [Am] **69**:32–38, 1987.

87    Coventry M, Ilstrup DM, Wallrichs SL: Proximal tibial osteotomy. A critical long-term study of eighty-seven cases. *Journal of Bone and Joint Surgery* [Am] **75**:196–201, 1993.

88    Yasuda K, Majima T, Tsuchida, T, Kaneda K: A ten to 15-year follow-up observation of high tibial osteotomy in medial compartment osteoarthrosis. *Clinical Orthopedics* **282**:186–195, 1992.

89    Ha'eri GB, Wiley AM: High tibial osteotomy combined with joint debridement: A long-term study of results. *Clinical Orthopedics* **151**:153–159, 1980.

90    Sprenger TR, Weber BG, Howard FM: Compression osteotomy of the tibia. *Clinical Orthopedics* **140**:103, 1979.

91    Kirgis A, Albrecht S: Palsy of the deep peroneal nerve after proximal tibial osteotomy. An anatomical study. *Journal of Bone and Joint Surgery* [Am] **74**:1180–1185, 1972.

92    Coventry MB: Upper tibial osteotomy for osteoarthritis. *Journal of Bone and Joint Surgery* [Am] **67**:1146. 1985.

93  LeMaire R: Etude comparative de deux series d'osteotomies tibales avec fixation par lame-plaque ou par cadre de compression. *Acta Orthopaedica Belgica* **48**:157, 1982.

94  Coventry MB: Upper tibial osteotomy for gonarthrosis. *Orthopedic Clinics of North America* **10**:91, 1979.

95  Enneking WF, Horowitz M: The intra-articular effects of immobilization on the human knee. *Journal of Bone and Joint Surgery* [Am] **54**:973, 1972.

96  Hall MC: Articular changes in the knee of the adult rat after prolonged immobilization in extension. *Clinical Orthopedics* **34**:184, 1964.

97  Johnson F, Leitl S, Waugh W: The distribution of load across the knee; a comparison of static and dynamic measurement. *Journal of Bone and Joint Surgery* [Br] **62**:346–349, 1980.

98  Burke JF: The effective period of preventive action in experimental lesions and dermal lesions. *Surgery* **50**:161–168, 1961.

99  Scuderi GR, Windsor RS, Insall JN: Observations on patellar height after proximal tibial osteotomy. *Journal of Bone and Joint Surgery* [Am] **71**:245, 1989.

100  Miura H, Kawamura H, Nagamine R *et al.*: Is patellar height really lower after high tibial osteotomy? *Fukuoka Acta Medica* **88**:261–266, 1997.

101  Katz MK, Hungerford DS, Krackow KA, Lennox DW: Results of total knee arthroplasty after failed proximal osteotomy for osteoarthritis. *Journal of Bone and Joint Surgery* [Am] **69**:225–233, 1987.

102  Windsor RE, Insall JN, Vince KG: Technical considerations of total knee arthroplasty after proximal tibial osteotomy. *Journal of Bone and Joint Surgery* **70**:544–555, 1988.

103  Staeheli JW, Gass JR, Morrey BF: Condylar total knee arthroplasty after failed proximal tibial osteotomy. *Journal of Bone and Joint Surgery.* [Am] **69**:28, 1987.

104  Marcacci M, Iacono F, Zaffagnini S, Marchetti PG: Total knee arthroplasty after proximal tibial osteotomy. *Chirurgia degli Organi di Movimento* **80**:353–359, 1995.

105  Takai S, Yoshino N, Hirasawa Y: Revision knee arthroplasty after failed high tibial osteotomy. *Bulletin, Hospital for Joint Diseases* **56**:245–250M, 1997.

106  Toskvig-Larsen S, Magyar G, Onsten I *et al.*: Fixation of the tibial component of total knee arthroplasty after high tibial osteotomy: a matched radiostereometric study. *Journal of Bone and Joint Surgery* [Br] **80**:295–297, 1998.

107  Marquet P: The treatment of choice in osteoarthritis of the knee. *Clinical Orthopedics* **192**:108–112, 1985.

108  Healy WL, Anglen JO, Wasilewski SA, Krackow KA: Distal femoral varus osteotomy. *Journal of Bone and Joint Surgery* [Am] **70**:102–109, 1988.

109  Edgerton BC, Mariani EM, Morrey BF: Distal femoral osteotomy for painful genu valgum. *Clinical Orthopedics* **288**:263–269, 1993.

110  Terry GC, Comino PM: Distal femoral osteotomy for valgus deformity of the knee. *Orthopaedics* **15**:1283–1290, 1992.

111  McDermott AGP, Finklestein JA, Farine I *et al.*: Distal femoral osteotomy for valgus deformity of the knee. *Journal of Bone and Joint Surgery* [Am] **70**:110–116, 1988.

112  Krackow KA: The treatment of unicompartmental knee disease. The case for osteotomy. *Orthopaedics* **17**:852, 1994.

113  McKeever DC: Tibial plateau prosthesis. *Clinical Orthopedics* **18**:86–95, 1960.

114 Marmor L: The modular knee. *Clinical Orthopedics* **94**:242–248, 1973.
115 Goodfellow JW, and O'Connor J: Clinical results of the Oxford knee. Surface arthroplasty of the tibiofemoral joint with a meniscal bearing prosthesis. *Clinical Orthopedics* **205**:21–42, 1986.
116 Stenstrom A, Lindstrand A, and Lewold S: Unicompartmental knee arthroplasty with special reference to the Swedish knee arthroplasty. Register Cahiers d'enseignement de la SOFCOT'61. Unicompartmental Knee Arthroplasty, pp. 159–162, 1996.
117 Scott RD: Mistakes made and lessons learned after 2 decades of unicompartmental knee replacement. Cahiers d'enseignement de la SOFCOT.61. Unicompartmental Knee Arthroplasty, pp. 163–166, 1996.
118 Miller RK, Carr AJ, Keyes GW *et al.*: Lateral unicompartmental replacement with the Oxford knee. *Journal of Bone and Joint Surgery* [Br] **75,Suppl.1**:65, 1993.
119 Lewold S, Goodman S, Knutson K *et al.*: Oxford meniscal bearing knee versus the Marmor knee in unicompartmental arthroplasty for arthrosis. *Journal of Arthroplasty.* **10**:722–731, 1995.
120 Gill T, Schemitsch EH, Brick GW, Thornhill TS: Revision total knee arthroplasty after failed unicompartmental knee arthroplasty or high tibial osteotomy. *Clinical Orthopedics* **321**:10–18, 1995.

# Con: Scott A. Brumby and Thomas S. Thornhill

The treatment of unicompartmental osteoarthritis (OA) of the knee is complex, controversial and requires a careful evaluation of the patient as well as an understanding of the available treatment options. It has been said that the controversy between high tibial osteotomy (HTO) and unicompartmental arthroplasty (UCA) should not exist, since both procedures have their own indications.[1] The majority of early clinical results for both UCA and HTO have been encouraging, but the mid-term results using certain criteria and implants are more variable. There are very few minimum 10 year follow-up reports that compare the results of UCA, HTO, and total knee arthroplasty (TKA). A great deal has been gleaned from the reports of poor mid-term results and these studies have been used to refine the indications for surgery; however, these reports should not be used to justify or criticize either procedure in general.

Unicompartmental OA may exist as a separate entity or may be the early presentation of tricompartmental OA. Between 3 and 30% of early failures of UCA and HTO are due to disease progression in the other two compartments, and in many cases it is difficult to predict which patients will progress to tricompartmental disease.[1-5] Unicompartmental OA may occur due to primary osteoarthritis, osteonecrosis, mechanical overload of one compartment following meniscectomy, laxity of the anterior cruciate ligament (ACL), intra-articular fracture with articular injury or incongruity, and lower limb malalignment.[6] Patients presenting with unicompartmental OA are usually younger and more active than patients with tricompartmental disease. The disease is often as a result of work- or sports-related injury and many patients will place high demand on the knee and wish to resume these activities. Inflammatory arthrosis such as

285

rheumatoid arthritis and the crystal arthropathies should not be considered candidates for UCA or HTO as disease progression is certain and poor results are likely in these groups with both techniques.

Initial management should consist of activity restriction, work modification, minor analgesics, nonsteroidal agents, and physical therapy. Unloading of the knee can be achieved with weight loss, and use of a cane or other walking devices. There is often a great individual variation in patient's pain, function, and disease. Arthroscopic knee surgery is indicated for treatment of associated mechanical symptoms of locking and giving way that may be due to degenerate meniscal tears and chondral flaps. Some have advocated arthroscopic lavage and debridement for treatment of early OA, but the results are variable and will provide only temporary relief. Although conservative measures and arthroscopy are used in the early stages, the natural course of unicompartmental OA is that of progression of disease with reduced function. Ultimately 70% of patients will require surgery[7] and the mainstay of surgical treatment includes UCA, HTO, and TKA.

The majority of the literature, and therefore of this contribution, is related to medial unicompartmental OA treated with valgus HTO of the proximal tibia, or medial UCA. Lateral unicompartmental OA may be treated with varus HTO of the proximal tibia, varus osteotomy of the distal femur, or lateral UCA. In this contribution, unless specified otherwise, unicompartmental OA, UCA, and HTO will refer to medial compartment OA with varus malalignment and the treatment of this condition.

Treatment should be tailored to the individual patient, and the decision-making process must take into account various patient factors, the patient's expectation's and likely satisfaction, technical skill of the surgeon, safety of the procedure, long-term survivorship, and ease of revision to TKA. Indications must be defined for both UCA and HTO, and they do not necessarily have to be the same. The surgeon treating unicompartmental OA must be confident in performing both of these procedures, understanding the indications and limitations of each procedure and the complications that may be present when TKA is required for failed UCA and HTO.

When assessing outcome studies it is important to differentiate between mean follow-up and minimum follow-up. For example, the proponents of HTO will highlight Insall's study[8] that showed 97% excellent or good results at 2 years decreasing to 85% at 5 years and 63% at a mean of 9 years. At first sight 63% pain free at a mean of 9 years appears to be a good outcome and would justify the use of HTO. However, if one looks closely, of the knees that had been followed for a minimum of 9 years only 37% were pain free. Moreover, in recent years Insall has abandoned HTO in favor of TKA even for unicompartmental disease (personal communication).

It is shortsighted to suggest that HTO is the best form of treatment for unicompartmental OA. HTO has a defined role in the management of deformity of the proximal tibia when the aim of the surgery is to correct deformity. Malalignment has been implicated and associated with OA,[9-11] but not all cases of unicompartmental OA are due to malalignment or deformity. Moreover it is not rational to create a bony deformity with an HTO if the malalignment is due to cartilage loss, tibial plateau bone loss, or ligament laxity. Coventry[12] has suggested that angulation creates and enhances abnormal loads on cartilage that results in OA; the rationale for HTO is to correct the abnormal loading. That paper also highlights the importance of dynamic loading and acknowledges that until dynamic loading can be accurately measured, we will only partially, and sometimes unsuccessfully, establish the foundations for treating unicompartmental OA. Several studies have supported this philosophy and suggested that there is not a simple correlation between bony angular deformity and compartmental loading of the knee; it has been shown that correction of malalignment as recommended from clinical studies may not result in significant unloading of the diseased compartment[13-15] and therefore the rationale for HTO is in question.

Our contention is that although HTO is a valuable surgical tool for treatment of unicompartmental OA, it is an insufficient bridge to gap the surgical indications for TKA and nonarthroplasty options in this patient population. UCA should be directed to that transitional group who, because of laxity associated with complete cartilage loss or early subluxation, is at risk for HTO failure but does not have sufficient disease or functional impairment to justify TKA. In addition, the long-term results of TKA performed for primarily unicompartmental OA are not known and may not equal that of TKA performed for multi-compartment OA in younger patients. Furthermore, this contribution will show that both UCA and HTO may provide good long-term results if selected for the correct indication and performed well.

## Surgical indications

The surgeon must correlate the history, examination, mechanical, and radiographic findings when deciding on the treatment options of UCA or HTO. Ideal indications for either UCA or HTO have been determined and modified, based on the analysis of successful and failed procedures. Many patients will not satisfy all criteria and the treating surgeon must make an informed judgement.

Several points should be considered when selecting patients for surgery:

* The patient has clinical symptoms localized to one compartment.
* The patient complains of severe activity related pain that results in reduced function.
* The patient's physiological age should be less than 70 years.
* The patient has a low ratio of body weight to ideal body weight.

- The patients expectations regarding work, general activity level, and wish to play sport are realistic for the procedure planned.
- The patient with an inflammatory arthrosis is not suitable for UCA and HTO and is best treated with TKA.
- Active infection should be excluded and is a contraindication to UCA, HTO, and TKA.

The indications for HTO have been defined and modified based on the review of failed HTO.[8,16–18] The current ideal preoperative criteria for HTO are:

- disabling knee pain due to early unicompartmental OA with deformity
- age less than 60 years
- normal body weight, defined as less than 1.32 times ideal body weight[18]
- the predominant deformity is in the tibia and is often evident as metaphyseal bowing
- ROM > 100°
- no fixed flexion deformity
- minimal lateral subluxation of the tibia with varus deformity or medial subluxation with valgus deformity
- intact collateral and cruciate ligaments (Mild instability due to loss of articular cartilage and stretch due to the deformity are not contraindications, but combined varus deformity and laxity of the ACL can be successfully treated with combined HTO and ACL reconstruction.)
- absence of severe bone defects or osteophytes
- minimal patellofemoral arthritis
- low adduction moment as evident by minimal varus thrust or by formal gait analysis.[19]

Preoperative planning of HTO is essential to ensure precise correction.[20–22] The aim of HTO is to correct deformity and unload the diseased compartment. Poor results of HTO have been associated with both overcorrection and undercorrection and there has been disagreement regarding the optimum alignment of the knee after HTO. Most reports suggest correction to 8–10° of anatomic valgus.[8,18] Coventry[23] has identified that postoperative correction greater than 8° valgus and normal body weight are the only two predictors of success. Arthroscopic assessment pre-HTO and post-HTO has shown repair of articular cartilage defects with fibrous tissue in the diseased compartment if the mechanical axis was corrected into the lateral compartment 30–40% beyond the center of the knee.[24]

Precise intraoperative measurement of correction is also required. Many techniques lack accuracy and are subject to confounding errors. Calculation of the size of wedge to remove in a closing wedge HTO using the "1 mm equals 1°" rule applies only to a tibia that has a mid-coronal diameter of 57 mm. Use of this rule in larger diameter tibias will result in undercorrection. Insall[8] noted that a 1 cm based wedge in a male will result in a correction of only 8°, not 10° as many surgeons would have planned. The width of the two saw cuts may induce an error of up to 4 mm to the base of the wedge (each saw cut will remove approximately 2 mm of bone). The level of the HTO with respect to the center of rotation of the deformity will also influence the alignment achieved; correction below the center of rotation of the deformity will result in undercorrection.[20] The use of angled cutting blocks has been shown to reduce these errors.[25]

Indications for UCA have been defined and modified by based on review of failed UCA.[1,26–32] The current ideal preoperative criteria for UCA are:

- disabling knee pain with unicompartmental disease
- physiological age greater than 60 years; Marmor[1] suggests greater than 50 years
- low level of activity; UCA is not recommended for young, active patients involved in heavy or repetitive manual activities
- Normal body weight (<82 kg), although weight is not a contraindication for Murray[32]
- no inflammatory component of the disease, minimal knee pain at rest
- range of movement (ROM) >90°
- flexion deformity <5–10°
- minimal subluxation
- intact ACL and collateral ligaments
- deformity <10° varus or 15° valgus; usually the deformity can be corrected manually.

Patients should first satisfy all preoperative criteria, and the surgeon should then be prepared to perform either a UCA or a TKA. At the time of surgery a decision is made whether to proceed with UCA or change to TKA depending on the operative findings. The intraoperative contraindications for UCA include:

- synovitis and effusion
- chondrocalcinosis or crystal arthropathy; this is not a contraindication for Murray[32]
- multicompartmental disease; small cartilage erosions or fibrillation in the opposite compartment are not a contra-indication
- normal patellofemoral joint; this is not a contraindication for Murray[32] or Marmor[1]
- deformity cannot be corrected with limited ligament releases
- deficient ACL
- opposite compartment meniscal disease.

Murray *et al.*[32] have stressed the importance of an intact ACL. A "normal" ACL was defined as one that retained its synovial covering and had no longitudinal splits. A deficient or damaged ACL has been associated with a high failure rate of UCA with the Oxford knee owing to tibial component loosening.

Despite the long-running controversy of UCA and HTO, no prospective, randomized trials have been performed to assess them. This is perhaps due to the widespread success of TKA and opposing views of proponents of either UCA or HTO.

Insall published his selection criteria and results of HTO[8] and in addition studied patient selection for UCA versus TKA[33] using Kozinn and Scott's criteria.[30] The HTO indications may be biased, as initially the options available were HTO or arthrodesis and the introduction of TKA resulted in redefining the role of HTO. The paper on criteria for UCA was performed at the time of arthrotomy for TKA and a decision was made whether UCA would be possible, although all patients received a TKA. They found that only 15% of patients presenting for TKA would have satisfied the criteria of visual assessment of unicompartmental articular cartilage changes at the time of arthrotomy and only 6% of patients satisfied all of the Kozinn and Scott criteria.

Some patients do not meet the criteria for either UCA or HTO and these should be considered for TKA; others satisfy the criteria for both UCA and HTO and thus create a dilemma. Surgeons have different approaches and options when performing UCA or HTO. In HTO a patient is selected on the basis of preoperative criteria, the amount of correction is calculated from preoperative radiographs, and the operation is performed. The postoperative correction at 1 year will determine the fate of the HTO.[18] A decision to perform a UCA gives the surgeon options at the time of the procedure. The patient is selected using the preoperative criteria, and then proceeds with UCA or changes to TKA depending on the operative findings.

## Operative planning

The mainstay of operative planning is plain radiography. All patients should have a standard weightbearing three-joint film (taken with the patella facing forward) and a 30° flexion weightbearing view to assess unicompartmental disease and lower limb biomechanics and to assist in the planning of UCA, HTO, and TKA. Several features are assessed:

- The relative disease involvement of each compartment as determined by joint space narrowing, hypertrophic spurring, and subchondral sclerosis.
- Subluxation of the knee joint is measured.
- Joint alignment is measured by constructing the mechanical axes of the lower limb bones (mechanical axis deformity).[20]

- Joint orientation is determined by constructing the lateral distal femoral angle (angle between a line drawn across the femoral condyles and the shaft of the femur) and the medial proximal tibial angle (angle between a line drawn across the tibial plateau and the shaft of the tibia).[20]

Bone scan has been suggested to aid in patient selection for HTO.[23,34] If there is increased uptake in the "normal" compartment in addition to the "diseased" compartment, one should be hesitant to perform an HTO or UCA.[23] Diffuse increased uptake around the knee may indicate a generalized inflammatory arthrosis, crystal arthropathy, or more extensive degenerative disease. There have been no studies reporting the sensitivity and specificity of bone scan in predicting the long-term success of HTO or UCA.

Standard magnetic resonance imaging (MRI) may be used to diagnose intra-articular pathology causing mechanical symptoms that may be treated by arthroscopy. Newly developed MRI cartilage sequences are currently being studied that assess gross morphologic defects in articular cartilage and the early changes of OA. These are currently experimental and may provide better patient selection in the future.

Gait analysis has been used in several centers to select patients for HTO based on measurement of adductor moments.[19,35,36] Although formal gait analysis is not standard practice in most centers, clinical observation of patient's gait can detect patients with high adductor moments evident as a varus or lateral thrust gait.

Low adduction moment has been suggested by one group of investigators as a predictor of success following HTO and may represent a positive compensatory mechanism to unload the diseased compartment by changing gait pattern.[19,36] A low preoperative adduction moment has been shown to be predictive of postoperative success up to 6 years after surgery regardless of preoperative knee score, initial deformity, postoperative correction, age, and weight. These findings have been recently contradicted using similar methodology.[35] In that study, postoperative correction was the only indicator of success following HTO and they suggested that low adduction moments may be associated with less severe disease and therefore better results. The usefulness of gait analysis and assessment of dynamic loading remains unclear, but more detailed review may improve the accuracy of patient selection for HTO.

Gait analysis has also been used to assess UCA and has been compared with TKA and normal knees.[37] Patients with a UCA had more normal knee kinematics when compared to TKA. Adduction moments were higher in the UCA group compared to TKA and correlated with postoperative varus alignment.

Arthroscopic assessment of the "diseased," "normal," and patellofemoral compartments is not a good predictor of success for HTO at minimum 5 year follow-up.[38]

## Technical aspects

It is widely assumed that static deformity at the level of the knee joint will result in abnormal load transfer to one compartment and this will result in the development of unicompartmental OA. The location and magnitude of the deformity determine the amount of angulation that will result in abnormal cartilage loading.[22,39] The theory of HTO is based on this premise and the hypothesis that correction or slight overcorrection of the deformity will change the load transmission in the diseased compartment and will reduce symptoms and slow or reverse disease progression.[17] Overcorrection may place more load through the normal compartment and if this increase is significant, may accelerate degenerate changes in the normal compartment. Many studies have highlighted flaws in the use of a static model for assessment of deformity and found the above theory to be incorrect.[13,14,19,36] Static assessment of deformity does not take into account the dynamics of gait, location, and movement of the body center of gravity, and internal forces due to ligaments, muscles, and the articular surfaces of the knee joint.

Harrington[13] found that during dynamic loading the knee joint force was shared between both compartments owing to the internal forces and the location of the joint force varied during the gait cycle. The resultant force was transmitted through the medial compartment for a significant part of the gait cycle for normal, varus and valgus deformities. It was observed that a large valgus angulation (20–30°) was required before the load was transmitted to the lateral compartment. Shaw and Molton[14] highlight many flaws in the theory used by advocates to support HTO and suggests that HTO must shift the dynamic axis laterally and a correction to 25° valgus is necessary to sufficiently unload the medial compartment.

Deformity due to collateral ligament and soft tissue laxity is difficult to assess and correct, but consideration of opening or closing wedge HTO or collateral ligament reconstruction should be made as these will influence collateral laxity. Balancing of the collateral ligaments is important for obtaining stability and restoration of the dynamic loading of the knee, however this subject has received little attention in the literature. Dugdale et al.[40] have suggested that each 1 mm of lateral tibiofemoral joint separation causes an additional 1° of varus angular deformity and this should be considered when calculating the HTO correction angle. Paley et al.[20] have clearly described the management of deformity based on bony deformity, collateral ligament laxity, and leg length discrepancies.

In 1965, Coventry[16] described six criteria for performing an HTO. Although these criteria were defined 35 years ago, most surgeons performing HTO still adopt Coventry's philosophical approach, which is that the HTO should:

* fully or slightly overcorrect the deformity

- be near the site of deformity
- involve bone that will heal rapidly
- allow early ROM and weightbearing
- allow for intra-articular assessment
- be relatively safe and simple.

However, there are several issues with some of these criteria.

- Full correction or slightly overcorrecting the deformity does not significantly unload the diseased compartment.[13,14]
- The exact position of the deformity must be defined. In some cases there is a metaphyseal bow and therefore the HTO is near the deformity and will primarily correct the deformity. However, in many cases the deformity is due to loss of cartilage, medial plateau bone loss or ligament laxity; in these cases HTO will create a secondary deformity and alter the joint line orientation.
- Although the surgeon may allow early ROM and restricted early weightbearing, studies have shown that gait does not return to the preoperative level until 12 months after the operation, unlike UCA and TKA where full ROM and weightbearing was usually allowed resulting in improved gait at 6 months after the operation.[41]

Coventry later documents that any internal derangement should be treated prior to HTO as postoperative stiffness has been a problem if arthrotomy is performed at the same time as HTO.[17] Others have suggested that arthroscopic assessment of the articular surface does not influence the results of HTO and that the decision to perform HTO is based on plain radiographs.[38]

The theoretical basis of HTO has some major deficiencies and controversies. More precise assessment techniques are required to document abnormal dynamic loading of the diseased compartment, calculate the level and amount of correction required, and assess the articular cartilage. Until these techniques are available, HTO will continue to be performed without any scientific basis. The result being, unpredictable results and early failure.

HTO not only affects the mechanical alignment of the lower limb, it also induces anatomical changes to the proximal tibia or distal femur, patella height, extensor mechanism alignment and collateral ligament tension that may cause problems immediately or later when TKA is required. HTO results in changes in the mechanics of the proximal tibiofibular joint either by disruption of the joint or fibula osteotomy.

A lateral closing wedge HTO will result in shortening of the lower limb, change of shape of the tibia metaphysis and alignment with the shaft, patella infera, LCL laxity, and increased Q-angle of the extensor mechanism. A medial opening wedge HTO will lengthen the lower limb, change the shape of the tibia metaphysis and alignment with the shaft, cause patella infera, further tighten the MCL, and increase the Q-angle of the extensor mechanism.

The philosophy of UCA is very simple and is less controversial than that of HTO. The main advantage of UCA is anatomical correction of knee joint deformity that is due to cartilage loss, tibial plateau bone loss, and ligament stretching without creating a secondary deformity. UCA should not be performed in knees where there is a significant primary deformity located in the metaphysis. UCA is performed to resurface the arthritic compartment of the knee and to re-establish the lower limb axial alignment. This is obtained by reconstructing the joint space gap and level with collateral ligament and flexion–extension balance. If the operation is performed correctly with stable and balanced ligaments, the kinematics and biomechanics of the knee are restored to near normal.

Minimal bone resection is performed, in fact less than with TKA, and UCA has a theoretical advantage of minimal anatomic changes to the proximal tibia and bone stock retention should revision to TKA be required. These advantages have not been proven in studies assessing failure of early designs with polyethylene wear and osteolysis; the results may be better with proven designs, improved polyethylene wear, and close surveillance with early revision at the first sign of failure.

Design rationale and surgical technique for UCA have already been described in detail.[30,42] The femoral component should be wide enough to cap the resurfaced condyle, be of a size that reproduces the AP dimensions of the femoral condyle, and adequately distributes the weightbearing forces and resists subsidence. The joint line level must be restored and therefore the distal femoral resection should equal the thickness of the component; in general 2–4 mm of bone from the distal femur is resected allowing for cartilage loss. The posterior condyle resection should equal the thickness of the component as cartilage loss is less in this area and it is better to resect too much of the posterior condyle than too little to avoid tightness in flexion. The femoral component should extend far enough anterior to cover the weightbearing surface of the tibia in full extension and should be recessed so as not to interfere with normal patellofemoral tracking. The tibial component must have at least 6 mm of polyethylene; either an 8 mm all-polyethylene component or a 8–10 mm metal-backed composite component. The tibia should be positioned such that there is contact with the cortical rim of the proximal tibia and be aligned with the femoral component through a full range of motion. Rotation of the components should be finally checked with the patella reduced in the trochlear groove. The tibial cut should be tilted to retain the posterior slope of the tibia specific for the knee. The tibial insert should adequately restore the normal joint line and correct the alignment towards but not beyond the neutral mechanical axis. As a general rule it is best to undercorrect by 3°.

Further advantages of UCA include the ability to improve knee range of motion and reduce pain by remove impinging osteophytes and intra-articular adhesions.[30] Postoperative immobilization is not required with UCA and bilateral procedures can be performed at the same sitting or during the same admission to hospital.[30] There is recent interest in performing UCA through a miniarthrotomy and as a day-case procedure, although long-term results are not yet available to recommend this approach.

UCA is a reconstructive procedure that restores the joint line, restores ligament tension, and does not effect the anatomy of the patella or extensor mechanism. The procedure does involve bone resection, although this is less than or equal to that performed during TKA. The desired alignment is so the mechanical axis is through the center of the knee.[30,43] Changes in anatomy are seen with failure due to component migration or osteolysis secondary to wear debris.

## Clinical outcome

It is important at this stage to compare the results of UCA and HTO with TKA. TKA is a successful operation for OA in older patients with several studies reporting 10–15 year survivorship of 90–95%;[44-46] on the basis of these results, many surgeons would suggest that unicompartmental OA is also treated best with TKA. However, there are few reports regarding TKA performed for OA in patients less than 55 years.[47-50] The results for young patients in general are skewed by the excellent outcome of TKA performed for juvenile rheumatoid arthritis and other inflammatory arthroses; the reports must therefore be reviewed with respect to OA if the findings are to be compared with UCA and HTO. Furthermore, there may be a selection bias as many young patients with unicompartmental OA may have been preferentially treated with a UCA or HTO on the basis of the recommended indications.

It can be expected that the patient younger than 55 years having a UCA or HTO will require conversion to TKA at some stage. The results of TKA performed primarily, after UCA, and after HTO may not be the same. Perhaps a more important outcome of UCA and HTO is the result of the first or second revision TKA performed after failure of the UCA, HTO, or primary TKA. There are no long-term detailed results of the outcome of revision TKA performed following HTO and UCA.

A problem facing many surgeons is the technically demanding procedure to convert a failed UCA or HTO to a successful TKA. There have been several reports of alternative surgical options for failed UCA and HTO. Abrasion arthroplasty is not a satisfactory salvage for failed HTO.[51] Revision of failed UCA to another UCA is in general not successful.[52] Revision of failed HTO to UCA has been performed. The current recommended treatment of a failed UCA or HTO would be revision to a TKA. It is important to have an understanding of the potential difficulties in revision of a failed UCA or HTO to TKA. A modern, modular revision TKA system with stemmed components and augmentation wedges and access to allograft bone is required to successfully treat potential bone deficiency and abnormal anatomy.

*Some technical points*

- A difficult exposure due to patella infera and collateral ligament contracture can be expected and an extensile exposure may be required. Available options include a quadriceps snip, quadriceps turndown, or tibial tuberosity osteotomy. Lateral release is often required.
- Attempt to lower the joint line if there is patella infera.
- Abnormal anatomy of the proximal tibia is common and may result in alignment and rotation difficulties.
- Bone deficiency is likely, therefore perform a minimal lateral tibial resection, consider wedges and bone graft.
- Posterior slope for the tibial resection should be set at 0°.
- Stemmed tibial components may be required.
- Peroneal nerve scarring and injury.

## Minimum 10 year results of HTO, UCA, and TKA

There are numerous reports dealing with new techniques of HTO, complications and early results (Table 11.4). There are similar reports for UCA with early results of new implant designs. Long-term, minimum 10 year results, are important when deciding on treatment options. We have been able to find only four published reports of minimum 10 year results of UCA, HTO, or TKA performed in young patients for unicompartmental OA.

**Table 11.4** The measured and predicted 10 year survivorship results for UNI, HTO and TKA in descending order of outcome success

| Reference | Procedure | 10 year survivorship | Follow-up (years) | Range (years) | 95% confidence interval |
|---|---|---|---|---|---|
| Murray et al. (1998)[32] | UNI | 98% | Minimum 5 | 5–14 | 93–100% |
| Diduch et al. (1997)[47] | TKA | 95% | Mean 8 | 3–18 | 63–100% |
| Capra and Fehring (1992)[73] | UNI | 94% | Mean 8 | | |
| Cartier et al. (1996)[54] | UNI | 93% | Minimum 10 | 10–18 | 80–100% |
| Ranawat et al. (1989)[49] | TKA | 91% | Mean 6 | | |
| Heck et al. (1993)[75] | UNI | 91% | Mean 10 | | |
| Duffy et al. (1998)[50] | TKA | 89% | Minimum 10 | 10–17 | |
| Bert (1998)[74] | UNI | 87% | Mean 10 | | |
| Scott et al. (1991)[2] | UNI | 85% | Minimum 8 | 8–12 | |
| Tabor and Tabor (1998)[80] | UNI | 84% | Minimum 5 | 5–20 | |
| Marmor (1988)[1] | UNI | 70% | Minimum 10 | 10–13 | |
| Coventry et al. (1993)[18] | HTO | 65% | Mean 10 | 3–14 | 52–78% |
| Rinonapoli et al. (1998)[53] | HTO | 55% | Minimum 10 | 10–21 | |
| Insall et al. (1984)[8] | HTO | 37% | Minimum 9 | 5–15 | |

Rinonapoli et al.[53] have published the only minimum 10 year results of HTO using the operative technique described by Insall.[8] They have reported 55% good to excellent results at minimum 10 years (range 10–21 years) and the subgroup with minimum 15 year follow-up had deteriorated to 46% good to excellent. Multivariate analysis of outcome demonstrated correlation only with time after surgery and no correlation between outcome and the amount of correction.

Marmor[1] has reported minimum 10 year results of 60 Marmor UNIs with 70% of patients having a satisfactory result. Only 7 patients were younger than 50 years. Failures were seen with loosening of thin polyethylene, obesity, inability to correct severe deformity, and patella impingement on the femoral component attributed to material or technical problems and improper patient selection. There was only 2 failures for progression of disease at 10 years after implantation. Marmor's paper was published in 1988 and has resulted in modifications to the implant design and indications for surgery.

Cartier et al.[54] followed 207 Marmor UNIs for a minimum 10 years (range 10–18 years) with a 93% 10 year survivorship (95% confidence intervals of 80–100%). Selection criteria were patients less than 70 years with a contraindication to HTO such as severe arthrosis, no deformity without metaphyseal bowing, pagoda shaped tibial plateaus, pseudolaxity due to osteophytes or bone stock deficiency, or AP translation of the tibia; in patients older than 70 years, a UCA was chosen in preference to a TKA. The results of UCA in the younger patients was not different to the older patients. Despite these excellent results, the authors still prefer to perform HTO in the younger patients.

Duffy et al.[50] have reported minimum 10 year follow-up of 74 TKAs for patients younger than 55 years and include 18 patients with a diagnosis of primary or post-traumatic OA. During the 10 year period, 3 revision procedures were performed, all in the OA group; one for ligament laxity, one for patella loosening, and one for polyethylene wear and femoral loosening. The 10 year survival with revision as the end-point was 89% in the OA group.

## HTO

The long-term results of Insall (1984) using a closing wedge proximal tibial HTO fixed in a plaster cast are often used to support HTO and describe the progression with time. At 2 years 97% had an excellent or good result; that decreased to 85% at 5 years and 63% at a mean of 8.9 years. Most other reports fail to mention an important finding from this paper:[8] only 37% of the knees that had been followed for a minimum of 9 years were pain free. They suggest that HTO should be reserved for patients less than 60 years who have a strenuous occupation or wish to continue playing sport.

Coventry has been performing closing wedge proximal tibial HTO fixed with staples for over 30 years, but hig group has published many excellent reports on the technique, indications, and results of

HTO unfortunately they have not published long-term results of the original or subsequent series. The most recent report in 1993,[23] at a median 10 years (minimum 3 years), documented 20 failures and identified the 2 factors that predicted success—body weight and postoperative correction. If at 1 year after surgery the body weight was less than 1.32 times the ideal weight and the valgus angulation was 8° or more, the survival probability was 90% at 5 years and 65 % at 10 years (95% confidence interval 52–78%). If at 1 year after surgery the body weight was more than 1.32 times the ideal weight and the valgus angulation was less than 8°, the survival probability was 38% at 5 years and 19% at 10 years.

Matthews et al.[55] reported the probability for continued useful function of the knee after HTO. The results showed a gradual deterioration with time with a chance of continuing satisfactory function of 86% at 1 year, 50% at 5 years and only 28% at 9 years. A greater chance of success was associated with younger age, lower body weight, and postoperative correction of 3–12° valgus from normal 5–7° anatomic valgus. Nonunion was treated with TKA in 4 patients.

Morrey[56] suggests that success is associated with young age, normal body weight, early OA changes, deformity due to metaphyseal bowing, low preoperative adductor moment, and correction to 3–6° of mechanical valgus. Ritter suggests that the reliable longevity of HTO is approximately 6 years.[57]

TKA after failed HTO has been reported by Staeheli et al.[3] where 35 patients were followed for a minimum 2.5 years. The main reason for revision to TKA was continued pain associated with progression of arthrosis (54%) or inadequate correction (29%). At the time of revision to TKA, the majority of patients had no subluxation, well-preserved lateral joint space, and an average of 3.5° of valgus. Patella infera was seen in only 11% and was mild. At a mean 44 months, 90% had an HSS good or excellent result. There were no difficulties with surgical exposure.

Amendola et al.[58] report on 42 patients that had a failed HTO converted to TKA. At minimum 2 year follow-up with 88% HSS good to excellent results. This group was compared to a historical control group and pain and function were similar, although the control group had slightly greater ROM. The preoperative alignment of the failed HTO group was 2° varus. They conclude that previous HTO does not alter the outcome of TKA in the short term.

Windsor et al.[59] reported 45 failed HTO revised to TKA and reviewed at a minimum 2 year follow-up with 80% HSS good to excellent results: 80% had patella infera, 47% required a lateral release, quadriceps turndown in 4%, and 22% required an extensive lateral collateral release. Loss of posterior tibial slope following HTO is highlighted in this paper and caution should be taken when resecting the tibia to prevent a large flexion gap.

Nizard et al.[60] report on 63 TKAs performed after failed HTO and compare them with a matched group of patients with primary TKA.

The failed HTO group had a higher rate of operative problems due to exposure and required 7 tibial tubercle osteotomies and 15 lateral releases. The clinical results at 4.6 years were not significantly different although the failed HTO group had more pain.

Katz et al.[61] report difficulty in exposure of failed HTO to TKA and results that approach but do not equal those of primary TKA. The HTO group had a preoperative average alignment of 6° valgus compared with 2° varus in the primary TKA group. Complications that occurred following the HTO such as peroneal nerve injury, reflex sympathetic dystrophy, retained hardware, abnormal proximal tibial anatomy, and extensor mechanism problems may compromise the result of TKA following failure of HTO.

Mont et al.[62] reviewed 73 TKAs (including those reported by Katz et al.[61]) after failed HTO at a minimum 2 years and performed a matched analysis with 2 groups of patients with TKA with similar deformity pre-TKA and pre-HTO. At their institution 8% of all TKA had prior HTO. Poor results were related to worker's compensation status, history of RSD, early onset, and no period of pain relief after HTO, multiple surgeries prior to HTO, and manual occupation.

### UCA

The early reports of UCA by Insall and Walker[26] and Laskin[63] were disappointing. However, both of these reports improved the selection criteria and knowledge regarding UCA. Insall and Walker[26] reported minimum 2 year follow-up on 24 UNIs. Patellectomy was performed in 63% of the patients at the time of UCA. Only 58% of the medial compartment UNIs had an excellent or good result. There were 3 of 19 (16%) medial compartment UNIs that required revision. Histology of the cartilage from the opposite compartment at the time of revision to TKA showed embedded polyethylene particles. All the lateral compartment UNIs had an excellent or good result.

Laskin[63] reported 22% revision at minimum 2 years with 37 Marmor UNIs. Poor results were associated with incorrect patient selection, disease progression in the opposite compartment, patellofemoral pain, and tibial component loosening. Laskin noted yellowing and fibrillation of the cartilage in the opposite compartment in almost every knee despite no radiographic changes. Embedded polyethylene particles were also noted on histology of the cartilage from the opposite compartment at the time of revision to TKA. Laskin also noted overcorrection in 4 of the 8 failed UNIs. It was interesting that the 3 patients with a lateral UCA had excellent results similar to that reported by Insall and Walker.[26]

Callahan et al.[64] have performed a meta-analysis of UCA and TKA. For UCA there were 2391 patients with a mean follow-up of 4.6 years. The overall complication rate was 18.5%, which was less than that reported for TKA. The revision rate was 9.2% for UCA, compared to 7.2% for TKA, and the results of UCA reported after 1987 showed improved results.

Data from the Swedish National Knee Arthroplasty Register has provided relevant information on UCA performed by many surgeons.[52] Some of this data has been reported in small studies from the individual institutions,[65,66] but the combined report provides an overall picture of UCA in the general community. Data was collected since 1975 and by the end of 1995, 1135 of 14 772 (7.7%) of UNIs had been revised; the main reasons for revision were implant loosening (medial UCA 45%, lateral UCA 31%) and joint degeneration (medial UCA 25%, lateral UCA 35%). The incidence of revision over the 10 year period (note: this is not survivorship or minimum 10 years) of the most common implants were Marmor (8%), St. Georg sledge (9%), Link (3%), PCA (16%), Oxford (9%), Brigham (3%). There was a higher rate of re-revision if a failed UCA was revised to a UCA rather than to TKA, leading to the conclusion that failed UNIs should be revised with TKA. The same institution has found that despite the higher revision rate of UCA compared to TKA, the predicted lifetime cost of a UCA was 57% of that of a TKA. They conclude that UCA can be recommended on the basis of cost-effectiveness as well as clinically.

Other data from the Swedish Knee Arthroplasty Project[5] has shown that the 5 year revision rate of the Marmor UCA has decreased from 11% to 5% and shown a continuous improvement with time. The design has remained constant over the study period and the improvement has been attributed to the learning curve, improved surgical skill, and improved patient selection. All the centers that were assessed were performing less than 50 UNIs per year.

Scott et al.[2] have reported minimum 8 year follow-up of the Brigham/PFC knee, previously reported at minimum 2 years.[67] Calculated survivorship was 90% at 9 years, 85% at 10 years, and 82% at 11 years; 87% had no significant pain at minimum 8 years. Schai et al.[68] have assessed 28 UNIs in patients younger than 60 years. Patients were selected as those less than 60 years who had a relative contraindication to HTO. Minimum 2 year results of 93% survivorship and 90% pain relief are similar to HTO but inferior to TKA.

High wear rates have been reported for early designs of the Brigham UNI[69] and the PCA UCA.[52,70,71] Possible failure mechanisms include inadequate polyethylene thickness, defects in the polyethylene due to sterilization, increased rotational freedom, reduced conformity, implant malalignment, and ACL laxity. Low wear rates have been reported with the Oxford UCA which is a fully congruent meniscal bearing implant[72] although there have been reports of higher revision rates due to dislocating meniscus, technical failure, and loosening.[65]

Murray et al.[32] have reviewed 143 Oxford fully congruent meniscal bearing UCA's at minimum 5 years and calculated 10 year cumulative survival rate of 98% (33 knees at risk, 95% confidence interval of 93–100%).

Capra[73] has reported predicted 10 year survivorship of 94% following a study with average 8 year follow-up. Bert[74] has reported

10 year survivorship of 87% following a study with a mean follow-up of 10 years.

The 10 year survivorship of a multicenter study[75] incorporating the results from Marmor[1] and Rougraff et al.[76] has been reported as 91%, declining to 81% at 12 years. Minimum 1 year,[70] 2 year,[77,78] and 4 year[79] reports have documented revision rates of 5–15% and good to excellent clinical results in 74–80%. The results of the Marmor UCA from other centers has been reported as 91% at minimum 5 years and predicted survivorship at 10 years of 84 ± 5%.[80]

Barrett et al.[4] reviewed 29 TKAs after failed UCA at a minimum of 2 years. In this study 93% were revised with a cruciate-retaining TKA and bone graft, augmentation with screws or cement, a long stem component, or a combination of these was used in 50% of cases. Bone graft, cement spacers, or metal wedges were used in 28% of cases to reconstruct bone defects. Tibial tuberosity steotomy was only required in one case. It was noted that failure of the UCA was related to a technical error or improper patient selection in 33%, and these errors would not occur using current criteria, implants, and surgical technique. The avoidable causes of failure included over-correction, undercorrection, femoral component malposition, and progression of disease.

Levine et al.[81] reviewed 31 TKAs after failed UCA at a minimum of 2 years. In 68% the reason for failure was polyethylene wear without component loosening and in 32% progression of disease at a mean of 5 years after UCA. Bone defects were managed with wedges (4 tibia, 2 femur) or cancellous grafts for contained defects. No structural grafts were required.

Chakrabarty et al.[82] report on 73 failed UNIs revised to TKA. In 64% there was either no defect or it was small and contained, presenting little problem. There was 75% excellent or good clinical function at an average of 5 years after revision to TKA.

## TKA

The largest series of TKAs in young patients with OA has been reported by Diduch et al.[47] with minimum 3 year (average 8 year) follow-up of 114 TKAs. They predict a 90% survival at 10 years (95% confidence interval of 63–100%). These results must be carefully interpreted, as the results are only accurate for the minimum 3 year follow-up, the rest are statistical predictions. Review of the Kaplan–Meier survivorship curves suggests progressive failure after 6 years with 8 year survival of 90%. The reasons for failure included infection, ligament laxity, polyethylene wear, and patella component loosening and it may be expected that failures due to polyethylene wear will increase with time. The clinical results for all reviewed knees were good or excellent.

Ranawat et al.[49] have reported average 6 year follow-up of 93 TKAs for patients younger than 55 years and 17 had a diagnosis of OA. The predicted survival at 10 years for revision or clinical failure was 91%.

## Comparative studies

Several studies have retrospectively reviewed HTO, UCA, and TKA in the management of unicompartmental OA. Newman et al.[83] have performed the only prospective, randomized trial of unicompartmental OA comparing UCA and TKA. There have been no long-term, prospective, randomized trials between UCA and HTO.

Newman et al.[83] have demonstrated superior results of UCA versus TKA in a prospective, randomized study at 5 years. The UCA group had lower perioperative morbidity, greater ROM, reduced hospital length of stay, and more excellent results. Revision rates and radiological evidence of loosening were low and were not different between UCA and TKA at 5 years.

Laurencin et al.[84] compared UCA versus TKA in the same patient performed during the same admission. They found that a UCA to have a subjectively better knee with less pain, and greater range of motion (ROM) than the TKA side. Rehabilitation seemed to be more rapid following UCA than TKA.[85] Rougraff et al.[76] found similar results suggesting that, with correct patient selection, UCA allows for reduced rehabilitation and a subjectively better knee than does TKA.

Broughton et al.[86] reported the 5–10 year results of a cohort of 121 patients that had either a St. Georg sledge UCA or an opening wedge HTO. The results of UCA (76% good) were better than HTO (43% good). Weale and Newman[87] reviewed the available patients from the same cohort at 12–17 years following surgery. They demonstrated superior results in the UCA group, 42% good results, that were maintained after a long follow-up period compared to 21% in the HTO group.

Ivarsson and Gillquist[41] studied early results in a small group of UCA and HTO patients. At 6 months after surgery, the UCA group had better quadriceps strength, gait parameters, Lyzholm scores, and improved activity levels. The HTO patients took 12 months to regain their preoperative quadriceps strength and at 12 months there was no change in their gait parameters or activity level. They concluded that UCA has faster rehabilitation and improved function.

The same group as reported by Levine et al.[81] was matched with 30 failed HTO requiring TKA and reported in a separate paper.[88] The HTO group had an average anatomic alignment at the time of revision to TKA of 7° valgus compared to 2° valgus in the UCA group. The Knee Society scores for the HTO group were significantly higher than for the UCA group and more osseous reconstructions were required in the UCA group. Difficulty with exposure and early failure of the TKA performed after UCA or HTO was not different. This is in agreement with other studies of failed HTO with minimal deformity.

Jackson et al.[89] compared the outcome of TKA following failed HTO and UCA. The group that had previous HTO had a higher incidence of deep infection and wound healing. In half of the UCA group there was significant bone loss from the medial tibial plateau. The clinical results before and after TKA were not different.

## Conclusion

The long-term outcome of HTO is clearly inferior to UCA and TKA. UCA in selected patients is supported by the reported minimum 10 year survivorship of 93% with a 95% confidence interval of 80%[54] and several reports of greater than 90% predicted 10 year survival.[32,52,64,73,75] TKA performed for OA in patients younger than 55 years has predicted 10 year survivorship of 90%, although the 95% confidence interval suggests results may be as low as 63%.[47] The outcome of HTO at minimum 10 years is pain free, good to excellent results in the order of 35–65% and the results tend to deteriorate progressively with time.[8,53,55] Although this may reflect selection of younger and more active patients in the HTO group, the published results available do not support the widespread use of HTO in the treatment of unicompartmental OA. In addition, the results of UCA are superior to TKA and HTO in terms of perioperative morbidity, faster rehabilitation, greater ROM, and a subjectively more normal feeling knee.

It is difficult to find any advantages in performing HTO except for buying time in the young patient who has an active occupation or continues to play sport. Even with this limited indication, rehabilitation, pain relief, function, and gait take more than 12 months to return to preoperative levels and pain relief is likely to be incomplete. The clinical literature on HTO technique and patient selection has changed little since Coventry's landmark paper of 1973[17] and the amount of correction, type of osteotomy, and method of fixation are the only variables that have been addressed in the recent clinical literature. It is unlikely that the results of osteotomy will improve unless patient selection and operative planning is modified by using new imaging modalities, better interpretation of gait analysis or techniques that improve bone healing, prevent disease progression, and more accurately realign the lower extremity.

The results for UCA and TKA have improved with time owing to improved patient selection, implant design, and surgical technique, whereas the results of HTO have not changed in the past 30 years. Furthermore, patients younger than 55 years at the time of the index operation should be aware that they will require one or several revision TKA procedures in their lifetime and the results following the first or subsequent revision are currently unknown.

Success of UCA has been associated with avoidance of thin (<6 mm) polyethylene, restoration to neutral alignment or slight undercorrection, and cementing both sides. Careful attention to ligament balancing, selection of a proven implant system, improved wear of current polyethylene inserts, and use of all-polyethylene patella components may improve the survival, but this remains to be proven. Certain designs have performed well whereas others have failed, and therefore implant selection is critical for success.

The main reasons for failure of UCA are aseptic loosening and osteolysis. The main difficulties encountered with failed UCA are related to delayed management of osteolysis owing to polyethylene wear. Regular radiographic review and early revision for polyethylene wear may allow for an easy revision procedure for liner exchange prior to component loosening or osteolysis. If detected early, most failures can be managed with a standard primary TKA system and bone defects will be contained and treated with minor cancellous bone grafting. In a small percentage of cases a dedicated revision TKA system with augmentation wedges or allograft will be required. It is suggested that a TKA system is used that allows progression from primary to revision components.

There are many conflicting reports of the technical difficulty, complication rate, and clinical outcome of TKA performed after failed HTO. The papers that report minimal difficulty[3,58] include many patients with inadequate correction and varus deformity at the time of TKA; this group as a whole had minimal deformity. Although persistent varus deformity may allow easy revision to TKA, it is associated with clinical failure of HTO. This group of patients is not representative of well-performed HTO patients with valgus correction. A more realistic picture of the difficulty of revising HTO to TKA will be found in studies that compare revision of HTO that were adequately corrected into 8° of valgus, that have functioned well for 10 years, and have then failed. If we look at papers where initial correction was adequate, we find that difficulty was experienced and was associated with patella infera, loss of posterior tibial slope, and abnormal proximal tibial anatomy.[59–62,89] This group more accurately reflects the greater difficulty in revising HTO to TKA, which is more complex than with primary TKA or UCA.

Overall, the results of revision TKA following HTO and UCA are similar but inferior to that of primary TKA. There is no comparative data available for the results of revision TKA for failed TKA in a subset of young patients. Following HTO where adequate valgus correction has been obtained, the anatomy of the proximal tibia is greatly altered, the extensor mechanism may be scarred, and there are many potential complications. Careful attention must be paid to the sagittal and coronal plane deformities that have been created by the HTO to ensure equal flexion–extension gaps and normal alignment and extensile approaches may be required. These difficulties are less of a problem with failed UCA, however bone deficiencies will need to be addressed if revising a component with osteolysis due to polyethylene wear.

Several comments should be repeated at this stage to reject the statement that unicompartmental OA of the knee is best treated by an HTO rather than UCA.

- It has been said that the controversy between HTO and UCA should not exist, since each procedure has its own indications.[1]

- The indications for HTO are limited. Following the proven success of TKA, HTO is currently indicated for patients who have an occupation requiring vigorous activity or who wish to continue to play sports.[8]
- HTO will provide only partial pain relief and only 37% of the knees that had been followed for a minimum of 9 years are pain free.[8] Many patients will not accept persistent pain.
- Coventry[23] has identified that postoperative correction greater than 8° valgus and normal body weight are the only two predictors of success.
- UCA is indicated for patients younger than 70, who are of normal body weight and are prepared to refrain from heavy activity and sports.
- UCA has a reported 10 year survivorship of 93% and several reports of greater than 90% predicted 10 year survival in selected patients.[17,52,54,64,73,75]
- TKA performed for OA in patients younger than 55 years has predicted 10 year survivorship of 90%.[47]
- There are superior results of UCA versus TKA in a prospective, randomized studies.[83,84]

Many questions remain to be answered and require carefully constructed prospective, randomized studies. The long-term clinical and functional outcome of young patients with unicompartmental OA at 30 years after initial UCA, HTO, or TKA followed by revision TKA is unknown. Until we understand the long-term outcome we can not unanimously support any of the techniques.

## Authors' recommendations

The following indications are common to both UCA and HTO. Patients outside of these indications should be treated with a TKA regardless of age and activity level:

- disabling knee pain with unicompartmental disease
- normal body weight
- ROM > 90°
- flexion deformity < 10°
- minimal subluxation
- intact ACL and collateral ligaments
- deformity <10° varus or 15° valgus.

If patients satisfy the above indications then consideration can be made for UCA, HTO, or TKA. all three have a role in the treatment of unicompartmental osteoarthritis. Factors that may influence the surgeon to select one option over another include:

*UCA*

- Physiological age less than 70 years
- female patients

- occupation of a sedentary nature and a low impact activity level
- deformity at the level of the knee joint due to cartilage loss, tibial plateau bone loss, or ligament laxity
- bone on bone arthritis.

It should be the aim to restore neutral alignment or undercorrect less than 3°. The surgeon should use an implant with proven long-term outcome. The implant should be made of cobalt–chrome and fixed with cement. The polyethylene should be more than 6 mm thick and be manufactured and sterilized in a manner to reduce wear.

## HTO

- Physiological age less than 50 years
- male patients
- occupation requiring vigorous activity or who wish to continue to play sports
- metaphyseal deformity
- low adductor moment on gait analysis.

It should be the aim to perform the osteotomy at the level of deformity and to correct to 8–10° of anatomical valgus. The osteotomy should be held with rigid fixation that allows for early range of motion.

## TKA

- Physiological age greater than 50 years
- inflammatory component to disease or significant rest pain
- generalized osteoarthritis
- not suitable for UNI or HTO.

It should be the aim to restore neutral alignment and balance of the knee to allow normal kinematics. The surgeon should use an implant with proven long-term outcome. The implant should be made of cobalt–chrome and fixed with cement. The polyethylene should be more than 6 mm thick and be manufactured and sterilized in a manner to reduce wear.

# References

1  Marmor L: Unicompartmental knee arthroplasty. Ten- to 13-year follow-up study. *Clinical Orthopedics* **226**:14–20, 1988.
2  Scott RD, Cobb AG, McQueary FG *et al.*: Unicompartmental knee arthroplasty. Eight- to 12-year follow-up evaluation with survivorship analysis. *Clinical Orthopedics* **271**:96–100, 1991.
3  Staeheli JW, Cass JR, Morrey BF: Condylar total knee arthroplasty after failed proximal tibial osteotomy. *Journal of Bone and Joint Surgery* [Am] **69**:28–31, 1987.
4  Barrett WP, Scott RD: Revision of failed unicondylar unicompartmental knee arthroplasty. *Journal of Bone and Joint Surgery* [Am], **69**:1328–1335, 1987.
5  Lewold S, Knutson K, Lidgren L: Reduced failure rate in knee prosthetic surgery with improved implantation technique. *Clinical Orthopedics* **287**:94–97, 1993.

6  Grelsamer RP: Unicompartmental osteoarthrosis of the knee. *Journal of Bone and Joint Surgery* [Am] **77**:278–292, 1995.

7  Odenbring S, Lindstrand A, Egund N *et al.*: Prognosis for patients with medial gonarthrosis. A 16-year follow-up study of 189 knees. *Clinical Orthopedics* **266**:152–155, 1991.

8  Insall JN, Joseph DM, Msika C: High tibial osteotomy for varus gonarthrosis. A long-term follow-up study. *Journal of Bone and Joint Surgery* [Am], **66**:1040–1048, 1984.

9  Tetsworth K, Paley D: Malalignment and degenerative arthropathy. *Orthopedic Clinics of North America* **25**:367–377, 1994.

10  McKellop HA, Llinas A, Sarmiento A: Effects of tibial malalignment on the knee and ankle. *Orthopedic Clinics of North America* **25**:415–423, 1994.

11  Eckhoff DG: Effect of limb malrotation on malalignment and osteoarthritis. *Orthopedic Clinics of North America* **25**:405–414, 1994.

12  Coventry MB: Upper tibial osteotomy for osteoarthritis. *Journal of Bone and Joint Surgery* [Am] **67**:1136–1140, 1985.

13  Harrington IJ: Static and dynamic loading patterns in knee joints with deformities. *Journal of Bone and Joint Surgery* [Am] **65**:247–259, 1983.

14  Shaw JA and Moulton MJ: High tibial osteotomy: an operation based on a spurious mechanical concept. A theoretic treatise [see comments]. *American Journal of Orthopedics* **25**:429–436, 1996.

15  Andriacchi TP: Dynamics of knee malalignment. *Orthopedic Clinics of North America* **25**:395–403, 1994.

16  Coventry MB: Osteotomy of the upper portion of the tibia for degenerative arthritis of the knee: A preliminary report. *Journal of Bone and Joint Surgery* [Am] 47:984, 1965.

17  Coventry MB: Osteotomy about the knee for degenerative and rheumatoid arthritis. *Journal of Bone and Joint Surgery* [Am] **55**:23–48, 1973.

18  Coventry MB, Ilstrup DM, Wallrichs SL: Proximal tibial osteotomy. A critical long-term study of eighty-seven cases. *Journal of Bone and Joint Surgery* [Am] **75**:196–201, 1993.

19  Prodromos CC, Andriacchi TP, Galante JO: A relationship between gait and clinical changes following high tibial osteotomy. *Journal of Bone and Joint Surgery* [Am], **67**:1188–1194, 1985.

20  Paley D, Maar DC, Herzenberg JE: New concepts in high tibial osteotomy for medial compartment osteoarthritis. *Orthopedic Clinics of North America* **25**:483–498, 1994.

21  Miniaci A, Ballmer FT, Ballmer PM *et al.*: Proximal tibial osteotomy. A new fixation device. *Clinical Orthopedics* **246**:250–259, 1989.

22  Murphy SB: Tibial osteotomy for genu varum. Indications, preoperative planning, and technique. *Orthopedic Clinics of North America* **25**:477–482, 1994.

23  Coventry MB: Alternatives to total knee arthroplasty. In *Total knee arthroplasty,* ed. JA Rand, pp. 67–83. Raven Press, New York, 1993.

24  Fujisawa Y, Masuhara K, Shiomi S: The effect of high tibial osteotomy on osteoarthritis of the knee. An arthroscopic study of 54 knee joints. *Orthopedic Clinics of North America* **10**:585–608, 1979.

25  Hofmann AA, Wyatt RW, Beck SW: High tibial osteotomy. Use of an osteotomy jig, rigid fixation, and early motion versus conventional surgical technique and cast immobilization. *Clinical Orthopedics* **271**:212–217, 1991.

26  Insall J, Walker P: Unicondylar knee replacement. *Clinical Orthopedics* **120**:83–85, 1976.

27  Marmor L: The modular knee. *Clinical Orthopedics* **94**:242–248, 1973.

28  Marmor L: Unicompartmental and total knee arthroplasty. *Clinical Orthopedics* **192**:75–81, 1985.

29  Thornhill TS, Scott RD: Unicompartmental total knee arthroplasty. *Orthopedic Clinics of North America* **20**:245–256, 1989.

30  Kozin SC, Scott R: Unicondylar knee arthroplasty. *Journal of Bone and Joint Surgery* [Am] **71**:145–150, 1989.

31  Chestnut WJ: Preoperative diagnostic protocol to predict candidates for unicompartmental arthroplasty. *Clinical Orthopedics* **273**:146–150, 1991.

32  Murray DW, Goodfellow JW and O'Connor JJ: The Oxford medial uni-compartmental arthroplasty: a ten-year survival study. *Journal of Bone and Joint Surgery* [Br] **80**:983–989, 1998.

33  Stern SH, Becker MW, Insall JN: Unicondylar knee arthroplasty. An evaluation of selection criteria. *Clinical Orthopedics* **286**:143–148, 1993.

34  Uematsu A and Kim EE: Role of radionuclide joint imaging in high tibial osteotomy. *Clinical Orthopedics* **144**:220–225, 1979.

35  Wada M, Imura S, Nagatani K *et al.*: Relationship between gait and clinical results after high tibial osteotomy. *Clinical Orthopedics* **354**:180–188, 1998.

36  Wang JW, Kuo KN, Andriacchi TP *et al.*: The influence of walking mechanics and time on the results of proximal tibial osteotomy. *Journal of Bone and Joint Surgery* [Am], **72**:905–909, 1990.

37  Chassin EP, Mikosz RP, Andriacchi TP *et al.*: Functional analysis of cemented medial unicompartmental knee arthroplasty. *Journal of Arthroplasty* **11**:553–559, 1996.

38  Keene JS, Monson DK, Roberts JM *et al.*: Evaluation of patients for high tibial osteotomy. *Clinical Orthopedics* **243**:157–165, 1989.

39  Kettelkamp DB, Chao EY: A method for quantitative analysis of medial and lateral compression forces at the knee during standing. *Clinical Orthopedics* **83**:202–213, 1972.

40  Dugdale TW, Noyes FR, Styer D: Preoperative planning for high tibial osteotomy. The effect of lateral tibiofemoral separation and tibiofemoral length. *Clinical Orthopedics* **274**:248–264, 1992.

41  Ivarsson I, Gillquist J: Rehabilitation after high tibial osteotomy and unicompartmental arthroplasty. A comparative study. *Clinical Orthopedics* **266**:139–144, 1991.

42  Barnes CL, Scott RD: Unicompartmental knee replacement. In *The Knee*, ed. WN Scott, pp. 1097–1103. CV Mosby, St. Louis, 1994.

43  Kennedy WR, White RP: Unicompartmental arthroplasty of the knee. Postoperative alignment and its influence on overall results. *Clinical Orthopedics* **221**:278–285, 1987.

44  Whiteside LA: Cementless total knee replacement. Nine- to 11-year results and 10-year survivorship analysis. *Clinical Orthopedics* **309**:185–192, 1994.

45  Ranawat CS, Flynn WF Jr., Saddler S *et al.*: Long-term results of the total condylar knee arthroplasty. A 15-year survivorship study. *Clinical Orthopedics* **286**:94–102, 1993.

46  Schai PA, Thornhill TS, Scott RD: Total knee arthroplasty with the PFC system. Results at a minimum of ten years and survivorship analysis. *Journal of Bone and Joint Surgery* [Br] **80**:850–858, 1998.

47  Diduch DR, Insall JN, Scott WN *et al.*: Total knee replacement in young, active patients. Long-term follow-up and functional outcome. *Journal of Bone and Joint Surgery* [Am] **79**:575–582, 1997.

48  Stern SH, Bowen MK, Insall JN *et al.*: Cemented total knee arthro-plasty for gonarthrosis in patients 55 years old or younger. *Clinical Orthopedics* **260**:124–129, 1990.

49  Ranawat CS, Padgett DE, Ohashi Y: Total knee arthroplasty for patients younger than 55 years. *Clinical Orthopedics* **248**:27–33, 1989.

50  Duffy GP, Trousdale RT, Stuart MJ: Total knee arthroplasty in patients 55 years old or younger. 10-to 17-year results. *Clinical Orthopedics* **356**:22–27, 1998.

51  Rand JA, Ritts GD: Abrasion arthroplasty as a salvage for failed upper tibial osteotomy. *Journal of Arthroplasty* **4**(Suppl):S45–S48, 1989.

52  Lewold S, Robertsson O, Knutson K *et al.*: Revision of unicompartmental knee arthroplasty: outcome in 1,135 cases from the Swedish Knee Arthroplasty study. *Acta Orthopaedica Scandinavica* **69**:469–474, 1998.

53  Rinonapoli E, Mancini GB, Corvaglia A *et al.*: Tibial osteotomy for varus gonarthrosis. A 10- to 21-year follow up study. *Clinical Orthopedics* **353**:185–193, 1998.

54  Cartier P, Sanouiller JL, Grelsamer RP: Unicompartmental knee arthroplasty surgery. 10-year minimum follow-up period. *Journal of Arthroplasty* **11**:782–788, 1996.

55  Matthews LS, Goldstein SA, Malvitz TA *et al.*: Proximal tibial osteotomy. Factors that influence the duration of satisfactory function. *Clinical Orthopedics* **229**:193–200, 1988.

56  Morrey BF: Upper tibial osteotomy: analysis of prognostic features: a review. *Advances in Orthopaedic Surgery* 213–222, 1986.

57  Ritter MA, Fechtman RA: Proximal tibial osteotomy. A survivorship analysis. *Journal of Arthroplasty* **3**:309–311, 1988.

58  Amendola A, Rorabeck CH, Bourne RB *et al.*: Total knee arthroplasty following high tibial osteotomy for osteoarthritis. *Journal of Arthroplasty* **4**(Suppl):S11–S17, 1989.

59  Windsor RE, Insall JN and Vince KG: Technical considerations of total knee arthroplasty after proximal tibial osteotomy. *Journal of Bone and Joint Surgery* [Am] **70**:547–555, 1988.

60  Nizard RS, Cardinne L, Bizot P *et al.*: Total knee replacement after failed tibial osteotomy: results of a matched-pair study. *Journal of Arthroplasty* **13**:847–853, 1998.

61  Katz MM, Hungerford DS, Krackow KA *et al.*: Results of total knee arthroplasty after failed proximal tibial osteotomy for osteoarthritis. *Journal of Bone and Joint Surgery* [Am] **69**:225–233, 1987.

62  Mont MA, Antonaides S, Krackow KA *et al.*: Total knee arthroplasty after failed high tibial osteotomy. A comparison with a matched group. *Clinical Orthopedics* **299**:125–130, 1994.

63  Laskin RS: Unicompartmental tibiofemoral resurfacing arthroplasty. *Journal of Bone and Joint Surgery* [Am] **60**:182–185, 1978.

64  Callahan CM, Drake BG, Heck DA *et al.*: Patient outcomes following unicompartmental or bicompartmental knee arthroplasty. A meta-analysis. *Journal of Arthroplasty* **10**:141–150, 1995.

65  Berry DJ: Epidemiology: hip and knee. *Orthopedic Clinics of North America* **30**(2):183–190, 1999.

66  Bergenudd H: Porous-coated anatomic unicompartmental knee arthroplasty in osteoarthritis. A 3- to 9-year follow-up study. *Journal of Arthroplasty* **10**(Suppl):S8–13, 1995.

67  Scott RD, Santore RF: Unicondylar unicompartmental replacement for osteoarthritis of the knee. *Journal of Bone and Joint Surgery* [Am] **63**:536–544, 1981.

68  Schai PA, Suh JT, Thornhill TS *et al.*: Unicompartmental knee arthroplasty in middle-aged patients: a 2-to 6- year follow-up evaluation. *Journal of Arthroplasty* **13**:365–372, 1998.

69  Palmer SH, Morrison PJ, Ross AC: Early catastrophic tibial component wear after unicompartmental knee arthroplasty. *Clinical Orthopedics* **350**:143–148, 1998.

70 Bartley RE, Stulberg SD, Robb WJ *et al.*: Polyethylene wear in unicompartmental knee arthroplasty. *Clinical Orthopedics* **299**:18–24, 1994.

71 Riebel GD, Werner FW, Ayers DC *et al.*: Early failure of the femoral component in unicompartmental knee arthroplasty. *Journal of Arthroplasty* **10**:615–621, 1995.

72 Psychoyios V, Crawford RW, O'Connor JJ *et al.*: Wear of congruent meniscal bearings in unicompartmental knee arthroplasty: a retrieval study of 16 specimens. *Journal of Bone and Joint Surgery* [Br] **80**:976–982, 1998.

73 Capra SW Jr., Fehring TK: Unicondylar arthroplasty. A survivorship analysis. *Journal of Arthroplasty* **7**:247–251, 1992.

74 Bert JM: 10-year survivorship of metal-backed, unicompartmental arthroplasty. *Journal of Arthroplasty* **13**:901–905, 1998.

75 Heck DA, Marmor L, Gibson A *et al.*: Unicompartmental knee arthroplasty. A multicenter investigation with long-term follow-up evaluation. *Clinical Orthopedics* **286**:154–159, 1993.

76 Rougraff BT, Heck DA, Gibson AE: A comparison of tricompartmental and unicompartmental arthroplasty for the treatment of gonarthrosis. *Clinical Orthopedics* **273**:157–164, 1991.

77 Sisto DJ, Blazina ME, Heskiaoff D *et al.*: Unicompartment arthroplasty for osteoarthrosis of the knee. *Clinical Orthopedics* **286**:149–153, 1993.

78 Klemme WR, Galvin EG, Petersen SA: Unicompartmental knee arthroplasty. Sequential radiographic and scintigraphic imaging with an average five-year follow-up. *Clinical Orthopedics* **286**:233–238, 1994.

79 Swank M, Stulberg SD, Jiganti J *et al.*: The natural history of unicompartmental arthroplasty. An eight-year follow-up study with survivorship analysis. *Clinical Orthopedics* **286**:130–142, 1993.

80 Tabor OB Jr., Tabor OB: Unicompartmental arthroplasty: a long-term follow-up study. *Journal of Arthroplasty* **13**:373–379, 1998.

81 Levine WN, Ozuna RM, Scott RD *et al.*: Conversion of failed modern unicompartmental arthroplasty to total knee arthroplasty. *Journal of Arthroplasty* **11**:797–801, 1996.

82 Chakrabarty G, Newman JH, Ackroyd CE: Revision of unicompartmental arthroplasty of the knee. Clinical and technical considerations. *Journal of Arthroplasty* **13**:191–196, 1998.

83 Newman JH, Ackroyd CE, Shah NA: Unicompartmental or total knee replacement? Five-year results of a prospective, randomised trial of 102 osteoarthritic knees with unicompartmental arthritis. *Journal of Bone and Joint Surgery* [Br] **80**:862–865, 1998.

84 Laurencin CT, Zelicof SB, Scott RD *et al.*: Unicompartmental versus total knee arthroplasty in the same patient. A comparative study. *Clinical Orthopedics* **273**:151–156, 1991.

85 Cobb AG, Kozin SC, Scott RD: Unicondylar or total knee replacement: the patients preference. *Journal of Bone and Joint Surgery* [Br] **72**:166, 1990.

86 Broughton NS, Newman JH, Baily RA: Unicompartmental replacement and high tibial osteotomy for osteoarthritis of the knee. A comparative study after 5–10 years' follow-up. *Journal of Bone and Joint Surgery* [Br] **68**:447–452, 1986.

87 Weale AE and Newman JH: Unicompartmental arthroplasty and high tibial osteotomy for osteoarthrosis of the knee. A comparative study with a 12- to 17-year follow-up period. *Clinical Orthopedics* **302**:134–137, 1994.

88 Gill T, Schemitsch EH, Brick GW *et al.*: Revision total knee arthroplasty after failed unicompartmental knee arthroplasty or high tibial osteotomy. *Clinical Orthopedics* **321**:10–18, 1995.

89  Jackson M, Sarangi PP, Newman JH: Revision total knee arthroplasty. Comparison of outcome following primary proximal tibial osteotomy or unicompartmental arthroplasty. *Journal of Arthroplasty* **9**:539–542, 1994.

89  Mont MA, Alexander N, Krackow KA *et al.*: Total knee arthroplasty after failed high tibial osteotomy. *Orthopedic Clinics of North America* **25**:515–525, 1994.

## Questions and answers

*Moderator:* Knee replacement performed after osteotomy has been shown to have results similar to that after a revision, not a primary. Since we know that at 10 years many osteotomies do fail and require conversion to a TKR, are we really doing the patient a service by doing the osteotomy in the first place?

*Dr. Hart:* Recent papers show that outcomes of TKA following HTO are no worse than after a primary TKA. Early procedures using inadequatefixation resulted in marked deformity which made TKA more difficult. Ken Krakow's argument quoted in my paper justified osteotomy as a better alternative to TKA in patients under 65 and I support this. Modern operations with improved technique, instrumentation and fixation devices give more precise results and, therefore, the need for "revision" TKA is likely to be less.

*Moderator:* Although using a plate gives better fixation of the osteotomy there is a real incidence of compartment syndrome with that method of care. Are there suggestions you can make to avoid this potential disastrous problem, Dr. Hart?

*Dr. Hart:* Compartment syndrome is recognized as a severe complication after high tibial osteotomy. The complication can be minimized by limited exposure by using a small but adequate plate, releasing the tourniquet before wound closure, careful postoperative assessment, the avoidance of plaster postoperatively, and the use of incomplete osteotomy with compression fixation. The use of epidurals postoperatively can confuse the diagnosis of compartment syndrome because of the relief of pain and induce sensory loss of weakness. Pressure monitoring should be performed if there is any doubt and decompression carried out if positive.

*Moderator:* A medial opening wedge has been suggested as the optimal way to perform a tibial osteotomy in that it doesn't cause shortening and may make the later TKR easier to do. Please discuss your thoughts about this technique. Please discuss your thoughts about this technique.

*Dr. Hart:* Medial wedge osteotomy for genu varum does have the potential to avoid shortening, but it is technically more difficult to achieve an accurate result. It requires bone graft or bone substitute to fill the defect which will increase the morbidity if taken from the iliac crest or the expense if allograft or bone substitute is used. Union is less certain and takes longer than with a closed wedge compression osteotomy. Weightbearing cannot be commenced as soon as with a closed wedge compression osteotomy and loss of correction is more likely to occur due to absorption of the graft. An opening wedge osteotomy can cause interference with the medial ligament and the pes anserinus, which is a potential disadvantage. All in all, this technique does have specific indications but is not preferred as the routine.

*Moderator:* Dr. Hart, what is your present alignment guide in correcting a varus knee using a high tibialosteotomy? Exactly how much tibiofemoral angulation do you personally desire to obtain?

*Dr. Hart:* I use a long alignment rod placed on the terminal head and the center of the talus under I.I. catheter. As indicated in my contribution we have estimated the amount of correction required in a series of patients with genu varum using Miniaci's technique and found that an average of 50° of correction beyond the mechanical axis is required with a narrow range of between 4° and 6°. This is in keeping with the findings of the long-term study of Yusuda *et al.* I would recommend aiming for a tibiofemoral angulation of 110° assuming that the mechanical anatomical axis is 60°, i.e., 50° of overcorrection. Where an osteotomy has been performed to protect a resurfaced area on the femoral condyle, less overcorrection may be acceptable.

# 12

*After the scar itself, the one factor that every patient who has undergone a total knee replacement will discuss is the range of motion. We are all striving to return our patients to a situation where their function will be maximized. More flexion often translates to a greater ability to perform a larger variety of activities. How, therefore, can we maximize flexion?*

# Range of motion after total knee replacement can best be obtained using a CPM machine

## Pro: Cecil H. Rorabeck and G. E. D. Howell

The concept of continuous passive motion (CPM) applied to joints of the extremities was first introduced to the clinical setting by Nickel in 1960 following synovectomy of the knee. Although cited by others, it was not reported.[1] It was Salter's experiments on rabbit models in the 1970s that brought the benefits of CPM to the world of orthopaedics.[2,3] Salter demonstrated that CPM aided healing of damaged articular cartilage and intra-articular fractures, and protected articular cartilage in septic arthritis.[19,20] Introduced into the clinical setting in the late 1970s for the treatment of osteochondral injuries and in the early 1980s for postoperative management of total knee arthroplasty, it is now most frequently used following total knee arthroplasty (TKA).

Early machines for CPM were primitive and invariably made from motorized braces or Thomas splints. Today's machines are triumphs of ergonometry and cost between $4000 and $8000. They are programmable and accurately reproduce the orthopaedic surgeon's desired movement for the patient. They may include ankle braces or mobilizers, and modularity allows one machine to be modified to fit a variety of patients. Their durability and adaptability allow repeated use on a large number of variable limb sizes and shapes. In short, they are patient-friendly and cost-effective.

The world of orthopaedics is divided on the efficacy of CPM. There are three opinions of postoperative CPM held by orthopaedic surgeons who regularly perform TKA. There are those who use CPM always, those that use it occasionally and those that never use it. We always use CPM and firmly believe that its use in the immediate postoperative period results in better knee flexion, early discharge from hospital, reduced requirement for manipulation, and increased patient satisfaction when compared to other postoperative TKA regimens.

## Discussion

Before the introduction of CPM in the immediate postoperative period, TKAs were managed by immobilization in extension. Although this was a tried and tested modality of orthopaedic management of various pathologies, dating back to Hippocrates, little science had been applied to the physiology of healing until the latter half of the nineteenth century.

Wolff's law states that collagen fibrils are laid down randomly during the healing process unless they are stressed.[4] Frank et al.[5] and Coutts et al.[6] proposed that the random laying down of collagen fibrils seen in postoperative TKA healing when the limb is immobilized in extension resulted in resistance to free movement. They believed that the use of CPM encouraged laying down ofinear collagen fibrils, reducing postoperative scar formation and thus increasing range of movement of prosthetic knees. Van Rooyan et al.'s experiments on rabbits in 1986 concluded that wound healing, in particular the structural orientation of collagen was better in limbs mobilized by CPM when compared to limbs that had been immobilized.[7] They believed that these conclusions were also applicable to humans. In 1983 Coutts et al.[8,9] studied two groups of patients, one receiving post TKA CPM and the other not. They suggested that CPM was advantageous as hospital stay was reduced, range of motion was regained earlier, their wounds healed better, patients were more satisfed, venous dynamics were improved, and an improved range of motion resulted.

In our practice we use a variety of knee implants inserted via a midline incision, with a tourniquet under spinal anaesthesia unless contraindicated. All femoral components are placed in approximately 3° of external rotation. Tibial components are placed in 3° of post-slope and externally rotated 3°. We commence CPM in the recovery room and mobilize the TKA passively between 70 to 100° of flexion as pain allows during the first 24 h. CPM is discontinued after the first 24 h and is augmented by physiotherapy. Patients ambulate on the first day postoperatively. Stair walking commences on day 4 and patients are discharged home on day 5 to the care of their own physiotherapist if

- there are no complications
- 90° of flexion has been obtained
- the patient is ambulatory with a cane or crutch
- the patient can ascend and descend stairs one at a time.

The literature concerning the use of CPM following TKA is confusing. Many studies have been retrospective and few use similar criteria for measurement of range of motion (active or passively). Little mention is made of preoperative range of motion, soft tissue releases performed during surgery, or the position of tibial and femoral components. All studies report on small cohorts and there is a paucity of prospective randomized clinical trials. It is however, clear that early use of CPM commencing immediately after TKA does not compromise full extension and improves flexion in TKA patients.[10-13] It probably reduces postoperative swelling, analgesia requirement, the incidence of manipulation for TKAs with reduced range of motion (ROM) and increases patient satisfaction. It may allow earlier early discharge from hospital as satisfactory postoperative 90° flexion is attained earlier and results in cost-effective TKA. Each of these points will be discussed separately.[10-13]

## Postoperative swelling

In our practice we have observed that patients mobilized following TKA using CPM have reduced knee swelling. These observations have also been recorded by Ritter et al.,[12] McInnes et al.[14] and Montgomery and Eliasson (1996).[15] Swelling inhibits flexion both by mechanical block and also due to pain. It is something that should be avoided in the postoperative period and to this end the use of CPM should be encouraged.

Ritter et al. in 1987[13] recorded the swelling observed at the center of the patella in 50 consecutive patients undergoing bilateral TKA. One knee was randomly assigned to the CPM and the other was not. Initially the knee randomized to the CPM had increased swelling (until day 2) but from day 2 to day 16 this was not the case. During this period, flexion was better in the knee treated with CPM. They stated that swelling was a cause of reduced motion and pain but did not comment upon patient satisfaction. All patients were hospitalized for an average of 8 days postoperatively or until flexion reached 70°.

McInnes et al.[12] in 1992 studied 93 patients undergoing TKA for osteoarthritis or rheumatoid arthritis in a randomized controlled study: 48 received standard postoperative physiotherapy and CPM as tolerated and 45 received postoperative physiotherapy alone. They identified a significantly reduced swelling ($p = 0.008$) in patients who had standard physiotherapy and CPM. This was most noticable in women.

Montgomery and Eliasson, in 1996,[14] studied 68 patients randomly assigned to either CPM or active physiotherapy following uncemented total knee arthroplasty. The group undegoing CPM had significantly reduced knee swelling as measured at the mid patella circumference when compared to the group receiving active physiotherapy.

## Postoperative analgesic requirements

In our practice we recognize that the analgesic requirements of patients who receive CPM post TKA is reduced. This is corroborated by the studies of Colwell et al.,[17] Coutts,[6] Frank et al.,[5] Harms and Engstrom,[10] McInnes et al.,[12] and Woods et al.[16]

Frank et al.[5] reviewed the physiology and therapeutic value of passive motion and concluded that the use of rhythmic motion inhibits the pain spasm reflex. Coutts[6] proposed that endorphin and encephalin production following movement as well as proprioceptive stimulation, may reduce postoperative pain levels. Colwell and Morris[17] studied 22 patients undergoing TKA and randomized into two groups. In 10 patients used as a control the limb was immobilized in extension for 3 days immediately following wound closure and straight leg raises, transfer and gait physiotherapy were commenced. The other group of 12 patients received CPM (range 0–40° on day 1 increasing 10° each day) in addition to the physiotherapy described for the controls. Analgesics were standardized into dose equivalencies and the CPM group required significantly less analgesia.

Harms and Engstrom[10] studied 113 consecutive patients undergoing TKA who were randomly allocated to a postoperative regime that did or did not include CPM.[11] They identified lower pain scores, using a visual analogue scale in patients receiving CPM when compared to those that did not. McInnes (in the previously described study[12]) reported reduced pain levels in patients treated post TKA with CPM which was significant.

## Reduced incidence of post-arthroplasty manipulation

The incidence of manipulation following TKA is difficult to assess as individual surgeons have different criteria for recommending the procedure, and indeed variable reduced range of motion at variable postoperative periods have been reported. It is our practice to avoid manipulation following TKA and since the use of CPM in our postoperative regimen we have not performed a single manipulation. McInnes et al.[12] reported that 8 out of 45 patients who did not receive CPM post TKA, underwent manipulation at less than 6 weeks for range of motion less than 50°. This compares to none out of 48 who did receive CPM. Romness and Rand[15] retrospectively studied 210 patients who underwent TKA; 94 received CPM as part of their rehabilitation programme. Of patients receiving CPM 1% required a manipulation whereas 4% of the control group required manipulation. Ververeli et al.[18] reported a 10% manipulation rate of 52 patients who did not receive CP post TKA compared to none of 51 patients who did receive CPM. The indications for manipulation were less than 50° of motion at day 10 postoperatively. The cost of these manipulations was estimated at almost $50 000.

## Improved range of motion

Many studies have demonstrated earlier flexion to 90° with the use of CPM.[1,8,19–22]

Goletz and Henry[20] studied, retrospectively, 19 patients who received CPM post TKA and compared them to 15 who did not. They identified that the group receiving CPM attained 90° of flexion at an average of 9 days whereas those that did not took an average of 16 days. Their study sample was, however, too small to demonstrate any statistical significance. Romness and Rand[15] demonstrated that 74% of patients receiving CPM attained 90° of knee flexion at the time of discharge compared to 60% of the group that did not receive CPM. Johnson[21] prospectively studied 102 patients post TKA randomized to receive CPM (50 patients) or immobilization (52 patients). He identified significantly increased flexion in the patients receiving CPM at 7, 10, 14 and 52 days. Harms and Engstrom in their 1991 study[10] noted similar findings.

In their cohort, range of motion was significantly improved at day 7 ($p$ = 0.001), at day 14 ($p$ = 0.001), and on discharge ($p$ = 0.005) in patients receiving CPM. They also noted that those patients with a primary diagnosis of rheumatoid arthritis did better than those with a primary diagnosis of osteoarthritis. They also identified improved active extension in the group receiving CPM. McInnes[12] in 1992 identified better postoperative flexion in the CPM treated group compared to the group that did not receive CPM (mean 82° versus 75°). This was statistically significant ($p$ = 0.004). Ververeli et al.[18] studied 103 patients in a prospective randomized trial, 51 of whom received CPM post TKA. At discharge on day 12 they identified significantly greater active flexion in those who had received CPM ($p$ = 0.0001). Montgomery and Eliasson[14] identified improved early knee flexion in the 34 patients who received CPM post TKA when compared to 34 that did not. Chiarello et al. [23] studied 46 patients post TKA. The patients were assigned to one of five groups which included no postoperative CPM or variable CPM regimes which had different daily increases in flexion or duration of daily CPM use. They concluded that when all CPM groups were compared to the control group (no CPM) active flexion was enhanced with CPM. There have been no long-term deleterious effects of early CPM and the improved gains in early motion noted in the CPM treated patients were maintained at 1 year review.5[6,9,21]

## Early discharge and cost benefits

Under our care, the average time to discharge post TKA is 5 days, our criteria being:

- a healing wound
- flexion to 90°
- ambulation using a cane or crutch
- ability to ascend and descend stairs independently
- no postoperative complications.

This, in part we believe, is due to early attainment of 90° of flexion using the CPM machine. Reduced hospitalization results in improved costings and the ability to perform more TKAs per annum.

Reduction of hospitalization between 1–6 days has been identified for patients receiving CPM as compared to controls that did not,[6,8,10,12–18,20,21,24] and this has obvious cost saving benefits.

Worland et al.[25] studied 103 consecutive TKA in 80 patients: 49 TKA's were randomized to home CPM and 45 to home physiotherapy. They demonstrated that even in the post-discharge setting CPM was cost effective. The cost of professional physiotherapy was almost twice that of CPM and the extensor lag, flexion, presence of knee flexion contracture and knee scores were not statistically different at 6 months post TKA.

## Patient satisfaction

Patients receiving post TKA CPM feel that they are taking an active role in their immediate postoperative management. They are comfortable and readily identify the improvement in motion from the calibration of the machine. Harms and Engstrom[10] concluded from their study of 113 patients that CPM appears to increase patients' confidence in the movement of their replaced joints.

## Potential disadvantages of CPM

We have not identified any negative factors associated with the use of CPM. Concerns about wound healing with early flexion beyond 40° using CPM have not been identified in our clinical practice. Goletz and Henry[20] reported 4 wound complications in 19 patients receiving immediate post TKA CPM initially at 0–30° increasing 15° per day. Three of these complications were superficial wound erythema and resolved when CPM movement was reduced and may be ascribed to the aggressive daily increase in CPM flexion employed in their study. One patient had avulsion of the tibial tubercle but further details are not presented. Johnson[21] studied 102 TKAs, 50 of whom received postoperative CPM. The remaining 54 were immobilized. He recorded transcutaneous oxygen tension either side of the wound on alternate days postoperatively. Reduced oxygen tension on both sides of the wound in patients receiving CPM was noted and was statistically lower when compared to the immobilized group. At day 7, reduced oxygen tension was noted only on the lateral wound aspect. However, he recorded that superficial infection occurred in 5% of patients receiving CPM and 10% of the patients that had been immobilized. This was not statistically significant. Yasher et al.[26] reported one case of wound necrosis in a group of 104 patients receiving CPM (70–100°) immediately postoperatively but this was thought to be due to a tight wound dressing. The patient ultimately required a gastrocnemius flap.

## Conclusions

CPM provides a safe, reliable adjunct to rehabilitation following TKA. It encourages early flexion and extension, which is maintained at 1 year. It is cost effective, reducing hospitalization and postoperative analgesic requirements with recognized patient satisfaction. There are few, if any, complications associated with its use and although it is not our current practice, it has potential benefits following discharge to the home setting.

## Summary

It would appear that the use of CPM, beginning in the recovery room between 70° and 120° of flexion and persisting overnight, is advantageous in improving patients' comfort, range of motion, and perhaps ambulation. There is no doubt, however, that at 6 weeks, most patients, whether they have had CPM or not, will do equally well. Although we had some concern initially, with the healing capacity of the wound, this has not in fact been an issue. It is important to note that a constricting dressing is not put around the limb and the dressing is changed the morning following surgery. Swelling is considerably reduced because the knee is held in flexion and there is considerably less "dead space" in which blood can accumulate. Provided the CPM using a high flexion protocol, is not continued beyond the first day, the possibility of the patient developing a flexion contracture is almost zero. On the other hand, if the high flexion protocol is continued, there is a risk of developing a flexure contracture. It is important to point out that not all patients are suitable for a CPM and in particular, the very bad valgus knee where extensive releases have been performed through a lateral approach, may be a relative contraindication. It is also important that the patient have good analgesia. This is normally accomplished through an epidural infusion or a PCA pump. If we can't get good pain control then the CPM will be discontinued. Concern has been expressed that high flexion CPM may result in an increased incidence of deep venous thrombosis. In a controlled randomized clinical study carried out at our institution, this has not been the case.

## References

1   Coutts RD, Kaita J, Barr R *et al.*: The role of continuous passive motion in the post-operative rehabilitation of the total knee patient. *Orthopaedic Transactions* **6**:277.

2   Salter RB, Simmonds DF, Malcolm BW *et al.*: The biological effect of continuous passive motion on the healing of full thickness defects in articular cartilage: An experimental investigation in the rabbit. *Journal of Bone and Joint Surgery* [Am] **62**:1232–1251, 1980.

3   Salter RB, Bell SR, Kelley FW: The protective effect of continuous passive motion on living articular cartilage in acute septic arthritis: An experimental investigation in the rabbit. *Clinical Orthopaedics and Related Research* **159**:223–247, 1981.

4   Forrester JC, Zederfeldt BH, Hayes TL *et al.*: Wolff's law in relation to the healing skin wound. *Journal of Trauma* **10**:770–779, 1970.

5   Frank C Akeson WH, Woo SLY *et al.*: Physiology and therapeutic value of passive joint motion. *Clinical Orthopaedics and Related Research* **185**:113–125, 1984.

6 Coutts RD: Continuous passive motion in the rehabilitation of the total knee patient, its role and effect. *Orthopaedic Review* 15:126–135, 1986.

7 Van Rooyan BJ, O'Driscoll SW, Dhert WJA. *et al.*: A comparison of immobilization and continuous passive motion on surgical wound healing in mature rabbits. *Plastic and Reconstructive Surgery* 78:360–66, 1986.

8 Coutts RD, Tooth C, Kaita J: The role of continuous passive motion in the rehabilitation of the total knee patient. In *Total knee arthroplasty—A comprehensive approach*, ed. D Hungerford, pp. 126–132. Williams and Wilkins, Baltimore, 1983.

9 Coutts R, Sharp D, Borden LS *et al.*: The effect of continuous passive motion in total knee rehabilitation. *Orthopaedic Transactions* 7:535, 1983.

10 Harms M, Engstrom B: Continuous passive motion as an adjunct to treatment in the physiotherapy management of the total knee arthroplasty patient. *Physiotherapy* 77:301–307, 1991.

11 Johnson DP, Eastwood DM: Beneficial effects of continuous passive motion after total condylar knee arthroplasty. *Annals of the Royal College of Surgical Engineering* 74:411–16, 1992.

12 McInnes J, Larson MG, Daltroy LH *et al.*: A controlled evaluation of continuous passive motion in patients undergoing total knee arthroplasty. *JAMA* 268:1423–1428, 1992.

13 Ritter MA, Campbell ED: Effects of range of motion on the success of a total knee arthroplasty. *Journal of Arthroplasty* 2:95–7, 1987.

14 Montgomery F, Eliasson M: Continuous passive motion compared to active physical therapy after knee arthroplasty. *Acta Scandinavia* 67:7–9, 1996.

15 Romness DW, Rand JA: The role of continuous passive motion following total knee arthroplasty. *Clinical Orthopaedics and Related Research* 226:34–7, 1988.

16 Woods L, Wasilewski SA, Healy W: The value of continuous passive motion in total knee arthroplasty. *Orthopaedic Transactions* 2:68, 1987.

17 Colwell CW and Morris BA: The influence of continuous passive motion on the results of total knee arthroplasty. *Clinical Orthopaedics and Related Research* 276:225–228, 1992.

18 Ververeli PA, Sutton DC, Hearn SL *et al.*: 1995 Continuous passive motion after total knee arthroplasty. *Clinical Orthopaedics and Related Research* 321:208–215.

19 Fischer RT, Kloter D, Bzdrya B *et al.*: 1985 Continuous passive motion following total knee replacement. *Connecticut Medicine* 49:498.

20 Goletz TH, Henry JH: Continuous passive motion after total knee arthroplasty. *South Medical Journal* 79:116–120, 1991, 1986.

21 Johnson DP: The effect of continuous passive motion on wound healing and joint mobility after knee arthroplasty. *Journal of Bone and Joint Surgery* [Am] 72:421–426, 1990.

22 Vince KG, Kelly MA, Beck J *et al.*: Continuous passive motion after knee arthroplasty. *Journal of Arthroplasty* 2 :281–284, 1987.

23 Chiarello CM, Gunderson L, O'Halleran T: The effect of continuous passive motion duration and increment on range of motion in total knee arthroplasty patients. *Journal of Orthopaedic Sports Physical Therapy* 25:119–127, 1997.

24 Maloney WJ, Schurman DJ, Hangen D *et al.*: The influence of continuous passive motion on outcome in total knee arthroplasty. *Clinical Orthopaedics and Related Research* 256:162–168, 1990.

25 Worland RL, Arredondo J, Angles F *et al.*: Home continuous passive motion machine versus professional physical therapy following total knee replacement. *Journal of Arthroplasty* **13**:784–788, 1998.

26 Yasher AA, Venn-Watson E, Welsh T *et al.*: Continuous passive motion with accelerated flexion after total knee arthroplasty. *Clinical Orthopaedics and Related Research* **345**:38–43, 1997.

# Con: Samuel R. Ward, Donald B. Longjohn, and Lawrence D. Dorr

## Historical perspective

Historically, postoperative management of TKA involved immobilization of the operated leg in a bulky dressing or a cylinder cast for up to 14 days.[1] This period of immobilization was thought to insure adequate healing of the skin and incision. ROM exercises were initiated after 10–14 days and 90° of flexion was to be achieved by discharge. This ROM milestone was felt to be sufficient for most activities of daily living. The need for a more aggressive range of motion program developed after connective tissue physiology literature introduced two concepts. One was that collagen deposition began around the second postoperative day and that peak collagen deposition occurred at days 5–7.[2] The second concept was that mechanical forces could regulate the orientation of new collagen deposits.[3] This knowledge stimulated change in postoperative care, and Coutts introduced the concept of early postoperative range of motion and the development of the CPM machine. Early studies comparing CPM machines to the traditional postoperative management favored use of the CPM.[4] Subsequent studies have shown that the duration of CPM use can be reduced to as little as 5 h per day,[5] and that early postoperative use of CPM produced more rapid gains in flexion without compromise of the surgical wound.[6]

## Purpose of postoperative rehabilitation

The purpose of postoperative rehabilitation is to optimize ROM, strength, and the gait pattern of the patient. ROM is necessary for proper gait, for arising out of chairs, in and out of cars, and proper use of stairs. Strength is necessary for all endurance activities. Gait re-education is necessary because the preoperative pattern for patients with arthritis is that of a stiff knee gait.[7] Correct full extension is necessary to allow proper loading of the limb at heel-strike and throughout stance or rapid fatigue of the quadriceps muscle and resultant increased energy consumption during gait will result.

One stride during normal gait is heel contact to heel contact and is divided into two periods—stance and swing. Stance compromises 60% of the duration of a single stride and places the largest force demand on the knee. Stance is subdivided into two tasks: weight acceptance which requires strong quadriceps activity to provide

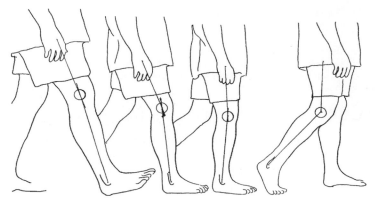

**Fig. 12.1**
Knee ROM during initial contact, loading response, mid-stance, and initial swing.

stability at the knee, and single limb support. Extension range is paramount for successful weight acceptance. If a flexion contracture greater than 10° is present, energy consumption during gait is significantly increased and rapid fatigue of the quadriceps occurs. The swing phase compromises 40% of a single stride, and has only one task which is limb advancement. This task places a much smaller muscle demand on the knee, but requires a large, rapid change in the flexion.[8] Flexion of 70° is important for the swing phase to be comfortable for the patient.

Weight acceptance and single limb support have been further subdivided into five phases: initial contact, loading response, mid-stance, terminal stance, and pre-swing.[8] (Fig. 12.1)

- During *initial contact*, the knee is close to full extension (approximately 5° of flexion) as the heel contacts the floor.
- *Loading response* is the phase of weight acceptance onto the stance limb. The knee flexes to 15° and the quadriceps acts eccentrically to counteract a vertical ground reaction of 120% of body weight.
- *Mid-stance* is characterized by knee extension close to 0° and a reduction in quadriceps muscle demand as the center of mass passes anterior to the knee axis of rotation.
- During *terminal stance*, the body continues to move forward with the knee remaining in extension with stability maintained by the ankle plantar flexors as they restrain the tibia from moving forward.
- *Pre-swing* is the transition from stance to swing and is characterized by the preparation of the stance limb to be advanced. Body weight is transferred onto the contralateral limb and the ipsilateral knee is flexed to 40°.[8]
- *Initial swing* places the greatest flexion demand on the knee (60–70°) as the foot is cleared for advancement.
- The remaining two phases of swing, *mid-swing* and *terminal swing*, are characterized by knee extension as the limb is brought forward. Because the knee is brought into extension by inertia, quadriceps activity is not seen until the end of terminal swing.[8]

322

The gait pattern following TKA is clearly pathological. It represents a classic pattern of quadriceps avoidance at the knee during stance. There is a reduction in knee flexion at loading response and initial swing. Although initially quite profound, this pattern has been found to persist to some degree for as long as 4–8 years.[7,9]

Quadriceps strength is therefore of greatest importance in the immediate postoperative period to allow knee control for the patient.

The in-hospital rehabilitation is the point of maximum intervention effectiveness for the physical therapist to establish ROM and strengthening, and to educate the patient in the correct program.

The controversy regarding postoperative rehabilitation for TKA is what is the most effective method for achieving rapid effective flexion and strength. This is so because at first, the most profound deviations from the normal gait pattern are lack of knee flexion torque in loading response, and lack of flexion in pre and initial swing. The lack of knee flexion torque is initially due to avoidance of knee flexion because of pain and quadriceps weakness. The lack of knee flexion at the end of stance and the beginning of swing is caused by lack of range of motion and pain.

## Current concept of postoperative rehabilitation

Optimization of ROM is a three-step process:

- firstly, passive knee flexion and extension are begun
- secondly the ease of movement through that arc of motion is improved
- finally, the strength available through the arc of motion is maximized and made effective.

This three-step process is done in the immediate postoperative period. The focus of therapy is for the patient to relearn and practice normal gait mechanics. This process begins with the use of active and passive ROM followed by isometric and active muscle strengthening and is completed when ROM and strength are coupled for complex tasks such as gait and stair navigation. Our experience is that active and active-assisted early ROM using the "sit and slide" provides a better outcome than the passive technique of the CPM machine. Our patients achieve ROM more quickly, with greater quadriceps strength, and this technique reduces both the length and cost of hospital stay.

Patients do not go home with full range of motion. On average, our patients have 80–85° of flexion with a 10° flexion contracture. This is adequate flexion for level gait, which requires 60–70° of flexion.[8] However, stair navigation needs 105° of flexion for a reciprocating pattern, and 105° for arising from a chair.[10] Lubenthal et al.[11] report that knee flexion for stairs requires only 85° of flexion, but does not give the stair height. What is most important is that the hospital discharge ROM is combined with satisfactory leg muscle strength and power for patients to utilize this range of motion. The patient can use only the range through which adequate strength and power is available. CPM machines (especially at home) are a negative technique for strengthening and training the quadriceps function. For the patient, they promote the concept that the machine will insure successful recovery.

## Technique of postoperative rehabilitation

Intraoperatively, the method by which the arthrotomy is repaired may affect postoperative range of motion. A tight closure with the knee in extension may lead to difficulty in achieving early flexion. On the other hand, closure of the arthrotomy with the knee in maximum flexion could result in an extensor lag. We initially place a single suture at the superior pole of the patella with the knee in extension and then flex the knee maximally to insure the extensor mechanism is not too tight (the suture does not break). With the knee flexed to about 100°, we suture the proximal corner of the quadriceps splitting incision and the peripatellar tissue to the inferior pole of the patella. We continue to close with the knee in flexion until the edges of the distal wound are parallel and not divergent, and then finish the proximal and distal wound closure in extension. Emerson et al.[12] have previously suggested that closure of the wound in flexion is preferred to promote earlier and easier postoperative flexion of the knee. Following closure of the arthrotomy, intraoperatively the knee should easily flex to maximum flexion under gravity alone. The anticipated postoperative flexion can thus be determined by allowing the knee to hang over the forearm of the surgeon.[13]

### Postoperative management for ROM

Postoperative management should begin on the same day as surgery. This is easiest for the patient if they have an indwelling epidural catheter through which morphine or fentanyl can be used for postoperative pain control. We do not recommend the use of "caine" drugs, such as bupivacaine or lidocaine (lignocaine), because of the risk of perineal nerve palsy. Physical therapy on the day of surgery consists of education, which includes isometric exercises for the knees and hips and active range of motion of the ankles for deep venous thrombosis prophylaxis. The patient also sits at the side of the bed and begins the "sit and slide" protocol for early ROM.

The sit and slide program has been described by Dorr and was initially termed the "drop and dangle" technique.[14] We now use the term "sit and slide" which is more accurate. The sit and slide technique is active-assisted ROM of the involved knee to approximately 70° of flexion with the foot in contact with the floor, then the hips slide forward with the foot firmly planted to achieve 90° of flexion (Fig. 12.2). This position is maintained to the tolerance of the patient as long as 20 min and is performed twice a day. If this position becomes intolerably painful, the knee is slowly extended for comfort and then the knee is again flexed to 90° for the completion

**Fig. 12.2**
'Sit and slide' at 90°.

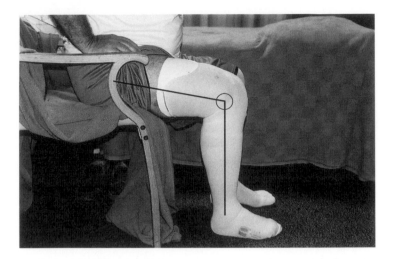

of the 20 min duration. Pain control is important and patients should be given pain medication 30 min prior to physical therapy.

*Restoration of strength with ROM*

The quintessential purpose of the rehabilitation technique is to incorporate restoration of strength with ROM. A CPM machine cannot do this. Any amount of ROM is useless unless the patient can effectively manage that range with muscle stability. Quadriceps strength must be emphasized and is facilitated by isometric "quad set" exercises performed hourly. The performance of these is difficult if the knee is in a CPM machine. Active quadriceps strengthening begins when pain control permits, and this may be 2–3 days following surgery.

Strength and ROM are integrated by the use of short arc knee extensions followed by long arc knee extension (Fig. 12.3). When these

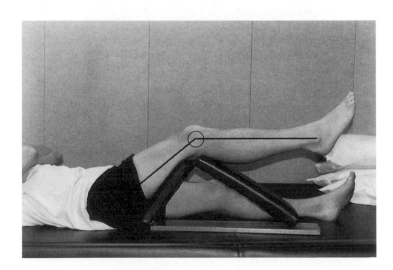

**Fig. 12.3**
Short arc quadriceps active exercise.

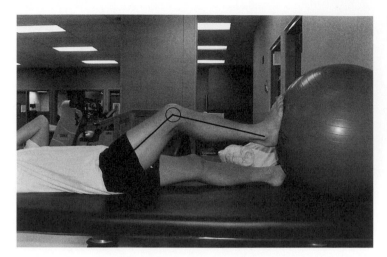

**Fig. 12.4**
Swiss ball extensions.

exercises are easily performed, closed chain quadriceps strengthening is initiated by the use of partial squats and knee extensions into an exercise ball (Fig. 12.4). When the patient reaches 80° using the sit and slide technique, active knee flexion and extension on a skateboard (Orthoskate, Expo Mfg., Los Angeles, CA) is introduced (Fig. 12.5) . Advanced knee exercises such as stationary bike active ROM, unilateral step-ups, and sports-specific exercises are started

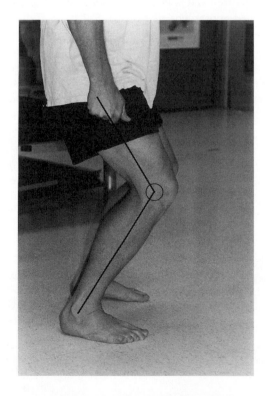

**Fig. 12.5**
'Sit and slide' with
Orthoskate.

6 weeks postoperatively. These exercises tend to aggravate knee edema in the early stages of rehabilitation, but are slowly incorporated in the later stages of rehabilitation.

## Discussion

There are two distinct advantages of rehabilitation techniques which do not use the CPM. The first is that the CPM overall is less effective in achieving the ultimate purpose of postoperative rehabilitation. The concept of early active and passive ROM without the use of a CPM has been effective and has proved that patients achieve similar motion results when ROM exercise is started early.[14–16] The sit and slide technique was compared to continuous passive range of motion by us with a randomized study of patients who were studied during their hospital stay and then at 3 and 6 months postoperatively.[14] There was no difference in knee flexion range of motion at discharge between the two groups, but the sit and slide patients had less extension lag (better strength), and were discharged 1 day sooner than the CPM group. This fact confirms that this technique is superior in initially integrating strength, motion, and function.

This superiority of rehabilitation is confirmed in a study by Ritter et al.[16] When comparing a technique similar to the sit and slide and the use of CPM, they found patients to have statistically identical knee ROM and a statistically smaller extension lag which suggests superior strength. These findings were identical to ours, as was the fact that they found that CPM patients had more flexion contractures postoperatively. Increased flexion contracture will reduce the efficiency of gait function. Furthermore, patients in the study of Ritter et al.[16] felt constrained by the use of the CPM machine.

Maloney et al.[15] found patients that did not use a CPM machine were discharged 2 days earlier. The study of Maloney et al., in combination with our findings of a discharge 1 day earlier, demonstrates the second advantage of the sit and slide technique which is a reduction in costs of rehabilitation by eliminating the CPM machine and reducing hospital stay. Finally, Lynch et al.[17] in a prospective randomized study could find no benefit for CPM use in reducing the prevalence of deep vein thrombosis. There are no advantages in the use of a CPM machine.

## References

1   Insall JN, Scott WN et al.: The Total Condylar knee prosthesis: a report of two hundred and twenty cases. *Journal of Bone and Joint Surgery* [Am] **61**:173–180, 1979.

2   Dunphy JE. Chemical and histochemical sequences in the normal healing of wounds. *New England Journal of Medicine* **253**(20): 847–851, 1955.

3   Amiel D, Woosty Harwood FL, Akeson WH: The effect of collagen turn-over in connective tissue: a biochemical/biomechanical correlation, *Acta Orthopaedica Scandinavica* **53**:325–332, 1982.

4   Coutts RD, Toth C *et al.*: The role of continuous passive motion in the rehabilitation of the total knee patient. In *Total knee arthroplasty: a comprehensive approach*, pp. 126–132. Williams and Wilkins, Baltimore, 1984.

5   Basso DM, Knapp L: Comparison of two continuous passive motion protocols for patients with total knee implants. *Physical Therapy* **67**(3):360–363, 1987.

6   Jordan LR, Siegel JL *et al.*: Early flexion routine. *Clinical Orthopaedics and Related Research* **315**:231–233, 1995.

7   Wilson SA, McCann PD *et al.*: Comprehensive gait analysis in posterior-stabilized knee arthroplasty. *Journal of Arthroplasty* **11**(4):359–367, 1996.

8   Perry J: *Gait analysis: normal and pathological function*, pp. 89–108, 228–230. Slack, Thorofare, NJ, 1992.

9   Bolanos AA, Coliza WA *et al.*: A comparison of isokinetic strength testing and gait analysis in patients with posterior cruciate-retaining and substituting knee arthroplasties. *Journal of Arthroplasty* **13**(8), 906–915, 1998.

10  Fleckenstein SJ, Kirby RL, MacLeod DA. Effect of limited knee-flexion range on peak hip moments of force while transferring from sitting to standing. *Journal of Biomechanics* **21**(11):915–918, 1988.

11  Lubenthal KN, Smidt GL *et al.*: Quantitative analysis of knee motion during activities of daily living. *Physical Therapy* **52**(1):34–43, 1972.

12  Emerson, RH Jr, Ayers CF, *et al.*: Surgical closing in primary total knee arthroplasties: flexion vs. extension. *Clinical Orthopedics* **331**:74–80, 1996.

13  Lee DC, Humedh, Scott RD, Sothers, K: Intraoperative flexion against gravity as an indication of ultimate range of motion in individual cases after total knee arthroplasty. *Journal of Arthroplasty* **13**(5):500–503, 1998.

14  Kumar PJ, McPherson EJ *et al.*: Rehabilitation after total knee arthroplasty a comparison of 2 rehabilitation techniques. *Clinical Orthopaedics And Related Research* **331**:93–101, 1996.

15  Maloney WJ, Schurman DJ *et al.*: The influence of continuous passive motion on outcome in total knee arthroplasty. *Clinical Orthopaedics and Related Research* **256**:162–168, 1990.

16  Ritter MA, Gandolf VS *et al.*: Continuous passive motion versus physical therapy in total knee arthroplasty. *Clinical Orthopaedics and Related Research* **244**:239–243, 1989.

17  Lynch AF, Bourne RB *et al.*: Deep-vein thrombusus and continuous passive motion after total knee arthroplasty. *Journal of Bone and Joint Surgery* [Am] **70**:11–14, 1988.

## Questions and answers

*Moderator:* Dr. Dorr, your original "drop and dangle" technique was an open chain type of motion while your new technique is closed chain. Why did you change?

*Dr. Dorr:* The original "drop and dangle" technique was not an open chain motion. The patient always has the operated foot in contact with the floor to avoid guarding. When patients "dangle" the operated leg, they tend to fire the quadriceps muscle group, increasing compression at the patellofemoral joint and the tibiofemoral joint and increasing pain. We abandoned the term "drop and dangle" and switched to "sit and slide" because it more accurately represents the exercise.

*Moderator:* Dr. Dorr, why does closing the retinaculum proximal to the patella in flexion, but the patella area in extension, eliminate the potential of extensor lag?

*Dr. Dorr:* This question does not accurately reflect the closure technique that we do. The closure technique has now been further described in the text above. The closure of the retinaculum adjacent to the patella is closed in flexion. Initially a single suture is placed at the proximal pole of the patella and the knee is taken to maximum flexion to insure that the extensor mechanism is not too tight. The knee is then closed in flexion at the proximal end of the wound because this had easier access and along the patella to the inferior pole of the patella. Distal closure is continued until the wound edges are parallel and the remainder of the closure is done in extension.

*Moderator:* One of my major concerns beginning flexion at high angles is the vascularity of the skin and potential wound healing problems. Would you please address this, Dr. Rorabeck.

*Dr. Rorabeck:* Clearly one of the potential concerns with high flexion relates to wound healing and, of course, oxygen retention plays a part in that. As you know, our protocol involves only a very light dressing with a dressing change being done on the morning of the first postoperative day. So far, at least, we haven't had any problems with wound healing that were attributable to this technique.

*Moderator:* We have talked about what angle to set the CPM machine. Are there any guidelines as to how fast to set the CPM machine?

*Dr. Rorabeck:* I'm not sure how fast or slow a CPM should cycle. However, generally, I would say that it should cycle very slowly. One wants to make sure that its not causing the patient undue discomfort, and our experience with the technique would suggest that they tolerate a slower cycle much better.

*Moderator:* Have you ever compared the motion obtainable by letting the knee flex passively after closure with that ultimately obtained by the patient?

*Dr. Dorr:* No, we have never done this comparison because it already has been performed by Dr. Richard Scott and his colleagues. The published study of Dr. Scott and his colleagues is referenced in the manuscript. (Lee DC *et al.*, *Journal of Arthroplasty* 1998;**13**:500–503)

*Moderator:* You have been using morphine for patient-controlled anesthesia (PCA). Why not bupivacaine or fentanyl?

*Dr. Dorr:* Mostly we use epidural analgesia and not PCA. For both the epidural and PCA we use both fentanyl and morphine. For some patients, morphine causes side-effects of pruritus and nausea which fentanyl does not. However, fentanyl does not give as good pain relief as morphine so some patients need the morphine for better relief. We do not use bupivacaine in epidurals because of the potential threat of peroneal palsy with the use of local anesthetics.

*Moderator:* I don't think that you are hinting that local anesthestics cause peroneal palsy. In theory, their presence may mask the symptoms of peroneal palsy although we routinely use them at HSS and have not noted this to be a real clinical problem.

*Moderator:* We have had problems using the CPM machine at night in that the patient's knee often moves from the axis point and as a result never comes out to full extension while in the machine. How do you avoid this, Dr. Rorabeck?

*Dr. Rorabeck:* I agree to some extent, with your point, namely that the patient often has difficulty coming out into full extension and therefore, may develop a fixed flexion deformity if the high flexion technique is used. I think that that is more likely to occur if the CPM machine is used for several days. Once again, I would emphasize, at our institution, that the CPM is put on in the operating room and removed the following morning. With that protocol, flexure contracture has not been a problem. What it does allow, however, is that on day 1, the patient is able to get 90° of flexion. This gives them considerable confidence and allows them to move along fairly quickly in their rehabilitation pathway.

*Moderator:* In your study, Dr. Dorr, were you using the CPM machine at night, and if not, why not?

*Dr. Dorr:* We do not routinely use the CPM machine at all. If a CPM was used, it was only for patients who had a VY-plasty and the machine was not used at night because patients report that they are unable to sleep. Our patients sleep with a knee immobilizer. There is an article by Basso and Knapp that supports not using a CPM at night with the patient still achieving an adequate number of treatment hours. However, this question is more appropriate for Dr. Rorabeck.

*Moderator:* There have been suggestions that the use of the CPM machine decreases the risk of thromboembolic disease. Do you agree, and if not, why not?

*Dr. Dorr:* The paper by Lynch *et al.*, which is by Dr. Rorabeck's group from Canada, clearly show in a prospective randomized study that there is no benefit for CPM for decreasing the risk of thromboembolic disease. There is a second article in the *Proceedings of the Knee Society* (ed Ran J. A., Dorr L.) entitled "Total arthroplasty of the knee," with the article by Goll S. R. *et al.* entitled "Failure of continuous passive motion for prophylaxis for deep venous thrombosis after total knee arthroplasty." Therefore, there is no literature support for a decrease of the risk of thrombophlebitis with the use of the CPM. Our protocol for DVT prophylaxis reflects our whole rehabilitation strategy which is early mobilization. Patients are fitted with pneumatic compression foot pumps which are used while they are in bed, and aspirin is given as an antithrombotic. Patients are mobilized the same day of surgery and progress to ambulation as soon as they can tolerate it, which is always by the second day. Beginning the first postoperative day, patients are up and out of bed at least twice a day with physical therapy, and once a day with occupational therapy. This is in addition to being out of bed with nursing.

*Moderator:* Are there any specific situations (revisions, ankylosed knees, etc.) in which you would consider the use of a CPM machine and knee replacement surgery?

*Dr. Dorr:* The "sit and slide" technique is used with the vast majority of primary TKAs, but an exception is included in the protocol. With both primary and revision TKA in patients who require a VY quadricepsplasty, or muscle flap coverage, a CPM is used in the first postoperative week up to 60° of flexion in an attempt to prevent suprapatellar pouch scarring so that range of motion is easier to achieve when active motion is allowed at 10 days postoperation.

*Moderator:* The same question for you Dr. Rorabeck, in a slightly different format. Are there situations in which you would *not* use a CPM machine?

*Dr. Rorabeck:* There may be some patients in whom the CPM is relatively contra-indicated. For example, a patient with an external rotation deformity always concerns me primarily because of potential pressure on the peroneal nerve. I've used it in patients with rheumatoid arthritis as well as with osteoarthritis, in patients on or off steroids, etc. I'm not aware of any particular problem with wound healing that has emanated from the use of the CPM machine.

*Moderator:* Have you done any patient satisfaction studies? Some patients like CPM because it feels "high tech."

*Dr. Dorr:* There were two opinions from patients. The patients with CPM machines did feel as though something was being done for them. However, the patients with the sit and slide technique liked the freedom to be able to have more bed mobility and more freedom to get in and out of bed. The preference of the patient can be almost completely controlled by the surgeon by the use of preoperative education in the technique that is going to be used and the reasons for the use of that technique.

*Moderator:* Have you found that you need more "hands-on" time with a therapist if you don't use a CPM machine?

*Dr. Dorr:* The first few days after surgery require more time with a physical therapist to insure that patients are performing the range of motion technique properly. After the first few days, patients are working on their ROM independently as they will be doing at home. The extra time from the therapist is offset by the time saved by nursing and the therapists placing and removing a CPM several times per day.

*Moderator:* Are you using epidural analgesic methods after surgery combined with CPM, Dr. Rorabeck?

*Dr. Rorabeck:* As our pool of anaesthetists is not uniform at our institution, the postoperative pain management is also not entirely uniform. Our preference is towards an epidural infusion but only approximately 40% of our patients receive an epidural infusion post-operatively. The others use PCA pumps and ketorolac tromethamine (Toradol). On occasion, the patient's pain does preclude the proper use of this machine. However, as the use of the machine has always been demonstrated by the patients preoperatively, it usually isn't a problem as it is only being used less than 24 h. I would be deceiving you, however, if I said that there are no patients in whom the CPM has to be discontinued because of pain. That certainly happens from time to time, and discontinuance of the machine is at the nurses' discretion.

*Moderator:* Dr. Rorabeck, do you think that the use of a CPM machine can adversely affect the incidence of thromoboembolic disease?

*Dr. Rorabeck:* Concern has been expressed that the risk of throm-boembolic disease may be higher in patients on the CPM primarily because of constriction of venous return. In a controlled randomized study done at our institution comparing the incidence of DVT with and without CPM, this has not been the case; the incidence of DVT is comparable in both groups. Part of the reason for this may be related to the fact that CPM was used for only a very short period of time. Perhaps with a longer application, there might have been an increased incidence, but we have no data in that regard.

Since this is my last question, I would like to summarize my thoughts, if you have no objection. As we all know, postoperative ROM depends, to a large extent, on preoperative ROM. Of equal importance, however, is the method of closure and I think both Dr. Dorr and I agree on that issue. It's absolutely imperative, intra-operatively, that the capsule and the extensor mechanism be closed very carefully and meticulously and once closure is complete, that the knee will flex fully without disruption of the suture line. To that end, I prefer to use a locking suture in the capsule and retinaculum and a running suture distally to insure a very tight reproducible closure. I think that if the surgeon either closes the knee in flexion or insures that the knee will fully flex intraoperatively, that the method of obtaining flexion postoperatively may be largely immaterial pro-vided the patient has adequate pain control.

I also believe, although I can't prove it scientifically, that one of the reasons why CPM works is related to the fact that the hematoma is less. This occurs because the "relative" joint space is lessened with the knee being in flexion and as a result, there is no place for the blood to go. One of the major factors which restricts patients obtain-ing maximum flexion relates to the development of a hematoma and this technique, although not perfect, seems to lessen the tendency towards the development of such hematomas. That, of course, can be negated if the anticoagulants get out of balance. Nevertheless, our CPM patients don't seem to have as large hemarthrosis on day 1 as our typical patient immobilized in extension would have.

## 13

*During revision total knee replacement, exposure is often difficult to obtain. Prior scarring, synovial hypertrophy, and metallosis can all combine to challenge even the most experienced total knee surgeon. Everting the patella may be difficult, if not impossible, using the standard techniques that we perform in primary knee replacement.*

# Proximal release procedures are the optimal way of increasing exposure during total knee replacement

## Pro: Jess H. Lonner and Richard D. Scott

Surgical exposure of the tight or scarred knee, during either primary or revision total knee arthroplasty (TKA), can be quite difficult. Patellar eversion and soft tissue mobilization to gain adequate exposure may be difficult with a standard medial parapatellar arthrotomy. It is paramount that extreme care is taken during surgical exposure to avoid compromise of the extensor mechanism, and particularly the patellar tendon insertion on the tibial tubercle.

Two basic surgical approaches are advocated to facilitate approach to the knee with restricted motion: a proximal quadricepsplasty or a tibial tubercle osteotomy. Quadricepsplasties may take on several forms, such as an inverted V-plasty (with or without advancement), a quadriceps snip, or a formal Coonse–Adams turndown. Both the proximal and distal ancillary procedures have proponents and are both effective, but our preference has been to address most of these knees with a proximal soft tissue release rather than with a tibial tubercle osteotomy because of its minimal morbidity and technical ease.

The modified inverted V-plasty, with or without eventual advancement of the extensor mechanism, as described by Scott and Siliski,[1] is our preferred technique. The proximal edge of the standard median parapatellar arthrotomy is diverted inferolaterally, at approximately a 30° or 45° angle, along the edge of the vastus lateralis insertion into the lateral retinaculum. In general the lateral limb of the inverted V-plasty need only be 1–2 cm, which allows preservation of the superior lateral genicular artery (Fig. 13.1). If there is any concern about excessive avulsion stress on the patellar tendon insertion, a smooth 1/8 inch (3 mm) pin is inserted through the tendon into the tubercle as a precaution.

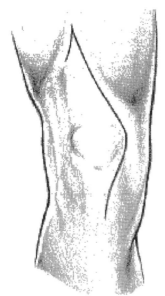

**Fig. 13.1**

Illustration of the inverted V quadriceps incision. The lateral limb is carried distally for 1–2 cm along the border of the vastus lateralis muscle (Reproduced with permission from Scott and Siliski[1]).

Some prefer to initiate the lateral limb of the inverted V-plasty more distal on the tendon, where the rectus tendon is more substantial and more easily repaired. This approach puts the superior lateral genicular artery at greater risk, with potential compromise in vascularity of the patella in the initial postoperative period.[2] However, the long-term clinical consequence of transecting the superior lateral genicular artery is uncertain.[3] During wound closure both the medial and lateral quadriceps incisions are sutured in an interrupted fashion. If no advancement is necessary to increase quadriceps excursion, the repair is anatomic and no modification of routine postoperative rehabilitation is necessary. If a VY-lengthening is required, active extension is withheld for 6 weeks, but isometric quadriceps exercises encouraged; flexion is limited to that achieved against gravity under anesthesia.

The quadriceps snip has been a more recent modification of the inverted V-quadricepsplasty.[4] It can achieve adequate exposure by a similar means while definitely preserving the superolateral geniculate vessel and allowing immediate and unprotected mobilization. In this technique, a standard medial parapatellar arthrotomy is extended proximally and laterally at a 45° angle, across the rectus femoris tendon (Fig. 13.2). If exposure remains difficult, the proximal limb may be extended by splitting the quadriceps muscle in line with the fibers of the quadriceps muscles and by adequate mobilization of periarticular soft tissues (i.e., releasing all adhesions). Additionally, a lateral retinacular release may further aid in exposure of the joint. The arthrotomy is sutured in a standard fashion, with closure of the proximal/oblique limb. Postoperative physiotherapy is not altered.

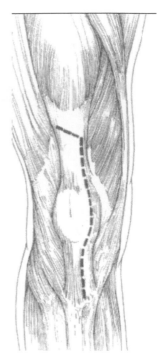

**Fig. 13.2**

Technique of the quadriceps snip.

The inverted V-plasty tends to be more versatile than the snip because of the ability to convert it to a formal VY-lengthening in the most ankylosed knees. It is also easier to suture the arthrotomy and seal the joint.

The complete patellar turndown, which is a modified version of the Coonse–Adams surgical approach, is the most extensile and extreme proximal quadriceps release for exposing the stiff knee.[5] In this approach, the proximal extent of the medial parapatellar arthrotomy is continued distally as an oblique, laterally directed limb that transects the entire rectus tendon, vastus lateralis tendon, and lateral retinaculum (Fig. 13.3). This approach tends to be reserved for severe tumor cases and we do not recommend it even for the most complex primary or revision TKAs. Patellar vascularity is definitely compromised by this technique. We recommend a tibial tubercle osteotomy if the previously described proximal releases are inadequate, rather than a quadriceps turndown. A VY advancement may be possible with the more conservative technique described by Scott and Siliski, but one must always weigh the risk of a residual extensor lag with a quadriceps lengthening against the possibility of residual flexion limitation that may otherwise result. Postoperatively protected gait is necessary with a knee immobilizer or locked brace until any extensor

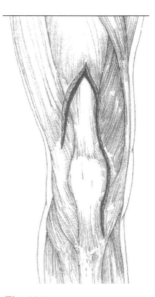

**Fig. 13.3**

Quadriceps turndown (Coonse–Adams).

lag improves, and flexion should be limited to 5° shy of what was achieved intraoperatively against gravity.

## Results of proximal quadriceps exposures

Scott and Siliski[1] reviewed the technique of modified VY-quadricepsplasty in seven patients. The authors reported an increase in average flexion arc from 25° preoperatively to 75° postoperatively. The average postoperative extensor lag was 8°. Windsor and Insall reported on 26 cases treated with a VY-quadricepsplasty, none of which had postoperative extensor weakness.[6] Reviewing 16 knees treated with VY-quadricepsplasty, Trousdale et al.[7] found reduction in quadriceps strength by Cybex testing compared to contralateral knees treated with standard median parapatellar approaches, but these differences were not statistically significant. Postoperative extensor lags in that series averaged 4° (range 0–20°). It was not mentioned whether there were contralateral extensor lags. Functional deficits were not significant in those with residual mild extensor weakness.[7] In a consecutive series of revision TKAs, treated with either quadriceps turndown or tibial tubercle osteotomy, Barrack et al.[8] found equivalent postoperative scores, but arc of motion was significantly greater in the quadriceps turndown group compared with the tibial tubercle osteotomy group ($p < 0.05$) (93° and 81° motion arcs, respectively). Extensor lag averaged 4.5° in the quadriceps turndown group, compared to 1.5° in the tibial tubercle osteotomy group. Forty-seven percent of patients treated with tibial tubercle osteotomy compared to only 36% treated with quadriceps turndown had difficulty climbing stairs, although this difference was not statistically significant. Additionally, a significantly higher percentage of patients in the tibial tubercle osteotomy group had difficulty kneeling and stooping compared to the other group (73% versus 43%, $p < 0.05$). Compared to a control group treated with either a standard approach or a quadriceps snip approach, the quadriceps turndown group of patients did not have a significantly higher degree of difficulty using stairs, kneeling, or stooping, compared to those patients in the control group. Quadriceps turndown patients also had equivalent satisfaction, pain relief, and return to activities of daily living compared to the control group and these ratings were significantly higher than observed in patients in the tibial tubercle osteotomy group.[8]

## Concerns with tibial tubercle osteotomy

Whiteside[9] has championed the extended tibial tubercle osteotomy for complex primary and revision TKAs, with excellent results. But although tibial tubercle osteotomy may be extremely effective for gaining exposure in the difficult primary or revision TKA, complications are of concern. Delayed union or nonunion may occur, and avulsion fractures (which may represent delayed union or nonunion) have been reported.[10] An additional concern, particularly when the distal aspect of the tibial tubercle osteotomy is not tapered, is that a tibial shaft stress riser may result, predisposing to fracture of the tibial shaft.[11] Finally, in the revision TKA with compromised tibial bone stock and perhaps just a thin shell of tibial tubercle remaining and a limited bed of trabecular bone, the osseous support and potential for nonunion remains a legitimate concern. Certainly in these cases with inadequate trabecular bony support, we advise against consideration for tibial tubercle osteotomy. Wolff et al.[12] reported on the results of tibial tubercle osteotomy in 26 knees and found complications occurred in 35% of patients: 23% had major nonmechanical complications including superficial skin necrosis or deep infection that required subsequent treatment, and 15% required further surgery for tibial tubercle osteotomy displacement or patella tendon rupture.

## Conclusion

The meticulous surgical approach to the complex primary or revision TKA is critical to ensure preservation of the integrity of the extensor mechanism. Both proximal and distal procedures to facilitate exposure are helpful in ensuring extensor integrity. Although some have reported mild extensor lags and quadriceps weakness with proximal releases, these risks seem to be quite limited in terms of functional limitations when compared to the far greater and more significant risks associated with tibial tubercle osteotomy. Patient satisfaction seems to be greater with proximal quadricepsplasties than with tibial tubercle osteotomy. The techniques of inverted V-plasty or quadriceps snips are technically easier than the distal procedure, and generally do not add significant morbidity to the surgical procedure.

## References

1   Scott RD, Siliski JM. The use of a modified VY-quadricepsplasty during total knee arthroplasty to gain exposure and improve flexion in the ankylosed knee. Orthopaedics 8:45–48, 1985.

2   Wetzner SM, Bezreh JS, Scott RD et al.: Bone scanning in the assessment of patellar viability following knee replacement. Clinical Orthopedics 199:215–219, 1985.

3   Ritter MA, Herbst SA, Keating EM et al.: Patellofemoral complication following total knee arthroplasties: Effect of a lateral release and sacrifice of the superior lateral geniculate artery. Journal of Arthroplasty 11:368–372, 1996.

4   Garvin KL, Scuderi G, Insall JN: Evolution of the quadriceps snip. Clinical Orthopedics 321:131–137, 1995.

5   Coonse K, Adams JD: A new operative approach to the knee joint. Surgical Gynecology and Obstetrics 77:344–347, 1943.

6   Windsor RE, Insall JN: Exposure in revision total knee arthroplasty. The femoral peel technique in orthopaedics. Techniques in Orthopaedics 3:1–4, 1988.

7   Trousdale RT, Hanssen AD, Rand JA, Cahalan TD. VY-quadricepsplasty in total knee arthroplasty. Clinical Orthopedics 286:48–55, 1993.

8  Barrack RL, Smith P, Munn B *et al.*: Comparison of surgical
   approaches in total knee arthroplasty. *Clinical Orthopedics*
   **356**:16–21, 1998.
9  Whiteside LA: Exposure in difficult total knee arthroplasty using tibial
   tubercle osteotomy. *Clinical Orthopedics* **321**:32–35, 1995.
10  Ries MD, Richman JA: Extended tibial tubercle osteotomy in total
   knee arthroplasty. *Journal of Arthroplasty.* **11**:964–967, £1996
11  Ritter MA, Carr K, Keating EM *et al.*: Tibial shaft fracture following
   tibial tubercle osteotomy. *Journal of Arthroplasty* **11**:117–119, 1996.
12  Wolff AM, Hungerford DS, Krackow KA, Jacobs MA: Osteotomy of
   the tibial tubercle during total knee arthroplasty. A report of
   twenty-six cases. *Journal of Bone and Joint Surgery* [Am]
   **71**:848–852, 1989.

# Con*: Leo Whiteside

The standard surgical approach to total knee replacement seldom is adequate for use in revision arthroplasty. Nevertheless, the standard approach generally is the first attempt at exposure, with final exposure achieved through an extension of the standard approach. All approaches to knee arthroplasty use the anterior route, and violate the quadriceps mechanism to some extent. The extensions of this approach all endanger quadriceps function, and must be used with caution. The skin and subcutaneous tissues also often are compromised from previous surgical procedures, and special techniques are required to avoid skin and fat necrosis. Obesity is one factor that impedes exposure of the knee in primary arthroplasty and causes even more problems with revision arthroplasty. Scarred subcutaneous tissue and overlying skin, a fibrotic quadriceps mechanism, and a shortened patellar tendon necessitate extensile exposure. In the nonobese patient whose subcutaneous tissue is not scarred densely to the underlying capsule, the quadriceps mechanism can be turned laterally for extensile exposure without extensive undermining. However, in obese patients the thick fibrotic adipose tissue layer that is directly adherent to the capsule and skin prevents the quadriceps mechanism from being folded laterally. This difficulty can be circumvented if subcutaneous undermining can be performed safely to allow placement of the quadriceps mechanism into a secure, subcutaneous pocket so that the entire wall of fat is not forcefully stuffed under the patella and quadriceps mechanism during exposure (Fig. 13.4).

The subfascial dissection technique makes exposure of the knee both safe and effective in the obese patient (Fig. 13.5). Subcutaneous fat receives its blood supply from vessels penetrating from the subdermal plexus and through anastomotic channels from vessels that penetrate through the deep infesting fascia of the lower extremity.[1]

*This contribution is adapted with permission from Whiteside LA: Surgical exposure in revision total knee arthroplasty, in Springfield DS (ed): *Instructional Course Lectures*, volume 46. Rosemont, IL, American Academy of Orthopaedic Surgeons. 1997.

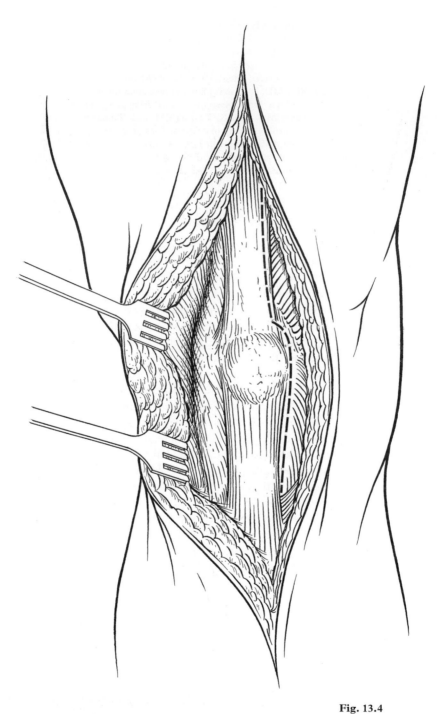

**Fig. 13.4**

Lateral subfascial dissection creates a pocket for the patella. (Reprinted with permission from the American Academy of Orthopaedic Surgeons).

These anastomotic channels can be severely disrupted by dissection into the subcutaneous fat for creation of a flap for exposure of the knee. Extensive subcutaneous fat necrosis can result, and dissection into this plane can cause overlying skin necrosis as well. However,

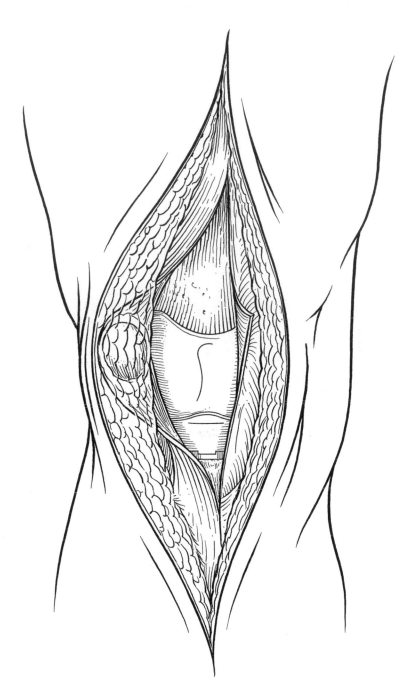

**Fig. 13.5**

Exposure of the obese knee. The patella is turned laterally into the subfascial pocket. (Reprinted with permission from the American Academy of Orthopaedic Surgeons).

dissection in the subfascial plane between the deep infesting fascia of the lower extremity and the capsule of the knee is relatively safe. Fairly extensive dissection can be done in this plane without significantly devascularizing the subcutaneous fat or overlying skin.[1] Exposure is achieved by incising directly through the subcutaneous tissue and deep investing fascia of the leg. Then, the dissection is directed laterally between the fascia and capsule of the knee approximately three finger breadths past the lateral edge of the patella. The patella is turned under the subcutaneous flap and into this pocket.

## Quadriceps transection exposure

Exposure in the presence of quadriceps contracture and fibrosis of the capsule and patellar tendon often requires additional surgical procedures as well as more extensive subfascial exposure. The classic exposure for extensive intraarticular work on the knee is the quadriceps turndown or VY plasty.[2] In this procedure the quadriceps inci-

**Fig. 13.6**
Outline for the quadriceps turndown (Coonse–Adams) approach to the knee. The standard medial parapatellar quadriceps-splitting approach is made, and then a lateral extension of the incision is made from above the patella to the joint line. (Reprinted with permission from the American Academy of Orthopaedic Surgeons).

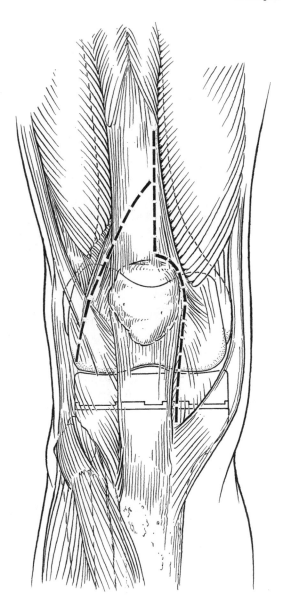

**Fig. 13.7**

Exposure of the knee with quadriceps turndown. Anterior knee exposure is excellent. The patella, patellar tendon, and fat pad form a large, poorly vascularized, distally based flap. (Reprinted with permission from the American Academy of Orthopaedic Surgeons).

sion is extended proximally with a downward incision across the top of the patella and through the lateral retinaculum to the joint line (Fig. 13.6). The patella and patellar tendon then become a distally based flap (Fig. 13.7). Excellent exposure can be achieved with this procedure, but extension lag is almost always reported in series results of the turndown or classic Coonse–Adams approach to the knee.[3] More recent reports by Barrack document a more ominous finding of avascular necrosis of the patella in one third of the knees in which a full turndown is done.[4]

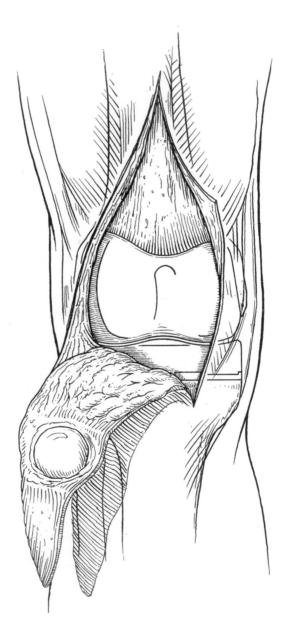

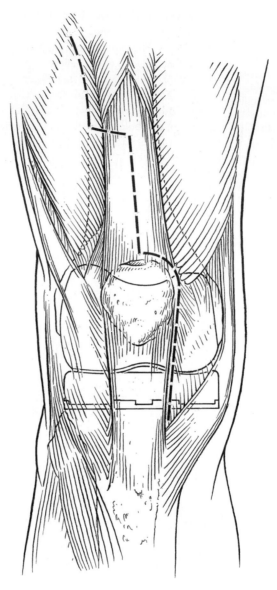

**Fig. 13.8**

The more commonly used transquadriceps approach to the knee is the so-called "quadriceps snip" procedure.[5] When the rectus tendon has been split in half as part of the approach to the knee, it adds little to the surgical procedure to transect the lateral half of the tendon. The standard incision is extended proximally along the main rectus tendon and then transversely into the vastus lateralis (Fig. 13.8). As the knee is flexed, the ends of the tendon and muscle fibers separate so that more slack is created in the quadriceps mechanism, and the patella can be retracted laterally more easily (Fig. 13.9). Complications with this procedure are few, and extension lag is uncommon. Normal rehabilitation can be prescribed, and splinting

Outline of the "quadriceps snip" for exposure of the knee. The quadriceps tendon is split in the initial approach. To gain further exposure, the remaining portion of the tendon is cut and the incision is allowed to extend further into the vastus lateralis. (Reprinted with permission from the American Academy of Orthopaedic Surgeons).

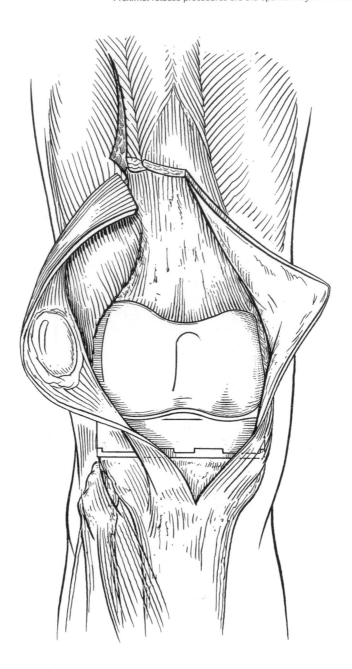

**Fig. 13.9**

Exposure of the knee with the quadriceps snip approach. The entire quadriceps, except for a portion of the vastus lateralis, has been transected. (Reprinted with permission from the American Academy of Orthopaedic Surgeons).

usually is not necessary. Because this procedure requires proximal extension along the quadriceps tendon, it cannot be used when a more medial approach has been made, such as the vastus medialis splitting or subvastus approach.

## Tibial tubercle osteotomy

Osteotomy of the tibial tubercle for extensile exposure into the knee is especially effective when extensive exposure to the lateral half of

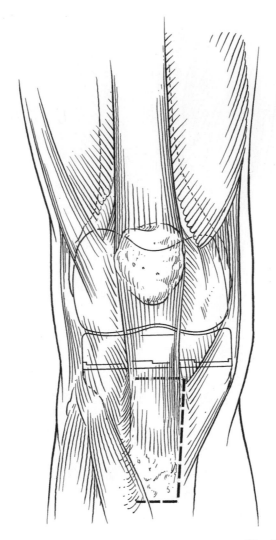

**Fig. 13.10**

Outline of the tibial tubercle osteotomy. The distal portion of the osteotomy is made with a saw, and the medial, superior, and lateral portions are made with a curved osteotome. Lateral soft tissue attachments are left intact. (Reprinted with permission from the American Academy of Orthopaedic Surgeons).

the knee is required, and when a medialis splitting or a subvastus approach has been made. This procedure offers the most extensive exposure to the knee in patients with severe quadriceps contracture, and it is especially useful in patients with fibrous ankylosis and with takedown of knee fusion.

A flap, approximately 4 cm long, measured from the top of the tibial tubercle, is elevated through a medial osteotomy that is carried transversely under the tubercle through the lateral cortex. (Fig. 13.10) A flap of bone 4 cm long, 2 cm wide, and 1 cm thick is elevated. The lateral attachments of the muscles and the periosteum are left intact. (Fig. 13.8) The stress riser effect of the osteotomy is minimized by making an oblique saw cut at the distal end of the osteotomized segment. The soft-tissue attachments between the fat pad and anterior tibia must be severed, and a small amount of the

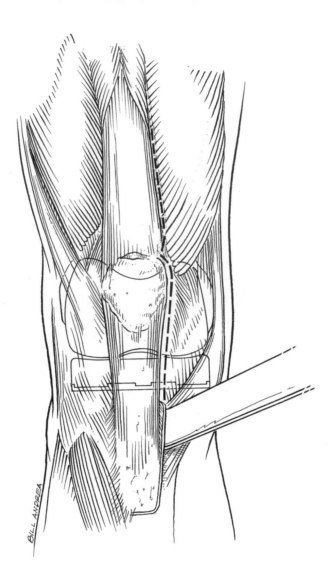

BILL ANDREA

**Fig. 13.11**

Outline of the incision used with tibial tubercle osteotomy exposure of the knee. The incision can be placed medially to the main quadriceps tendon, and can be allowed to extend proximally in line with the fibers of the vastus intermedius. The osteotomy is made from the medial side to maintain the lateral soft tissue hinge. (Reprinted with permission from the American Academy of Orthopaedic Surgeons).

anterolateral capsular attachment of the tibia must be released to allow the quadriceps mechanism to turn laterally. Where there is dense contracture of the quadriceps group, an extended incision proximally is necessary. (Fig. 13.11)

When the tubercle osteotomy is used for exposure of the knee, it is not necessary to transect the main quadriceps tendon. Instead, the proximal incision is allowed to follow the line of the vastus medialis fibers above the vastus medialis obliquus (Fig. 13.12). The nerve and blood supply to the vastus medialis enter from the posterior edge, so the muscle-splitting incision does not compromise healing and function of the muscle. Often the quadriceps mechanism is tightly adherent to the anterior aspect of the femur, and must be dissected carefully from the bone to allow the quadriceps to be turned laterally;

347

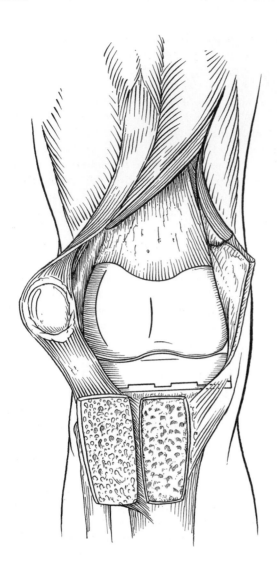

**Fig. 13.12**

Exposure of the knee with tibial tubercle osteotomy. The interval between the vastus medialis and vastus medialis obliquus has been split in line with the muscle fibers. The lateral soft tissue attachments to the tibial tubercle are oriented longitudinally, so the bone fragment does not slip proximally. (Reprinted with permission from the American Academy of Orthopaedic Surgeons).

however, it is not necessary to transect any of the lateral aspect of the quadriceps mechanism. The lateral soft-tissue attachments to the tibial tubercle allow the bone flap to turn laterally while maintaining its blood supply. These fibers also maintain attachment of the bone fragment and prevent its proximal migration.

Careful reattachment of the tibial tubercle osteotomy will avoid fracture of the proximal pole of the osteotomized fragment. Because the lateral, soft-tissue hinge has been left intact, the lateral edge does not need to be fixed. However, the medial edge requires firm attachment to bone. When screws are used to reattach this segment, they must be placed through the central or medial aspect of the fragment to be effective. Drill holes in this area significantly weaken the bone fragment, and often cause fractures. The proximal screw hole, placed in the soft cancellous bone of the tubercle, is especially vulnerable to fracture. Severe extension lag can result if a fracture occurs through the proximal pole, and surgical repair is difficult. Fixation of the tibial tubercle with wires, however, is highly effective and is safe from fracture. The drill holes are placed along the lateral edge of the tibial tubercle and matching drill holes—offset approximately 1 cm distally—place the wires so that they pull obliquely downward across almost the entire width of the tibial tubercle. When these wires are twisted and tightened, semirigid fixation of the tubercle is achieved. Despite the less than rigid fixation, healing occurs in virtually all cases. Fracture of the proximal pole of the tubercle has not occurred in more than 200 surgical exposures with this technique.[6,7] and only minimal, clinically insignificant slippage of the tubercle fixation has occurred in a few cases.[5,6] Fracture of the tibia has occurred, however, and is associated with a tibial tubercle bone segment of longer than 4 cm.[7,8] When a short stem is used on the tibial component, the tibial tubercle osteotomy causes concentration of stress in the anterior tibial cortex, and increases the risk of fracture. However, too short an osteotomy fragment often can be associated with fracture of the tubercle fragment itself.[9] A tubercle segment measuring about 4 cm is recommended.

## Intraosseous exposure

When infection is present, or on rare occasions in which long stems have been cemented into the femur and tibia, intraosseous exposure must be achieved to remove the implants and to debride thoroughly. Anterior exposure of the distal half of the femur can be achieved easily through the quadriceps split approach described earlier. Once subperiosteal exposure is achieved, the anterior cortex is drilled to outline an anterior slot osteotomy. The bone segment is removed with a straight osteotome, and lifted directly anteriorly. This direct approach to the cemented stem and polymethylmethacrylate allows safe removal of the implant and thorough debridement of the bone. The bone is then repaired by replacing the removed segment and securing it with circumferential cables to create a strong construct that can accept a tight-fitting stem and withstand early weightbearing loads.

Extended intraosseous tibial exposure can be achieved through the tibial tubercle osteotomy, and through extensions of this osteotomy distally. Cable reconstruction of the anterior tibial slot is more difficult because passing wires and cables around the tibia is more dangerous than the same procedure done with the femur. A long stem that completely bypasses the tibial osteotomy creates a safer construct for early load bearing.

## Closure

Management of skin closure after revision total knee replacement is sometimes the most challenging aspect of this surgical procedure. A thin subcutaneous or subcuticular closure over implants is inade-

349

quate surgical technique, and will result in a high rate of deep infection. In cases of severe loss of skin and subcutaneous tissue, medial and lateral gastrocnemius flaps are necessary to secure adequate vascularized coverage of the capsule and underlying implants.

## Summary

Extensile exposure is one of the crucial skills for managing the challenges presented by revision TKA. Full exposure is necessary to perform the intricate bone and ligament work, and short incisions combined with a timid approach to the quadriceps mechanism will result in inadequate reconstruction of the knee. Repair and reconstruction of the fascial, subcutaneous, and cutaneous tissues to achieve closure are separate and equally important skills.

## Acknowledgment

The author appreciates the assistance of William C. Andrea MA CMI with the illustrations, and Diane Morton MS with the manuscript preparation.

## References

1   Hallock GG: Salvage of total knee arthroplasty with local fasciocutaneous flaps. *Journal of Bone and Joint Surgery* [Am] **72**:1236–1239, 1990.
2   Coonse K, Adams JD: A new operative approach to the knee joint. *Surgical Gynecology and Obstetrics* **77**:344–347, 1943.
3   Trousdale RT, Hanssen AD, Rand JA, Cahalan TD: V-Y quadricep-splasty in total knee arthroplasty. *Clinical Orthopedics* **286**:48–55, 1993.
4   Barrack RL: Specialized exposure for revision total knee arthroplasty: quadriceps snip and patellar turndown. *Journal of Bone and Joint Surgery* [Am] **81**:138–141, 1999.
5   Garvin KL, Scuderi G, Insall JN: Evolution of the quadriceps snip. *Clinical Orthopedics* **321**:131–137, 1995.
6   Whiteside LA: Exposure in difficult total knee arthroplasty using tibial tubercle osteotomy. *Clinical Orthopedics* **321**:32–35, 1995.
7   Whiteside LA, Ohl MD: Tibial tubercle osteotomy for exposure of the difficult total knee arthroplasty. *Clinical Orthopedics* **260**:6–9, 1990.
8   Ritter MA, Carr K, Keating EM *et al.*: Tibial shaft fracture following tibial tubercle osteotomy. *Journal of Arthroplasty* **11**:117–119, 1996.
9   Wolff AM, Hungerford DS, Krackow KA, Jacobs MA: Osteotomy of the tibial tubercle during total knee replacement. *Journal of Bone and Joint Surgery* [Am] **71**:848–852, 1989.

## Questions and answers

*Moderator:* Dr. Whiteside, do you believe that a quadriceps snip really weakens the quadriceps? Is there any hard scientific evident to support this?

*Dr. Whiteside:* Yes, I believe a quadriceps snip weakens the quadriceps. Cutting across a muscle weakens it. It would require a lot of data to convince me otherwise.

*Moderator:* Dr. Whiteside, do you ever perform a quadriceps release?

*Dr. Whiteside:* No, but I did when I was in the Army. We all found that cutting through the quadriceps in young soldiers invariably weakened the muscle. I think that all muscles are weakened when they are cut in two. Can you imagine transecting the abductors to expose the hip?

*Moderator:* Most of the time, Dr. Scott, you will perform the VY plasty just to enable exposure. Are there times, however, where you will advance or transfer the VY flap?

*Dr. Scott:* In a knee with substantial flexion limitation resulting from scar and contracture, one might consider a VY quadriceps advancement. If one does choose to advance the quadriceps to enhance flexion, advancement should be no more than 1 cm. Otherwise there is a risk of an iatrogenic residual extensor lag and gait dysfunction. It is our contention that a quadriceps release is helpful for exposure of the stiff knee, but once a well positioned arthroplasty is implanted, most patients are better off with full extension and persistent flexion limitations, rather than a clinically significant extensor lag and enhanced flexion.

*Moderator:* You have spoken in the past, Dr. Whiteside, about how a tibial tubercle osteotomy can be "adjusted" so as to overcome a quadriceps contracture in a tight knee. Just how far can you proximally advance the tubercle and are there any surgical tips related to this?

*Dr. Whiteside:* The tubercle can be advanced 1–1.5 cm proximally, but this should be done only when the patellar tendon has shortened pathologically or the tubercle has previously been transferred distally. If the contracture is in the quadriceps, raising the tubercle will weaken the quadriceps muscle further. Transferring the tubercle distally can be done to treat patella alta associated with extension lag. This has been fairly effective in cases of elongation of the patellar tendon caused by injury.

*Moderator:* You allude to the problem with thin skin over the proximal tibia. In the face of that, Dr. Whiteside, would you consider a proximal release procedure in order to obviate having to place subcutaneous wires in the proximal tibia?

*Dr. Whiteside:* No, I would work through the available skin, and consider a flap if necessary.

*Moderator:* Dr. Scott, what do you mean by mobilization of the periarticular tissues?

*Dr. Scott:* When we say mobilization of periarticular tissues we mean incising the lateral patellofemoral synovial ligaments; excising scar

351

from the medial and lateral gutters, infrapatellar fat pad, inter-condylar notch, and suprapatellar pouch; removing hypertrophic osteophytes; balancing the collateral ligaments; and releasing muscular adhesions.

*Moderator:* How often during revision surgery do you have to perform a tubercle osteotomy? One gets the feeling that you do it in every case. Is that so?

*Dr. Whiteside:* No, I osteotomize the tubercle only when exposure requires it. This amounts to about 30% of revision knee cases and 1% of primary knee cases.

*Moderator:* Dr. Scott, When you are performing a VY plasty there is a small narrow tongue of soft tissue superiorly. Are you not worried about the vascularity to this small flap? Have there been any problems clinically?

*Dr. Scott:* In the technique of the inverted V quadricepsplasty the proximal apex of soft tissue is in theory hypoperfused for some period of time. Some of the vascularity may be preserved if the superior lateral geniculate vessels are intact. In theory, though, this area of tissue may have its blood supply compromised even using a standard medial arthrotomy when a lateral retinacular release is performed (with or without sacrifice of the lateral geniculate vessels). Although we cannot document scientific data that specifically addresses whether vascularity of this tongue of tissue is compromised by this approach, it is probably clinically unimportant in the majority of cases. We have not observed problems clinically with this approach that would suggest problematic ischemia or necrosis.

*Moderator:* You seem to indicate that if a VY plasty is insufficient you can then progress on with a tibial tubercle osteotomy. Doesn't that leave you with almost a free piece of quadriceps having been released both proximally and distally? Have you ever done this, and what were the results?

*Dr. Scott:* It would be very unusual to require both an extensive proximal release and tibial tubercle osteotomy for exposure. In rare occasions, however, an inverted V quadricepsplasty or a quadriceps snip can be safely combined with a tubercle osteotomy, provided the superior lateral limb of the incision is less than 2 cm and the superior lateral geniculate vessels are preserved. A tubercle osteotomy would not be recommended in the presence of more extensive turn-down-type procedures because of the significant risk of jeopardizing extensor mechanism function, compromising vascularity, and leaving an extensor mechanism that effectively functions like an auto- or allograft. Neither of us has ever combined the two.

*Moderator:* There are two very distinct situations, Dr. Scott, in which someone might do a quadriceps release. The first relates to safely everting the patella. The second is in a knee that has a markedly restricted range of motion preoperatively. Do you have different algorithms in these two situations and what are they?

*Dr. Scott:* There are several circumstances in which starting with a tibial tubercle osteotomy may be more helpful than a quadriceps release. The authors' primary indication for a tibial tubercle osteotomy is a case in which a lateral subvastus approach is utilized (in order to remove a lateral plate for instance or to perform a simultaneous corrective osteotomy). In such cases a tibial tubercle osteotomy is advisable to facilitate exposure and lyse adhesions (Lonner JH *et al., Journal of Arthroplasty* 1999;**14**:969–975; Lonner JH *et al., Journal of Bone and Joint Surgery*, in press March 2000). We would also consider this option for complex primary TKAs with severe patella infera, although we do not recommend addressing the infera with more proximal reattachment of the tubercle. We do not recommend tibial tubercle osteotomies for revision arthroplasty in the setting of severe osteolysis and anterior metaphyseal bone loss because of concern about limited surface area that the thin cortical shell of bone has available for healing. We also advise against tubercle osteotomy in primary TKA performed for post-traumatic arthrosis resulting from a highly comminuted tibial plateau fracture because of concern about compromised bone stock. Finally, atrophic or compromised soft tissues, superficial to the tibial tubercle, should discourage use of the tibial tubercle osteotomy.

*Moderator:* Dr. Scott, you mention that you check passive gravity flexion at surgery as a test of how you can move the knee after the operation. Does this passive gravity flexion have any relationship to the eventual motion obtained by patients?

*Dr. Scott:* I have previously reviewed the value of intraoperative flexion against gravity as a predictor of ultimate motion (Lee DC *et al., Journal of Arthroplasty* 1998;**13**:500–503). In an analysis of 364 primary TKAs comparing preoperative and intraoperative flexion to postoperative flexion at a minimum 2 year follow-up interval, 55% of knees had postoperative flexion within 10° of their preoperative flexion and 97% had postoperative flexion within 10° of their intraoperative flexion against gravity with the capsule repaired. Particularly in those patients who had less than 85° of preoperative flexion, intraoperative motion against gravity was noted to be a better predictor of ultimate motion than the preoperative flexion arc.

# 14

*Over 95% of all total knee replacements performed worldwide have a fixed polyethylene surface, either modular or nonmodular. There is, however, a school of thought that states that one can obtain better range of motion and decreased polyethylene wear by maximizing congruity and allowing the tibial polyethylene to be mobile in its base plate.*

# A fixed-bearing implant is optimal for most total knee replacements

## Pro: Timothy Wright

The design of any total joint replacement must provide appropriate joint function and range of motion, transfer the large loads that cross the joint from the implant components to the surrounding bone, and allow for long-term use without severe wear to the implant surfaces. For total knee replacements, these design objectives compete with one another. For example, providing adequate varus–valgus and rotational laxity to a knee replacement requires less than fully conforming joint surfaces, resulting in reduced contact areas and higher contact stresses than if the surfaces remained more closely matched in their shapes. Thus, a compromise must be sought between function and wear resistance.

### The case for fixed-bearing implants

For fixed-bearing knee replacements, rational solutions to these competing objectives have led to bicondylar geometries with curved surfaces in both the anteroposterior (AP) and medial–lateral directions (Fig. 14.1). Appropriate choices for radii of curvature for the tibial and femoral components minimize contact stresses while providing adequate constraint.[1,2] Analytical studies have demonstrated that the choices of medial–lateral radii on the tibial plateau and the femoral condyle have a very large effect on contact stresses. The AP radii do not affect contact stresses nearly as much (Fig. 14.2), giving the designer considerable latitude in seeking optimal compromises between important attributes such as torsional stiffness, rotational laxity, and wear.[2,3]

Range of motion for fixed-bearing total knee replacements is provided by the implant geometry. Placing the location of the low point, the so-called equilibrium position, posteriorly assures that the femur will remain posterior on the tibial plateau as compressive loads are

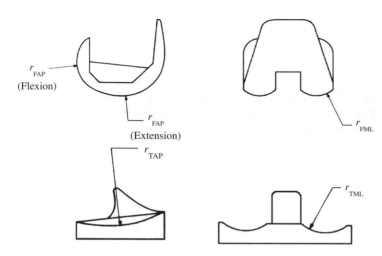

**Fig. 14.1**

The geometry of the articulating surface of a fixed-bearing knee implant[1] can be described by two radii on the tibial plateau (AP and medial–lateral) and three radii on the femoral component (two AP, one in extension and one in flexion, and one medial–lateral).

applied across the joint. The clearance that posterior contact provides between the posterior femoral condyles and the posterior tibial plateau in flexion allows the implant a range of motion in excess of 120°. To assure posterior movement of the femur in flexion, posterior-stabilized components with a cam and post mechanism can be used.[4] The conformity between the articulating surfaces interacts with the posterior stabilization mechanism to assure adequate roll-back of the femur during flexion.

One need only examine the clinical results of fixed-bearing implants to understand how well these designs have met the objec-

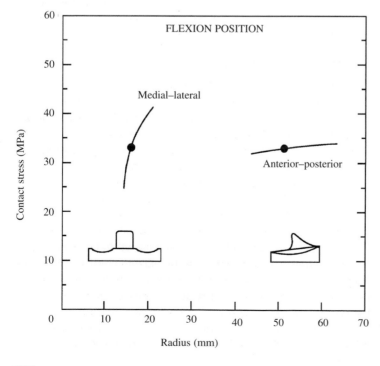

**Fig. 14.2**

The contact stress between fixed-bearing components such as those shown in Fig. 14.1 is much more sensitive to changes in the medial-lateral radii than in the AP radii with all other radii held constant.[2,32]

**Table 14.1** Clinical data for fixed bearing knee replacements (taken from references 5 and 6)

| Design | Follow-up (years) | Survival (%) |
|---|---|---|
| Total Condylar | 21 | 90.8 |
| Insall–Burstein PS all poly | 16 | 94.1 |
| Insall–Burstein PS metal-backed | 14 | 98.1 |
| Insall–Burstein PS modular | 10 | 93.6 |
| Optetrak | 2 | 100 |

tives of function, load transfer and wear resistance. Fixed-bearing knee replacements have demonstrated the best clinical results to date (Table 14.1), beginning with the original Total Condylar design with a 91% survival at 21 years follow-up,[5] and continuing with the modern Hospital for Special Surgery design with 100% survival at 2 years.[6] Even in younger patients (less than 55 years of age), the clinical results have been impressive, with 96% survival at 10 years[7] and 87% survival at 18 years.[8]

Reproducible function is provided by predictable, controlled posterior rollback of the femur on the tibia in the posterior-stabilized versions of fixed-bearing implants. The rollback designed into the implant matches that experienced clinically as verified with *in vivo* fluoroscopic studies.[9] As fixed-bearing designs have improved, the range of motion has increased from about 90° for the Total Condylar[10] to 115° for the Insall–Burstein Posterior Stabilized design.[4] Aseptic loosening is rare, as is severe wear damage, which has been observed only rarely and only after very long periods of implantation.[11,12]

## The case against mobile-bearing implants

Despite the excellent clinical success with fixed-bearing knee implants, clinicians and implant designers continue to strive for even more naturally functioning and wear-resistant knee replacements, particularly for use in younger patients. A solution that has gained increased attention is that of mobile-bearing knee replacements. The goal of a mobile-bearing knee replacement is to separate the movement needed for function from the movement between the articulating surfaces. This is achieved by having two articulations, one between the femoral and tibial components and a second between the tibial component and a base plate fixed to the tibia (Fig. 14.3). The mobile nature of the tibial component, either as a meniscal type bearing or a medial pivot bearing, is intended to allow the soft tissues (muscles and ligaments) around the joint to provide more control and constraint to joint motion than in a fixed-bearing implant. The intended goals are to allow for more natural joint kinematics, while also allowing the articulating surfaces to be more conforming than in a fixed-bearing knee, leading to larger contact areas, lower contact

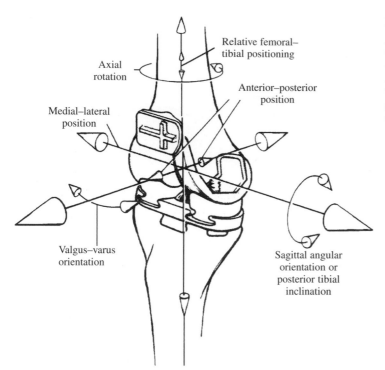

Axial rotation

Relative femoral–tibial positioning

Anterior–posterior position

Medial–lateral position

Valgus–varus orientation

Sagittal angular orientation or posterior tibial inclination

**Fig. 14.3**

Mobile-bearing knee implants, such as the New Jersey low contact stress design,[15] have an additional moving interface between the polyethylene tibial insert and the metallic tibial tray.

stresses, and presumably better wear resistance.[13,14] Unfortunately, a number of disadvantages have arisen from the clinical use of mobile-bearing knee designs. These include abnormal kinematics, dislocation and fracture of implant components, and osteolysis secondary to polyethylene wear.

### Abnormal kinematics

At least three factors contribute to abnormal kinematics. The first factor is the conformity between the femoral and tibial articulating surfaces. Supposedly a primary advantage for mobile bearing[15] is that the femoral and tibial articulating surfaces can have a single matching radius (since the additional mobile-bearing interface allows for movement). In meniscal-bearing designs,[16] however, this configuration results in too great a posterior displacement of the tibial mobile-bearing during flexion (Fig. 14.4). Therefore, meniscal-bearing designs have femoral components with multiple radii (much like fixed-bearing designs). A major advantage is thus significantly compromised, leading John Insall to reflect that such a design, "because of its lack of flexion congruence, may behave more like the total condylar prosthesis than a true meniscal-bearing type."[17]

Conformity between the articulating surfaces is also a potential problem in the kinematics of medial pivoting designs. In these types of implants, the medial femoral condyle and tibial plateau geometries are made highly conforming; in the extreme case, the geometry is a ball and socket similar to a total hip design with a large femoral diam-

**Fig. 14.4**

With a single radius on the femoral component of a meniscal-bearing implant, the tendency is for excessive posterior movement of the femur on the tibia in flexion.[16]

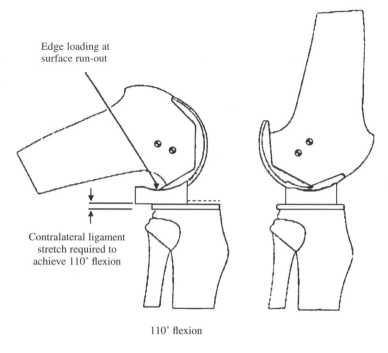

Edge loading at surface run-out

Contralateral ligament stretch required to achieve 110° flexion

110° flexion

eter. The presumption for medial pivoting designs is that proper surgical placement of the components will assure that the knee will pivot around the center of rotation of this conforming joint on the medial plateau. Of course, if the components are placed inappropriately, the medial pivot constraint will not match normal knee kinematics. In such cases, the tibial polyethylene socket will not be strong or stiff enough to constrain the knee joint against such inappropriate kinematics, leading most probably to severe polyethylene deformation, wear, and subluxation of the joint. Even if the components are properly placed, abnormal or unexpected knee motions could put unacceptable loads on the conforming surfaces. The situation is analogous to that of the original Total Condylar design from two decades ago, for which failures due to anterior subluxation of the femur on the tibia were common. In these cases, the anterior polyethylene lip of the tibial component underwent massive gross deformation as the femur subluxed through it.

A second factor contributing to abnormal kinematics in mobile-bearing designs is the impediment to motion that can result from the ingrowth of soft tissue around the components. Such ingrowth has been a problem in the patellofemoral joint of posterior-stabilized fixed-bearing knees,[18] though design improvements have essentially eliminated the problem (T. Sculco, personal communication). When motion is restricted at the mobile-bearing surface, the effect is to raise the joint line. An elevated joint line in a design intended to work with normal ligamentous constraints can be problematic, as has been noted for posterior cruciate retaining fixed-bearing knee implants.

The third factor also involves soft tissues; because of the complexity of mobile-bearing designs and because of their reliance on soft tissues for constraint, soft tissue balancing can be more complex than with a fixed-bearing design.

Measurements in the laboratory using cadaver knees have demonstrated abnormal kinematics for meniscal-bearing implants, most notably increased AP laxity.[19] Abnormal kinematics have also been demonstrated in clinical tests. Ten patients were asked to perform a simple function (a deep knee bend), while the relative motion between the knee components was monitored fluoroscopically.[20] In half of the patients, no motion was noted at the mobile-bearing, but in the other five patients, the femur moved anteriorly with respect to the tibia as the knee flexed (Fig. 14.5). Similar studies with normal knees and knees replaced with a posterior-stabilized fixed-bearing knee demonstrate a natural rollback of the femur on the tibia as flexion progresses.[9] These *in vivo* studies underscore the fact that soft tissues and the remaining (altered) knee anatomy cannot be relied upon to provide natural function. Similar unpredictable results have been shown for posterior cruciate ligament sparing devices that employ unconstrained geometries in hopes that the remaining ligaments and soft tissues will provide normal function.[21]

## Dislocation and fracture

Dislocation of mobile bearings from the tibial tray and fracture of the mobile bearings have been significant clinical problems. Unconstrained motion of meniscal bearings can cause them to dislocate or sublux from the metal base plate.[22] Besides causing a

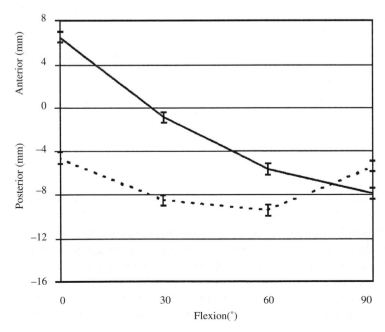

**Fig. 14.5**

Fluoroscopic studies of deep knee bends performed by normal individuals (solid line) and by patients with a meniscal-bearing knee implant (dotted line) showed dissimilar movements of the femur relative to the tibia. In the normal knee, the femur moves posteriorly on the tibia as the knee flexes, whereas in the knee replaced with a meniscal bearing implant the femur moves anteriorly.[20]

**Fig. 14.6**

Too great a movement of the polyethylene meniscal bearing can cause the bearing to be loaded like a cantilever beam. This situation creates high stresses at the base of the cantilever that in turn causes fracture of the polyethylene.[23]

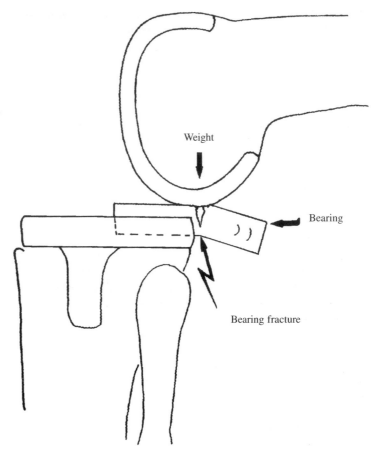

Weight

Bearing

Bearing fracture

**Table 14.2** Fracture and dislocations of mobile-bearing knee replacements

| Source | Design | No. of knees | No. fractured or dislocated |
|---|---|---|---|
| Buechel and Pappas[15,26] | LCS | 357 | 8 |
| Bourne et al.[27] | Oxford | 67 | I |
| Minns[28] | Minns | 165 | 8 |
| Bert[24] | LCS | 43 | 4 |
| Weaver et al.[23] | LCS | 56 | 5 |
| Anonymous[29] | LCS | 100 | 4 |
| Jordan et al.[30] | LCS | 473 | 12 |
| Huang et al.[25] | LCS | 276 | 8 |
| Total | | 1537 | 50 (3.3%) |

significant functional deficit, subluxation can leave the polyethylene meniscal bearing unsupported under the application of large cyclic and static joint loads,[23] causing fracture (Fig. 14.6). A review of the literature shows that of more than 1500 reported clinical cases of mobile-bearing implants, the rate of dislocation or fracture exceeds

3% (Table 14.2). More disturbing, dislocations and fractures continue to be reported, even after long-term follow-up of as long as 8 or 9 years.[24,25]

## Wear

Wear of the ultra high molecular weight polyethylene (UHMWPE) surfaces of fixed-bearing knee replacements typically occurs as delamination and pitting, rather than as the abrasive and adhesive wear that is commonly observed in total hip replacements.[31] The type of wear depends on the contact mechanics.[1,32] In total knee replacements, for example, the functional need for less conforming joint surfaces than in total hip replacements results in smaller contact areas and greater contact stresses. The contact area in knee replacements moves across the surfaces of the polyethylene components to a much greater extent than in hip replacements, so that points on and near the surfaces experience a wide range of cyclic stress.[32,33] The cyclic stresses in turn lead to the initiation of surface and subsurface cracks that grow to form pits and delamination. In total hip replacements, contact areas are much larger and surface kinematics are more confined. Wear in total hips occurs as the removal of much smaller particles from the surface,[31] primarily through abrasion against the matching metallic surface.

In mobile-bearing knees, a second wear-prone articulation exists between the flat surfaces of the polyethylene and metal components that form the mobile bearing. For these highly conforming surfaces, adhesive and abrasive wear dominate. The contact areas of the bearing surfaces are usually large, but nonetheless the resulting stresses and sliding distances are adequate for abrasive and adhesive wear to occur and, like in total hip replacements, to generate large numbers of submicron debris particles. Unfortunately, laboratory and clinical evidence demonstrate that smaller particles cause a more biologically insidious reaction, leading to osteolysis.[34,35]

Indeed, long-term follow-up of meniscal-bearing knee replacements shows osteolysis as a significant cause of premature failure.[25] The release of critical amounts of debris from the types of large, flat surfaces could occur without significant changes in the component thickness.[36] The contact area on the backside of a mobile-bearing knee is typically larger than the contact surface between the femoral and acetabular components of a total hip replacement. Thus, smaller changes in thickness in the case of the mobile-bearing knee would still produce comparable volumes of wear debris, and thus it may be difficult to appreciate that substantial wear has occurred based simply on radiographic studies.

Laboratory data from knee joint simulators bear out the propensity for mobile-bearing knees to generate more debris than fixed-bearing implants.[37] This type of simulator is aimed at applying the appropriate kinematics, cyclic load, environment, and soft tissue constraint to mimic the *in vivo* situation. Wear is measured as weight loss from the

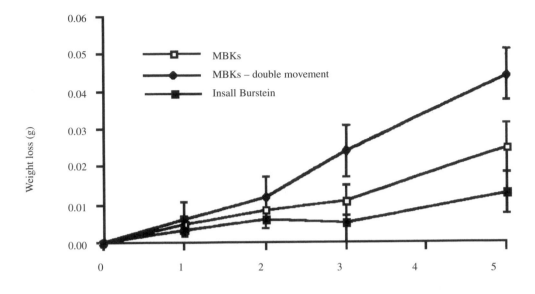

Number of cycles (millions)

**Fig. 14.7**

Wear, as measured by the weight of polyethylene lost from the tibial insert as a function of the number of cycles of testing in a knee joint simulator, was significantly greater for a mobile-bearing implant (MBK, open squares on figure) compared to a fixed-bearing implant (Insall–Burstein, black squares). The greater wear occurred regardless of whether or not greater motion ("double movement") was allowed in the meniscal-bearing implant (black circles).[37]

component as a function of the number of cycles of load that the polyethylene component experiences in the test. In a head to head comparison between a fixed-bearing design, the Insall–Burstein Posterior Stabilized, and a mobile-bearing design, the MBK, the fixed-bearing design demonstrated less wear, even when the mobile-bearing design was restricted to move less than might be expected *in vivo* (Fig. 14.7).

The greater wear in mobile-bearing designs could be a result of both the extra articulation and the joint surfaces themselves. The use of multiple radii in the femoral component of many mobile-bearing designs makes the articulation geometry similar to fixed-bearing designs. Even though contact areas are generally larger in a mobile-bearing design, contact stresses are comparable if not larger than many fixed-bearing designs at certain portions of the range of motion[14] and are more adversely affected by rotational malalignment than fixed-bearing designs.[15] Thus, these designs may not possess the intended advantage of increased wear resistance over fixed-bearing designs.

The use of a single radius, as in some medial pivot mobile-bearing designs, is not necessarily a solution to this problem. Again, a more conforming articulation combined with a large radius of curvature simply increases the propensity for abrasive wear because the product of surface velocity and load is quite high. The probability, therefore, that mobile-bearing designs will fare better than fixed-bearing designs is remote, especially considering that fixed-bearings designed to resist wear have demonstrated long-term clinical success with no evidence of wear-related failures.[5,32]

## Summary

The disadvantages (abnormal kinematics, dislocation and fracture, and polyethylene wear) of mobile-bearing knee designs, together with their failure to demonstrate better function even after long-term clinical use, show that contemporary mobile-bearing knees have not met the intended design goals. Longer follow-up, exceeding 20 years, may show mobile-bearing knees to have exceptional longevity, perhaps beyond that of fixed-bearing knee replacements. But given the clinical data thus far, this outcome seems unlikely. Together with the increased cost of mobile-bearing implants (with prices from several hundred dollars to over a thousand dollars more than fixed-bearing implants), the lack of superior performance has lead some orthopedic surgeons to abandon use of mobile-bearing knees until further design improvements are developed.[38] Such improvements must rely on a better understanding of how soft tissues (including muscles) and knee implant designs interact to control loads and function in the knee joint.

## Acknowledgements

The author wishes to acknowledge the helpful discussions with Dr. Thomas Sculco from Hospital for Special Surgery and Dr. Gary Miller from the University of Florida.

## References

1   Bartel DL, Bicknell VL, Wright TM: The effect of conformity, thickness, and material on stresses in UHMWPE components for total joint replacement. *Journal of Bone and Joint Surgery* [Am] **68**:1041–1051, 1986.

2   Burstein AH, Wright TM: *Fundamentals of orthopaedic biomechanics*, pp. 203–218, Williams and Wilkins, Baltimore, 1994.

3   Bartel DL, Rawlinson JJ, Burstein AH *et al.*: Stresses in polyethylene components of contemporary total knee replacements. *Clinical Orthopedics* **317**:76–82, 1995.

4   Insall JN, Lachiewicz PF, Burstein AH: The posterior stabilized condylar prosthesis: a modification of the total condylar design. Two to four-year clinical experience. *Journal of Bone and Joint Surgery* [Am] **64**:1317–1323, 1982.

5   Font-Rodriguez D, Scuderi GR, Insall JN: Survivorship of cemented total knee arthroplasty. *Clinical Orthopedics* **345**:79–86, 1997.

6   Gradisar I, Burstein AH, Petty W, Miller G: Clinical performance of Optetrak total knee prosthesis. Proc 1999 EFORT Meeting, Brussels.

7   Ranawat CS, Padgett DE, Ohashi Y: Total knee arthroplasty for patients younger than 55 years. *Clinical Orthopedics* **248**:27–33, 1989.

8   Diduch DR, Insall JN, Scott WN *et al.*: Total knee replacement in young, active patients. Long-term follow-up and functional outcome. *Journal of Bone and Joint Surgery* [Am] **79**:575–82, 1997.

9   Dennis DA, Komistek RD, Colwell CE Jr *et al.*: In vivo anteroposterior femorotibial translation of total knee arthroplasty: a multicenter analysis. *Clinical Orthopedics* **356**:47–57, 1998.

10  Insall JN, Hood RW, Flawn LB, Sullivan DJ: The total condylar knee prosthesis in gonarthrosis. A five to nine-year follow-up of the first one hundred consecutive replacements. *Journal of Bone and Joint Surgery* [Am] **65**:619–628, 1983.

11  Colizza WA, Insall JN, Scuderi GR: The posterior stabilized total knee prosthesis. Assessment of polyethylene damage and osteolysis after a ten-year-minimum follow-up. *Journal of Bone and Joint Surgery* [Am] **77**:1713–1720, 1995.

12  Li EC, Ritter MA, Montgomery T *et al.*: Catastrophic failure of a conforming type of total knee replacement. A case report. *Clinical Orthopedics* **333**:234–238, 1996.

13  Matsuda S, White SE, Williams VG II *et al.*: Contact stress analysis in meniscal bearing total knee arthroplasty. *Journal of Arthroplasty* **13**:699–706, 1998.

14  Szivek JA, Anderson PL, Benjamin JB: Average and peak contact stress distribution evaluation of total knee arthroplasties. *Journal of Arthroplasty* **56**:953–963, 1996.

15  Buechel FF, Pappas MJ: The New Jersey low-contact-stress knee replacement system: Biomechanical rationale and review of the first 123 cemented cases. *Archives of Orthopedic and and Trauma Surgery* **105**:197–204, 1986.

16  Pappas MJ, Buechel FF: On the use of a constant radius femoral component in meniscal bearing knee replacement. *Journal of Orthopaedic Rheumatology* **7**:27–29, 1994.

17  Insall JN: *Surgery of the knee*, pp. 696–698, Churchill Livingstone, New York, 1993.

18  Markel DC, Luessenhop CP, Windsor RE, Sculco TA: Arthroscopic treatment of peripatellar fibrosis after total knee arthroplasty. *Journal of Arthroplasty* **11**:293–297, 1996.

19  Matsuda S, Whiteside LA, White SE, McCarthy DS: Knee stability in meniscal bearing total knee arthroplasty. *Journal of Arthroplasty* **14**:82–90, 1999.

20  Stiehl JB, Dennis DA, Komistek RD, Keblish PA: In vivo kinematic analysis of a mobile bearing knee prosthesis. *Clinical Orthopedics* **345**:60–66, 1997.

21  Stiehl JB, Komistek RD, Dennis DA *et al.*: Fluoroscopic analysis of kinematics after posterior cruciate retaining knee arthroplasty. *Journal of Bone and Joint Surgery* [Br] **77**:884–889, 1995.

22  Bert JM: Dislocation/subluxation of meniscal bearing elements after New Jersey low-contact stress total knee arthroplasty. *Clinical Orthopedics* **254**:211–215, 1990.

23  Weaver JK, Derkash RS, Greenwald AS: Difficulties with bearing dislocation and breakage using a movable bearing total knee replacement system. *Clinical Orthopedics* **290**:244–252, 1993.

24  Bert JM: Delayed fracture of meniscal bearing elements in total knee arthroplasty. *Journal of Arthroplasty* **11**:611–612, 1996.

25  Huang CH, Young TH, Lee YT *et al.*: Polyethylene failure in New Jersey low-contact stress total knee arthroplasty. *Journal of Biomedical Materials Research* **38**:153–160, 1998.

26  Buechel FF, Pappas MJ: New Jersey low-contact-stress knee replacement system: ten year evaluation of meniscal bearings. *Orthopedic Clinics of North America* **20**(2):147–177, 1989.

27  Bourne RB, Rorabeck CH, Finlay JB, Nott L: Kinematic I and Oxford knee arthroplasty. A five to eight year follow-up study. *Journal of Arthroplasty* **2**:285–291, 1987.

28  Minns RJ: The Minns meniscal knee prosthesis: Biomechanical aspects of the surgical procedure and a review of the first 165 cases. *Archives of Orthopaedic and and Trauma Surgery* **108**:231–235, 1989.

29 Audience participant, Instructional course: Primary total knee arthroplasty (K Vince, Chair), Annual Meeting of the AAOS, Atlanta, 23 February, 1996.

30 Jordan LR, Olivo JL, Voorhorst PE: Survivorship analysis of cementless meniscal bearing total knee arthroplasty. *Clinical Orthopedics* **338**:119–123, 1997.

31 Wright TM: Biomaterials and prosthesis design in total knee arthroplasty. In *Orthopaedic knowledge update: hip and knee reconstruction*, ed. JJ Callaghan *et al.*), pp. 263–268. American Academy of Orthopaedic Surgeons, Rosemont, IL, 1995.

32 Bartel DL, Rimnac CM, Wright TM: Evaluation and design of the articular surface. In *Controversies of total knee arthroplasty*, ed. V Goldberg, pp. 61–73. Raven Press, New York, 1991.

33 Walker PS, Sathasivam S: The design of guide surfaces for fixed-bearing and mobile-bearing knee replacements. *Journal of Biomechanics* **32**:27–34, 1999.

34 Hirakawa K, Bauer TW, Stulberg BN *et al.*: Characterization of debris adjacent to failed knee implants of three different designs. *Clinical Orthopedics* **331**:151–158, 1996.

35 Wright TM Goodman SB: *Implant wear: the future of total joint replacement*. American Academy of Orthopaedic Surgeons, Rosemont, IL, 1996.

36 Argenson J, O'Connor JJ: Polyethylene wear in meniscal knee replacement. A one to nine-year retrieval analysis of the oxford knee. *Journal of Bone and Joint Surgery* [Br] **74**:228–232, 1992.

37 Bell CJ, Walker PS, Sathasivam S *et al.*: Differences in wear between fixed bearing and mobile bearing knees. *Transactions of the Orthopaedics Research Society* **24**:962, 1999.

38 Rorabeck CH: Fixed versus mobile bearings: Clinical difference? Presented at the 10th Holiday Knee Course (R Laskin, Chair), New York, 3 December, 1998.

# Con: Frederick F. Buechel

Despite the complacence of many orthopedic surgeons to the contrary, fixed-bearing tibial components are not ideal for most total knee patients. Mobile-bearing tibial components that maximize the bisperical surface congruity of the femoral component during the stance phase of gate, while minimizing the torsional constraints, represent the optimal implants for most total knee patients. Although this view was held by the minority of surgeons 10 years ago, it has become the dominant view of enlightened surgeons as we enter the year 2000.

The reason for the shift from fixed-bearing to mobile-bearing technology has been documented mechanical superiority and improved long-term performance. In this contribution I discuss the natural evolution of mobile bearings from fixed bearings, on the basis of sound mechanical engineering principles and long-term clinical results.

## Design rationale for mobile-bearing knee replacement

Engineering analysis predicts improvement in wear properties if surface congruity can be maintained in metal-plastic bearing surfaces.[1] Incongruent surfaces, such as found in fixed-bearing knee replacements, overload the plastic[2–4] and can lead to fatigue wear

**Fig. 14.8**

Flat-on-flat, fixed bearing tibial component revised for surface fatigue failure, cracking and delamination with metal-on-metal articulation after only 24 months.

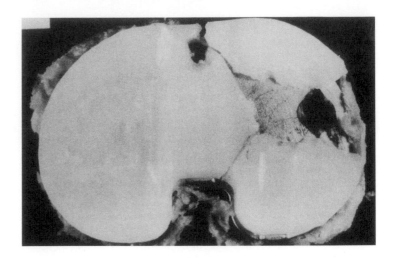

with delamination of the plastic surface in only a few years.[3] Flat-on-flat, fixed-bearing designs can increase wear even more due to edge loading during condylar lift-off, which occurs during the stance phase of gait (Fig. 14.8).[5]

Knee joint bearings need spherical surfaced geometry to maintain congruity during condylar lift-off. Such surfaces provide the most wear resistance and are considered ideal from a mechanical engineering standpoint.

A design dilemma occurs in knee joint replacement however when spherical surfaces are used without rotational or transitional ability. Such spherical fixed bearings overload the fixation interfaces by shear thus causing early loosening, a result seen clinically in the Geomedic total knee of the early 1970s.[6]

The introduction of mobile bearings in the mid-1970s was an attempt to overcome the limitations of completely incongruent bearings, which would wear out sooner, and fully congruent bearings, which would loosen sooner. By allowing congruency and mobility, wear resistance and improved fixation became achievable. Thus, mobile bearings became established as having ideal stress and movement capabilities from both engineering and kinematic perspectives (Fig. 14.9).[7,8]

## Contact stress analysis of knee replacement

Mechanical engineering design of knee joint replacement devices requires a thorough knowledge of anatomy, kinematics, bearing materials, and load limits of these materials. The industrial load limit for UHMWPE has been defined as 10 MPa of contact stress.[9] The medical load limit for repetitive loadbearing activities has been defined as 5 MPa of contact stress.[1,11] Such load limits impose restrictions on tibiofemoral and patellofemoral design geometries to provide sufficient congruity to maintain low contact stresses

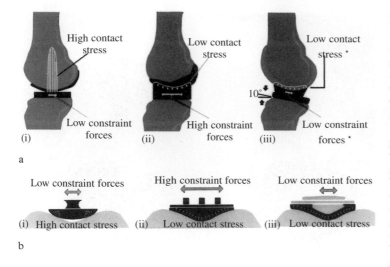

a

b

**Fig. 14.9**
(a) Comparison of total knee stress patterns versus movement: (i) mobility without congruity; (ii) congruity without mobility; (iii) mobility with congruity (ideal stress and movement conditions). (b) Comparison of patellofemoral stress patterns versus movement. (i) incongruent contact, fixed bearing—mobility without congruity; (ii) congruent contact, fixed bearing—congruity without mobility; (iii) congruent contact, rotating bearing—mobility with congruity (ideal stress and movement conditions).

(<10 MPa). Failure to maintain low contact stresses (<10 MPa) results in catastrophic, accelerated, fatigue-type wear rather than mild, slower, abrasive-type wear.

Evaluation of tibiofemoral and patellafemoral bearing geometries during walking and routine activities of daily living (Fig. 14.10) demonstrates the ability of mobile-bearing geometries to maintain safe contact stress (<5 MPa), whereas fixed-bearing geometries are constantly overloaded (>10 MPa). This basic engineering analysis lends important credibility to the mobile-bearing concept for enhancing long-term wear resistance while demonstrating a fatal flaw in fixed bearings, which remain overloaded and in danger of accelerated wear.

## Mechanical simulation of knee replacements

To understand wear mechanisms and predict the future outcome of a knee prosthesis, mechanical simulation of walking loads for 10 years is quite useful and recommended before general release of such a device.[8,10] It has been postulated that 1 million gait cycles represents approximately 1 year of walking in an elderly adult, so 10 million gait cycles at 2–3 times body weight load would provide 10 year walking simulation. A useful simulator, however, needs to provide axial rotation and translation as well as condylar load flucuation to approximate the normal torsional, translational, and condylar lift-off functions of the human knee.

A uniaxial knee simulator, which continuously rolls in one direction without translation, rotation or lift-off, can give deceptive results. Once started, such a simulator allows the bearing surfaces to "bed-in" to each other, which increases conformity and slows down the wear process. This type of simulation can give erroneous wear data and should be used with caution, especially with incongruent joint designs.

**Fig. 14.10**

(a) Tibiofemoral implant contact stress patterns: (i) area contact (3.9 MPa); (ii) double curve line contact (13 MPa); (iii) point contact (25 MPa); (iv) flat-on-flat line contact (32 MPa). (b) Contact stress values in tibiofemoral implants. (c) Surface geometrics of various patellofemoral implants at 30° of flexion).

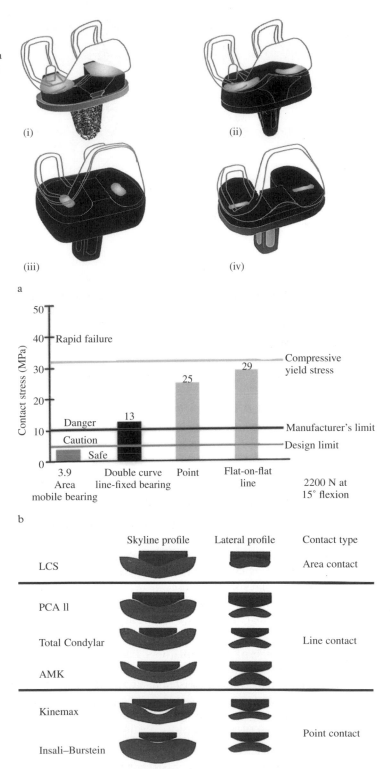

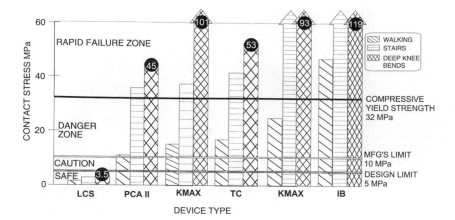

d

**Fig. 14.10**

(d) Contact stress values in various patellofemoral implants.

Knee joint replacement simulation was carried out and presented in 1992 to determine the volumetric wear of mobile-bearing and fixed-bearing knee replacements using a multiaxial simulation with fluctuating varus–valgus loads.[11] The data in this study suggests that mobile bearings wear six times less than incongruent fixed bearings, even though the mobile bearings have upper and lower articulating surfaces, whereas the fixed bearings are wearing only on their upper surface. The preferred wear pattern seen was of mild, abrasive nature in mobile bearings and a delaminating, fatigue pattern in the fixed bearings, as predicted by contact stress analysis.

## Retrieval studies of knee replacements

Analysis of well-functioning knee replacements that suddenly fail or are retrieved at autopsy represents the most important study to determine the relative wear of one design compared to another, so that design and material improvements can be considered for the future. *In vivo* performance of knee replacements retrieved after 5–10 years can be compared to simulator studies to corroborate or negate the mechanical simulation data. Well-designed knee implants should demonstrate mild but progressive abrasive wear patterns during both simulation and *in vivo* use.

Mobile bearings have generally demonstrated this mild, abrasive wear behavior after long-term *in vivo* use, even when compromised by gamma irradiation in air and poor quality polyethylene (Fig. 14.11).[2] Fixed-bearings designs have shown less satisfactory *in vivo* performance, which has been catastrophic when poor-quality polyethylene has been gamma-irradiated in air and used in a flat-on-flat bearing configuration.[2]

## Clinical evaluation of knee replacements

Patient perception of knee function following knee joint replacement goes to the heart of the matter. A successful knee replacement from a patient's perspective would be one that allows painless, near normal

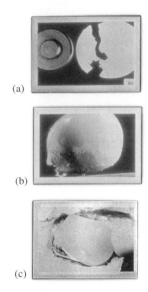

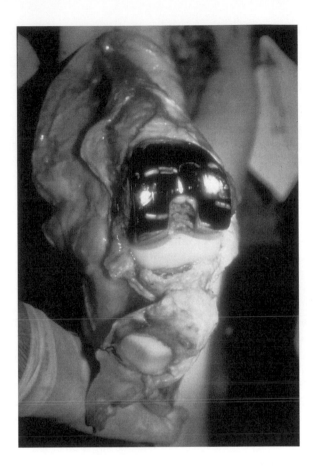

**Fig. 14.11**

(a) Postmortem retrieval of a
well functioning rotating platform device after 16 years' use
with a minimal abrasive wear
seen on all bearing surfaces.
(b) Comparison of fixed-
bearing and rotating-bearing
patella components after revision (fixed bearings) and postmortem retrieval (rotating
bearing): (a) 2 years, point
contact; (b) 3 years, line
contact; (c) 10 years, rotating-
bearing area contact.

function for the rest of his or her life. If the patient is 80 years old and
relatively inactive, this formula for success may be achieved by either
a fixed-bearing or a mobile-bearing knee replacement. For younger
patients under the age of 70, however, increased activities result in
increased loads and increased number of knee flexion cycles. Wear is
related to the number of cycles and the amount of load (contact
stress). A proper knee prosthesis should be able to withstand at least
10 years of active use, before wearing out or suffering a mechanical
failure. During this time interval 90% of patients should feel that
they have satisfactory function and score in the good or excellent
range on a documented knee scoring scale.[12,13] Such objective evidence allows comparison of various devices over time and provides
an important outcome measure.

Several mobile-bearing knee replacement studies have documented greater than 90% clinical success over a 10 year period using
the same prosthesis that remains commercially available.[14–17]

Fixed-bearing knee replacements have not demonstrated similar
success. Although mid-term and long-term studies of various fixed-
bearing knee implants have shown promise,[18,19] design changes have

occurred because of some inherent wear, loosening or instability problem that was uncovered, leaving these designs as historical relics of orthopedic joint development.

## Survivorship analysis of knee replacement

Long-term survivorship of an implant for 10 years or more in 90% of patients without a revision for any reason has been advocated as a criterion for success.[20] Several fixed-bearing implants have documented such success.[18-20] However, once this 10 years success was achieved these fixed-bearing designs were abandoned because of some clinically unacceptable problem, such as wear loosening, poor motion, or instability. Few, if any, fixed-bearing designs are promoted in their original form after 10 years.

Mobile bearings, on the other hand, have demonstrated improved 10 year survivorship over fixed bearings in several studies[15,17] without change to the initial design configuration. In fact, the original articulation of the current mobile-bearing knee system has not changed since its introduction in 1977. A currently available bearing can be exchange for a worn one in a 20 year old implant, since the metallic geometry and articulating features remain unchanged.

Survivorship of an implant relies on a host of mechanical and biological factors. Infection and implant failure will cause revision surgery to adversely affect overall survivorship. Lowering contact stress (< 5MPa) to minimize wear and providing bearing motion to reduce loosening problems have been essential ingredients for increasing implant survivorship.

## Conclusions

After a thorough analysis of the factors influencing the longevity of knee joint replacement, I conclude that mobile-bearing designs that lower contact stresses below 5 MPa using spherical articulating surfaces are optimal for most total knee replacement patients.

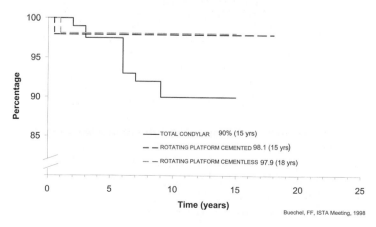

**Survivorship of TKR**

TOTAL CONDYLAR    90% (15 yrs)
ROTATING PLATFORM CEMENTED 98.1 (15 yrs)
ROTATING PLATFORM CEMENTLESS 97.9 (18 yrs)

Buechel, FF, ISTA Meeting, 1998

**Fig. 14.12**

Long-term survivorship comparison of fixed-bearing (Total Condylar, solid line) and mobile-bearing (rotating-platform, dashed line[19]) knee replacements.

This conclusion is supported by simulator studies that document six times more volumetric wear with incongruent fixed bearings than with congruent mobile bearings.[11] It is also supported by retrieval studies that document linear, abrasive wear patterns in mobile bearings as opposed to fatigue–delamination wear patterns seen in fixed bearings.[22] Further support is given by long-term clinical studies which demonstrate good or excellent clinical results in more than 90% of mobile-bearing knees followed for 10 years or more[14–17] and survivorship studies which document greater than 90% survivorship after more than 15 years using the same implant geometry that remains currently available (Fig. 14.12).[17]

Fixed-bearing knee designs have failed to remain available after 10 years in their original geometry due to problems of wear, loosening, poor motion, or instability. Also, osteolysis from wear debris is commonly seen in long-term fixed-bearing knee replacements[23] but is extremely uncommon in long-term mobile-bearing knees.

After more than 20 years of positive clinical experience it is now recommended that mobile-bearing knee replacement be considered the current standard for reproducible and dependable long-term knee replacement results.

# References

1   Pappas MJ, Makris G, Buechel FF: Biomaterial for hard tissue applications. In *Biomaterial and clinical applications: Evaluation of contact stresses in metal-plastic knee replacements*, ed. PG Pizzoferrato *et al.*, pp. 259–264. Elselvier, Amsterdam, 1987.

2   Collier JP *et al.*: The biomechanical problems of polyethylene as a bearing surface. *Clinical Orthopedics* **261**:107–113, 1990.

3   Engh GA Dwyer DA, Hares CK: Polyethylene wear of the metal-backed tibial components in total and unicompartmental knee prosthesis. *Journal of Bone and Joint Surgery* [Br] **73**:9–17, 1992.

4   Landy M, Walker PA: Wear in Condylar replacement Knees. A 10 year follow-up. *Transactions of the Orthopedics Research Society* **10**:96, 1985.

5   Dennis DA, Komistek RD, Hoff WA, Gabriel, SM: In vivo knee kinematic derived using an inverse perspective technique. *Clinical Orthopedics* **331**:107–117, 1996.

6   Riley D *et al.*: Long term results of Geomedic total knee replacement. *Journal of Bone and Joint Surgery* [Br] **67**:548–550, 1985.

7   Schlepkow P: The LCS knee kinematics in comparison with kinematic behavior of the natural joint. LCS Users Symposium, Frankfurt, Federal Republic of Germany, 30 September, 1989.

8   Pappas MJ, Buechel FF: Wear in prosthetic knee joints. Scientific exhibit presented at the 59th Annual Meeting of the American Academy of Orthopaedic Surgeons, Washington DC, 20–25 February, 1992.

9   Hostalen GUR: Hoechst aktiengellschaft, Frankfurt, Germany 1982, p. 22.

10  Buechel FF: Guidelines for choosing a joint replacement implant. *Orthopaedics Review* **16**:5, 1987.

11  Pappas MJ Makris G, Buechel FF: Wear in prosthetic knee joints. Scientific exhibit, 59th Annual Meeting of the American Academy of Orthopaedic Surgeons, Washington DC, 1992.

12  Buechel FF: A simplified evaluation system for the rating of knee func-
    tion. *Orthopaedics Review* 97–101, 1982.

13  Insall JN, Dorr LD, Scott RD and Scott WN: Rationale of the Knee
    Society Clinical Rating System. *Clinical Orthopedics* **248**:13–14,
    1989.

14  Jordan LR, Olivo JL, and Voorhorst. P.E: Survivorship analysis of
    cementless meniscal bearing total knee arthroplasty. *Clinical
    Orthopedics* **338**:119–123, 1997.

15  Sorrells RB: Primary knee arthroplasty long-term outcomes: The Rotation
    Platform mobile bearing TKA. *Orthopedics* **19**:793–796, 1996.

16  Keblish PA, Varma AK, Greenwald AS: Patellar resurfacing or retention
    in total knee arthroplasty: A prospective study of patients with bilat-
    eral replacements. *Journal of Bone and Joint Surgery* [Br] **76**:421,
    1994.

17  Buechel FF: Long-term results of total knee replacement: Mobile
    Bearing total knee replacement. *Orthopaedic knowledge update: hip
    and knee*. American Academy of Orthopaedic Surgeons, Rosedale,
    IL (in press 1999).

18  Ranawat CS, Flynn WF, Saddler S *et al.*: Long term results of the Total
    Condylar knee arthroplasty: A 15 year survivorship study. *Clinical
    Orthopedics* **286**:94–102, 1993.

19  Scuderi GR, Insall JN, Windsor RE *et al.*: Survivorship of cemented
    knee replacements. *Journal of Bone and Joint Surgery* [Br]
    **71**:789–803, 1989.

20  Buechel FF, Pappas MJ: Long-term survivorship analysis of cruciate
    sparing versus cruciate-sacrificing knee prosthesis using meniscal
    bearing. *Clinical Orthopedics* **260**:162–169, 1990.

21  Ritter MA, Campbell E, Faris P, Keating ME: The AGC 2000 total
    knee arthroplasty with and without cement. *American Jcounral of
    Knee Surgery* **2**:160, 1989.

22  Collier JP, Mayor MB, McNamara JL *et al.*: Analysis of the failure of
    122 polyethylene inserts from uncemented tibial knee components.
    *Clinical Orthopedics* **273**:232–242, 1991.

23  Insall JN: Adventures in mobile bearing knee design: A mid-life crisis.
    Presented at the 14th Annual Current Concepts in Joint
    Replacement, Orlando, Florida, 12 December, 1997.

## Questions and answers

*Moderator:* Dr. Buechel, how much congruity is really necessary in
a mobile-bearing knee? Some mobile-bearing knees have a J shaped
femoral component with congruity predominately in extension,
whereas others have a uniradius femoral component attempting to
gain congruity through a greater flexion arc. Which is better, if either,
and why?

*Dr. Buechel:* Maximum congruity of a mobile-bearing surface with
the largest surface area possible should be designed for the most
repetitive and highest peak loads in the knee, which are found during
the stance phase of gait (0–30° of flexion). Other less frequent
loading positions which don't involve peak impact loading, such as
rising from a chair, should have as much congruity as possible to
avoid fatigue, but should allow full flexion. Additionally, the
patellofemoral articulation must be considered to avoid overload of

this articulation during walking, squatting, or stair-climbing. As such, the J-curve type femoral component can give perfect congruity for the patellofemoral joint during all phases and the tibiofemoral joint during the entire stance phase of gait.

*Moderator:* It has been said that the particles generated in a mobile-bearing knee are the small ones that, at least in hips, can lead to osteolysis. Is this really true, and if so, will osteolysis be a problem in mobile-bearing knees?

*Dr. Buechel:* Polyethylene wear debris of small particle size is associated with increased osteolysis in hips after 5–10 years of active use. It will likely occur in mobile-bearing knees if a long enough interval of use is seen. After 20 years, however, we have not seen osteolysis as a major concern in mobile-bearing knees. It's incidence has been less than 0.5% in my experience. Perhaps the large volume of synovial tissue in the knee accepts these small particles to a greater degree than the hip, so that osteolysis in the knee is delayed.

*Moderator:* Dr. Wright, the medial pivot knee has been espoused as being the proper configuration for a knee prosthesis. Why do you think designers of medial pivot knees feel so strongly about their efficacy?

*Dr. Wright:* I would guess that they believe there are two overriding advantages over conventional fixed-bearing implants. One is the possibility for more natural function and the other is for better wear resistance. Without repeating the information and opinions presented in my contribution, I would point out that the first belief presupposes that patients with fixed-bearing knees do not function appropriately (a difficult belief to back up with functional or clinical outcome data). It also assumes that the knee will function normally given no constraints from the design, so that the clinically proven approach of controlling function with help from the geometry of the implant surfaces can be sacrificed (again a difficult belief to support with kinematic data). The other belief, better wear resistance, may be totally incorrect given the predilection for more conforming, ball-and-socket surfaces to suffer abrasive wear, releasing small debris particles that are known to be effective osteolysis generators.

*Moderator:* I know that you are not a surgeon, but as a bioengineer, do you feel that soft tissues be appropriately balanced for a mobile-bearing knee to function properly?

*Dr. Wright:* As a biomedical engineer and not an orthopedic surgeon, I'll answer this question only on the condition that you ask Dr. Buechel a complicated question about stress distributions or wear mechanisms in polyethylene! Seriously though, I believe the answer is a definite yes, at least for treating knees without considerable deformity or conditions such as trauma that might disrupt soft tissue function. My concern for the present is that we simply do not have enough information on knee kinematics that could be used in designing an appropriate mobile bearing and in developing appropriate surgical techniques (component placement, component orientation, and soft tissue balancing). This will not always be the case. Recent work combining fluoroscopic and gait analyses, efforts aimed at measuring joint loads *in vivo* using instrumented knee implants, and the availability of ever more detailed and robust dynamic computer models for the knee will all combine to give us the necessary tools to attack this problem. My concern is that we're racing into mobile-bearing designs without first obtaining and then considering this information (and a way to incorporate it into rational design goals). If I'm right, we will witness unacceptably high failure rates in these designs.

*Moderator:* You have said that your prosthesis has not changed over the past 10 years, Dr. Beuchel. Has your surgical technique changed, however? Have your indications changed?

*Dr. Buechel:* The LCS prosthetic knee design has not changed its articulating surface geometry for more than 20 years. The surgical technique remains similar today as 20 years ago, using a tibial cut first approach, balancing the flexion gap while rotating the femur into proper external position, and then balancing the extension gap by distal femoral resection. Some instruments have been refined over the years, but the indications for surgery also remain the same–end stage arthritis, unresponsive to medical or other surgical means.

*Moderator:* Dr. Wright, if wear could be decreased (say for instance by the use of ceramic rather than cobalt surfaces) do you think your negative feelings about mobile-bearing prostheses would change?

*Dr. Wright:* The answer is maybe and the reasons are as follows. Clinical data with alternative bearing materials in total hip replacements, where such bearing materials are intended to reduce abrasive wear, are not all that convincing in terms of long follow-up series demonstrating reduced incidence of osteolysis. Nonetheless, if such materials (including new forms of cross-linked UHMWPE), proved to be clinically advantageous for conforming surfaces, then these materials might be of benefit in mobile-bearing designs. However, because these alternative materials are only beneficial for reducing abrasive wear (that is, in conforming geometries), they would be of no benefit in a less conforming case, for example, the lateral condyle of a medial pivot design. This is the same reason alternative bearing materials have never proven beneficial in fixed-bearing knees, which by design are less conforming.

*Moderator:* You have been talking almost exclusively about a rotating platform design. Have you abandoned the meniscal bearings? If not, what are your present indications for one type over another?

*Dr. Buechel:* Rotating platforms have outperformed meniscal bearings over the past 20 years, mostly because of inferior grade polyethylene materials gamma-sterilized in air, which have caused a 2–4%

meniscal bearing wear or fracture, but less than 0.5% wear in rotating platforms. They appear to be less sensitive to wear. Currently, gas plasma or ethylene oxide sterilization of high quality UHMWPE seems to minimize these wear problems.

*Moderator:* What are your feelings about the mobile-bearing patellar prosthesis, Dr. Wright?

*Dr. Wright:* I feel quite strongly that mobile-bearing patellar implants serve no purpose and, in fact, create more problems than they are intended to solve. The design rationale is similar to that for the tibiofemoral joint: reduce the constraint provided by the implant with an additional mobile articulation, thus allowing the remaining natural structures to dictate joint function. But the clinical function of fixed-bearing patellar implants, whether a simple dome shape or more anatomical, is quite good by all reports. Besides, the function of the patellofemoral joint in a total knee probably has more to do with soft tissue function, particularly the quadriceps muscle, and thus with surgical technique than with implant design. Furthermore, the anatomy simply doesn't allow sufficient space to design the additional articulation. For that matter, space doesn't exist to design even an additional fixed articulation (just recall the clinical performance of fixed-bearing metal-backed patellar implants). Thus, mobile-bearing patellar implants such as the LCS have polyethylene and metal components that are quite thin, making them especially susceptible to excessive wear and disarticulation, especially if they fail to remain mobile while implanted.

*Moderator:* It has beens said that implanting a meniscal-bearing knee is more difficult for the average orthopedist than implanting a fixed-bearing knee. Any thoughts about this? It has been said that flexion space balancing is more critical.

*Dr. Buechel:* Inserting a mobile-bearing knee is actually easier than implanting a fixed-bearing knee. The tibial component can be placed centrally on the berst bone without being exactly oriented, since the mobile bearing will self adjust to the proper axial alignment. The remainder of the technique is the same as in fixed-bearing knee replacement.

*Moderator:* What I am really asking is, for the average orthopedist who is implanting 10–20 knee replacements each year, mainly in patients over the age of 70, is there a real advantage in using a mobile-bearing prosthesis.

*Dr. Buechel:* There are two great advantages in using a mobile-bearing prosthesis for the orthopedist who is implanting only 10–20 knee replacements per year in patients over the age of 70. Firstly, the technique of implanting the prosthesis is easier, so the surgeon should be able to finish a well-aligned procedure in less time than a fixed-bearing knee that requires extra diligence in correctly aligning the axial rotation of the tibial component. Secondly, the surgeon can depend on the mobile-bearing prosthesis to last for the next 18 years in over 97% of cases based on survivorship data. This means that when their elderly patients are most vulnerable, they won't be needing revision total knee surgery before they die.

*Moderator:* I appreciate that, but for fairness I must point out that the long-term survivorship of fixed-bearing knees in the age group over 70 is just as long, if not longer, and that the overwhelming number of these patients (nearly all) also won't need a revision before they die. Likewise, I personally feel that the ease of rotary alignment in a mobile-bearing knee is easily offset by the greater diligence that is necessary to balance the flexion space when using a mobile design. At least in my experience, many surgeons have more difficulty with flexion space balancing than do with tibial component rotation.

# 15

*Outcome measurement is as important for the clinician in a small private practice as it is for the professor in the large university. Unless we can describe our results properly and adequately, patients, government, insurance companies, and colleagues will have no true idea of what we are doing and how we are truly benefiting patients and society as a whole.*

# Outcome measurement in total knee replacement

John P. Davis

Patient outcome measurement has become a high priority throughout the healthcare industry. Fueled by concerns for quality versus cost, healthcare providers have determined that outcome data collection and subsequent management is necessary to support treatment decisions and differentiate levels of care. In theory, outcome measurement in the patient with total knee replacement (TKR) surgery can assist the surgeon in the planning of care, empower the patient to make educated decisions in determining treatment options, and assure that quality is provided across the entire continuum.

Total knee surgeons have been involved in outcome measurement through clinical research since the first TKR was performed over 30 years ago. Recent trends show a demand for a more detailed and formalized process. Collection of pertinent information will help the clinician keep up with demands made from within the rapidly changing managed care environment. Insurers, implant designers, and the patients themselves are requesting more and more detailed outcome information. Physicians need to make an internal assessment of their existing practice patterns to ensure that they are managing their outcomes and that the associated operational costs will enable the delivery of efficient care in the next millennium.

An outcomes program implies that a process is in place to track progress while monitoring the level of quality from one point in time to another. Although its origins were in research, outcome measurement has now evolved into a practice for all providers. The expansion of information systems has raised expectations of many within the physician practice setting. The ability to capture and manage large volumes of data has also altered the competitive playing field. A key to future survival of the total knee specialist is efficient and effective management of TKR quality information.

The purpose of this chapter is to heighten the awareness of outcome management in the TKR community. A message should be given that the collection of information does not have to be a time-consuming and expensive process. On the contrary, if the process is set up correctly and information technology is utilized appropriately, it can save time by improving efficiency and save money by reducing expenses.

Hopefully, the concepts presented here will reaffirm the efforts of those with an outcome system already in place. For those who have not yet begun, perhaps this will provide information to help choose a more reliable path. The overall goal is to provide the reader with a more definitive picture of the outcomes movement by providing a practical template demonstrating how volumes of total knee specific information can be collected, analyzed, and effectively incorporated into a quality program.

## Outcomes research

Some believe the history of outcomes management stems from the pioneering work of John Wennberg and associates in 1973[1] who looked at the health services delivery process and sought to understand the process of care in hospitals and to explain the differences across small geographic areas. Others feel that the historical roots of outcomes and medical effectiveness research rest in the general health service research. Outcomes research is described as one thin slice of this larger body of investigation that serves to document, analyze, and prescribe the structure, process and outcomes of medical and public healthcare in various cultures, legal and geographic jurisdictions, and countries.

Three important factors that stimulated the emergence of outcomes research are the rapidly rising cost of healthcare, variations in practice patterns, and deficiencies in clinical research methods.[2] Additional motivating factors driving the outcome movement to a nonresearch practice include competition, public concern, and policy intervention for quality assurance and improvement.

Over time, orthopedic clinical research widened its focus from review of the outcome of a procedure to the improvement of health and well being of the patient after treatment. The orthopedic community must understand that appropriate studies of outcome are needed to demonstrate how much musculoskeletal procedures improve the quality of life and that these procedures are, therefore, economically worthy of continued support by government and by private insurance carriers.[3]

## Concept of outcomes

Orthopedic outcomes are specific to the medical condition and the surgical intervention and deal with intended and unintended consequences of treatment. Outcomes today include health-related quality of life (HRQL), patient and provider satisfaction, economic efficiency, as well as symptom reduction, return to work, and improved clinical indicators. Outcomes research requires the commitment of various skills to identify these outcomes conceptually and then to operationalize measurements, so that studies can be accomplished to confirm or reject hypothesized relationships between interventions, covariates, and these outcomes, while severity and comorbidity are held constant.[4]

A more detailed understanding of the conceptual framework of outcome research is presented in Fig. 15.1. A key element that must be emphasized is the feedback loop from patient's outcomes to inputs. Hence, the outcome of one patient–provider interaction affects all that follows. Continuity of care is critical to both quality and effectiveness. By tracking the outcomes of one's own practice, one can learn from the experience of many patients and use this information to ascertain that the response of this particular patient is below the normal response to therapy. This implies that practice data could generate within-practice patterns that might improve diagnosis and treatment. Moreover, if these data are standardized and aggregated over several practices, the learning can be even greater.[5]

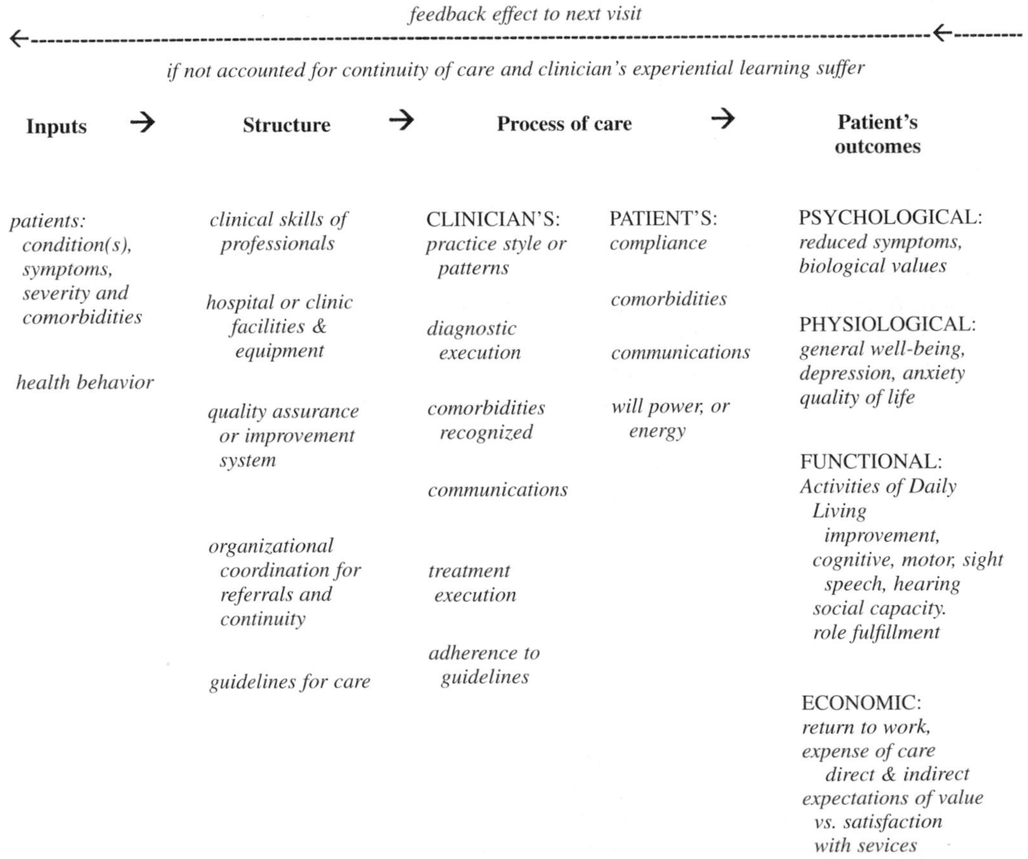

**Fig. 15.1**

Conceptual model for orthopedics outcomes research. Adapted from Bradham.[1]

*feedback effect to next visit*

←--------------------------------------------------------------------------------------------------←---------

*if not accounted for continuity of care and clinician's experiential learning suffer*

| Inputs → | Structure → | Process of care → | | Patient's outcomes |
|---|---|---|---|---|
| *patients:* *condition(s),* *symptoms,* *severity and* *comorbidities* | *clinical skills of* *professionals* | CLINICIAN'S: *practice style or* *patterns* | PATIENT'S: *compliance* | PSYCHOLOGICAL: *reduced symptoms,* *biological values* |
| | *hospital or clinic* *facilities &* *equipment* | *diagnostic* *execution* | *comorbidities* *communications* | PHYSIOLOGICAL: *general well-being,* *depression, anxiety* *quality of life* |
| *health behavior* | *quality assurance* *or improvement* *system* | *comorbidities* *recognized* *communications* | *will power, or* *energy* | FUNCTIONAL: *Activities of Daily* *Living* *improvement,* *cognitive, motor, sight* *speech, hearing* *social capacity.* *role fulfillment* |
| | *organizational* *coordination for* *referrals and* *continuity* | *treatment* *execution* | | |
| | *guidelines for care* | *adherence to* *guidelines* | | ECONOMIC: *return to work,* *expense of care* *direct & indirect* *expectations of value* *vs. satisfaction* *with sevices* |

Applying the concept to the typical total knee practice is better explained in the following examples. Inputs include the patient's condition, symptoms and co-morbidities taken from a comprehensive medical history, assessment, and physical examination during the initial evaluation. Knee-specific instruments used to collect information to measure levels of pain, range of motion, mobility, and other clinical findings as well as demographic information help lay the foundation of the outcome process.

Structure is a step in the process that addresses practice guidelines for care, equipment, and environment. A process that is written and communicated to the team has a better chance of being consistently adhered to.

- What is needed, where, and by whom is the care to be provided?
- Are protocols or pathways in place?
- Does the hospital, clinic, office and radiology department understand and utilize the total knee routine or protocol?
- Are the care providers delivering expert care?
- Is there a mechanism in place to address areas for improvement?

The structuring of the process includes when, where, and what data is collected. The procedure for office visits (Fig. 15.2) shows that data forms are presented to patients along the pathway to collect quality information specific to the diagnosis. The flow diagram helps with identification and clarification of communication and accountability patterns throughout the procedure. Process flow variance or breaks in communication can be easily recognized and corrective actions to address staff members or process issues can be initiated as needed. These internal steps address care consistency and demonstrate ongoing continuous quality improvement.

The process of care also involves input from both the surgeon and patient. Communication again is a key component.

- Does the surgeon communicate the plan of care effectively to other staff?
- Are the surgeon's style, diagnostic ability, and treatment execution effective?
- Is the patient able or motivated to participate in his or her own care?
- Is the patient compliant with recommended therapeutic treatment plans?
- Does the patient comply with scheduled appointments?

All of these questions address process effectiveness. Without the office's staff's strict attention to detail, the active participation of patients and families, and excellent communication, the process will often fall prey to administrative pitfalls including duplication of services, time wastage, and their associated additional costs and frus-

**Fig. 15.2**

Feedback effect to next visit.

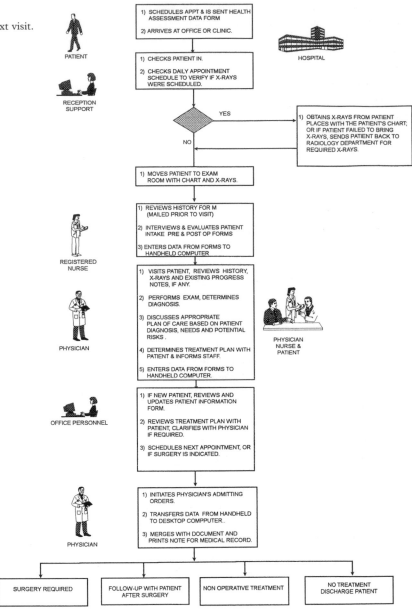

trations. A patient satisfaction survey to elicit comments and feedback along the care pathway can assist with problem identification for process improvement.

TKR patient outcomes are categorized as physiological, psychological, functional, and economic. All of these categories have measurable components. Physiological outcomes are measured by reduction of symptoms (reduced pain an improved mobility), psychological by general wellbeing and quality of life scores

383

(depression/social interaction), functional by activities of daily living (walking, bathing and dressing) and economic by return to work and overall expense of care.

Does pain, range of motion, and function improve after surgical intervention? Ongoing assessment and collection of data triggers the feedback mechanism and keeps the process circling in a continuous loop. Conceptually, the process itself is relatively uncomplicated. Implementation of the process is the tricky aspect and if it is done without proper planning, it can become time consuming and costly. When done correctly, however, the long-term value of operational efficiency and patient satisfaction justifies the initial dedication of time and start-up costs.

Pertinent data collection with easy storage and retrieval of information is a vital component to the patient care process. Figure 15.2 describes steps taken by the nurse and physician with respect to data entry. The specific data items collected are discussed in greater detail later on in this chapter.

## TKR outcome research

TKR surgery has become a common procedure. In 1996, according to the National Center for Health Statistics,[4] 245 000 TKR procedures were performed in the USA alone. This was an increase of 30 000 from the year before. The research potential on such a volume is staggering, yet to date there has been little success with creating a meaningful national data repository. This will change as information systems become more integrated and clinicians become more comfortable with sharing information.

Current outcome research includes methods such as analysis of large databases, small-area analysis, structured literature reviews (meta-analysis), prospective clinical trials, decision analysis, and guideline development. Clinical research should ideally be prospective and should employ modern statistical and assessment tools.[2] Retrospective studies depend on record retrieval and are generally not as accurate. However, there is a place for them in tracking nonresearch items especially if the data collection and process is consistent.

For years total knee outcomes focused primarily on the procedure and technique and not the improvement of health and wellbeing of the patient. Tools used were designed to collect specific patient functional items. Some tools deployed a rating system to compare results across time. Drake et al.[5] looked at different rating systems used to assess outcomes and found 34 different systems represented in the literature from 1972 to 1992. They found great variability in the design and utilization of rating systems. This diversity made comparisons and aggregate research virtually impossible. The need to establish the use of a uniform instrument was and continues to be an ongoing concern.

Kettlekamp and Thompson[6] noted that a uniform rating system was of great importance. The criteria for developing this uniform rating system included:

- using important measurable characteristics of the knee
- avoiding arbitrary assignment of point values
- relating the total points derived from the scoring scale to the clinical results
- using clinical variables that could be easily quantified
- simplicity.

The ability to compare outcomes across studies of TKR is important for a number of reasons. The aforementioned concern for cost and improvement of quality tops the priority list. This dichotomy is reinforced when we look at how physicians and patients compare risks and benefits of TKR with other therapeutic options. Will a course of anti-inflammatory medication and physical therapy provide enough of improvement in the patient's quality of life? Does sacrificing the PCL, or size of polyethylene, make a significant difference? Is there a cheaper way to provide care with similar outcomes? The patient's clinical characteristics after the intervention need to be better understood.

Lastly, the future design of new prostheses and surgical techniques are based on outcome results. A comparison can only be made when you study similar parameters under similar conditions over similar time frames. Trends and quality practice can be identified with statistically significant numbers. Consistent measures are needed to compare outcomes because you can't make comparisons without it. You can not compare apples to oranges.

## Data collection

Historically, rating systems similar to the Hospital for Special Surgery (HSS) knee score were used to collect knee specific data. Drake's study[5] found that this system was the one most frequently used throughout their literature review. The typical outcome process, again primarily for research, included reviewing data that was collected at time of the patient office or clinic visit. The pre- and post-procedure information was embedded in a written or dictated progress note and later extracted from the office and or hospital record. These predominantly retrospective reviews required many hours of research time and relied on the resourcefulness of many staff members.

Ideally, clinical research should be conducted prospectively, through randomized clinical trials. However, it is not always possible to randomize patients for many kinds of medical and surgical treatments, and there are several other study designs that can reasonably effectively control for various biases. It is extremely difficult to recover valid and accurate outcome information from records that were not set up for the purpose of a specific study.[2]

The Knee Society Clinical Rating Score and Medical Outcomes Study 36-item short-form health survey (SF-36) health survey are examples of tools that have been generally accepted as standards for use in the TKR community. The widespread use of these data tools has resulted in the proliferation of TKR research. This research has lead to rapid growth and advancements in implant designs, materials and surgical techniques, and has also contributed to the validation of TKR as a cost-effective and worthwhile treatment option.

Many important steps to an outcome process revolve around data collection. The choice of data tools, methods of collection, and delegation of appropriate personnel are integral decisions. Having a consistent process with a quality improvement feedback mechanism as previously outlined is crucial (Figs 15.1, 15.2). The outcome process is not merely the collection of data. It also involves practice management and operational issues related to the handling and delivery of forms at specific timed intervals. Data analysis and interpretation should be built into the system design. Action plans can be initiated to facilitate quality improvements at any point along the continuum of care.

Anticipated cost, insufficient time, and limited computer expertise seem to be common barriers to an outcomes program. Costs include possible additional staffing, the purchasing of computer hardware and software, and training. Additionally, lack of universally standardized data tools, evidenced by the numerous rating systems available, continue to be a concern and the most likely drawback to implementation. It is easy to procrastinate and rationalize putting off data collection until a better tool is developed or until the price of computers declines. This is probably a mistake as it will be difficult to justify the care you provide today to the many interested healthcare parties. Some of these barriers have become less of an issue as hospitals, vendors, insurers, and specialist associations offer programs to assist their clinicians.

It seems obvious that TKR clinicians should decide the course of treatment for their patients. These decisions are grounded in education and new concepts and trends demonstrated in published literature. Peer and professional organizations like the American Knee Society have established overall guidelines of care. New ideas and treatment modalities are implemented only after clinical research is approved, tested, and validated. It is absolutely imperative that more TKR surgeons become involved with outcome collection, and share the information. A growing fear is that in the absence of significant data from clinicians, the external market forces will utilize their own, less reliable, and less pertinent data to make clinical practice policy decisions.

TKR surgeons need to define the standard core data set. This has been debated for years and is still undecided. For all practical purposes, complication rates including infection, deep vein thrombosis, and fracture are standards observed by everyone. Length of stay data, for example, may be relevant to the hospital administrators and insurers, but less relevant to the implant designers. TKR data necessary for medical publication in peer-reviewed journals generally requires specific clinical scores, but these scores may not be requested at all by insurers. The decision to use one data tool over another has come down to an individual choice. Only data with value should be collected. The collection of unimportant data is a colossal waste of time and resources.

Other factors to consider before choosing data instruments are validity and reliability. To be useful, the data collection techniques and the rules for converting responses to numbers must produce information that is not only relevant, but also correct.[7] Two crucial aspects of correctness are reliability, the extent to which measures give consistent or accurate results, and validity, the extent to which the results pertain directly to the desired attribute or characteristic being measured.

As mentioned, TKR outcomes can be separated into functional, clinical, and quality of life measurements. Drake et al.[5] reported that many assessment tools are used around the world and global standardization seems very unlikely in the near future. With this in mind, the combination of tools that includes knee selective items, overall health assessment, and a generalized satisfaction survey should be considered. The American Knee Society clinical and roentgenographic rating systems, SF-36, and an expectation or satisfaction questionnaire will satisfy many needs and provide a comprehensive framework to measure TKR patient outcomes.

## The American Knee Society clinical rating system

The American Knee Society clinical rating system is used and accepted worldwide. It measures important knee characteristics including pain, function, and range of motion. The scores ascertained with this tool help monitor the technical aspect of knee surgery and when used in conjunction with the SF-36 instruments, it paints a more complete outcomes picture.

Insall et al.[8] described the rationale for the Knee Society clinical rating system in 1989. He felt that the knee rating and functional assessment should be separate. With regard to the knee assessment, it was decided that only the three main parameters of pain, stability, and range of motion should be judged and that flexion contracture, extension lag, and misalignment should be dealt with as deductions (Table 15.1).

Konig et al.[9] discussed the need for a dual rating system to eliminate the declining scores associated with patient infirmity that are found in assessment systems by aggregating functional and joint parameters to a global score. They concluded that both scores improve up to 2 years postoperatively. The knee score then reaches a plateau with a constant rate, whereas functional rating declines. It is

**Table 15.1** American Knee Society knee score

| Patient category | |
|---|---|
| A | Unilateral or bilateral (opposite knee successfully replaced) |
| B | Unilateral, other knee symptomatic |
| C | Multiple arthritis or medical infirmity |

|  | Points |  | Points |
|---|---|---|---|
| *Pain* | | *Function* | |
| None | 50 | Walking | 50 |
| Mild or occasional | 45 | Unlimited | 40 |
|   Stairs only | 40 | >10 blocks | 30 |
|   Walking and stairs | 30 | 5–10 blocks | 20 |
| Moderate | | Housebound | 10 |
| Occasional | 20 | Unable | 0 |
| Continual | 10 | Stairs | |
| Severe | 0 | Normal up and down | 50 |
| *Range of motion* | | Normal up; down with rail | 40 |
| (5° = 1 point) | 25 | Up and down with rail | 30 |
| *Stability (maximum movement* | | Up with rail; unable down | 15 |
|   *in any position)* | | | |
| Anteroposterior | | Unable | 0 |
|   <5 mm | 10 | Subtotal | – |
|   5–10 mm | 5 | *Deductions* (minus) | |
|   10 mm | 0 | Cane | 5 |
| Mediolateral | | Two canes | 10 |
|   <5° | 15 | Crutches or walker | 20 |
|   6–9° | 10 | Total deductions | – |
|   10–14° | 5 | Function score | – |
|   >15° | 0 | Subtotal | – |
| *Deductions* (minus) | | | |
| Flexion contracture | | | |
|   5–10° | 2 | | |
|   10–15° | 5 | | |
|   16–20° | 10 | | |
|   >20° | 15 | | |
| Extension lag | | | |
|   <10° | 5 | | |
|   10–20° | 10 | | |
|   >20° | 15 | | |
| Alignment | | | |
|   0–4° | 0 | | |
|   5–10° | 3 points each degree | | |
|   11–15° | 3 points each degree | | |
| Other | 20 | | |
| Total deductions | – | | |
| Knee Score—(If total is a minus number, score is 0) | | | |

Source: Insall *et al.*[8]

assumed that advanced age and its concomitant disease deteriorate function.

The Knee Society rating system is a valuable instrument because its data items are knee selective. The questions of reliability and validity were addressed by Drake et al.[5] They determined that this and other current knee rating systems probably satisfy the needs which they were originally conceived—to provide orthopedic surgeons with an estimate of their technical success in TKR. It does not however meet the reliability, validity, and measurement precision necessary to address more detailed questions concerning patient outcomes.[5]

Peer-reviewed journals currently consider this tool a requirement for publication. Until a more valid instrument is designed, tested, and implemented it will continue to be used as a primary method to assess knee function. Again, one should realize that ideally, the concomitant use of other tools is needed to complete the total outcome picture. At present there is a multicenter evaluation by the Knee Society to test the validity of the rating system.

## The Knee Society TKR roentgenographic evaluation and scoring system

Ewald's report[10] on behalf of the Knee Society encouraged the uniform reporting of the results of TKR. It was realized that no ideal rating system existed, but the need for many to use one so that relative comparisons could be made was significant. This enabled comparisons to be made between institutions as well as different implants.

The evaluation and scoring includes component position, leg and knee alignment, and the prosthesis–bone interface or fixation is reviewed on anteroposterior (AP), lateral, and patella skyline or Merchant view radiographs. The tibial interface is evaluated in the AP and lateral views and the femoral interface in the lateral view. The patella is evaluated in the Merchant view.

Zones are delineated and numbered accordingly in all views. Location and number of zones are established by the prime developers of any particular knee design and should follow these guidelines. The scoring system for each of the three components is determined by measuring the width of the radiolucent lines for each of the zones in millimeters for each of the three components. The total widths are added for each zone each of the three prostheses. This total produces a numerical score for each component. A high score signifies possible or impending failure.

## Medical Outcomes Study 36-item short-form health survey (SF-36)

The SF-36 was constructed by Ware et al.[7] from the Medical Outcomes Study in 1992 to satisfy minimum pyschometric standards necessary for group comparisons involving generic health concepts.

This comprehensive short form with only 36 questions yields an 8-scale health profile as well as summary measures of HRQOL.

The SF-36 is referred to as a generic measure because it assesses health concepts that represent basic human values that are relevant to everyone's functional status and well-being. Generic health measures assess HRQOL outcomes, namely, those known to be most directly affected by disease and treatment.

Naughton and Shumaker[11] concluded that the assessment of HRQOL in orthopedic interventions provides rich information regarding the effect of treatments on patients' daily lives. In general, HRQOL refers to an individual's overall sense of well being—physically, socially, and emotionally. In orthopedic conditions, Wright[12] argues that there are four primary aims at to orthopedic treatments:

- to preserve life
- to treat symptoms or complaints such as pain and functional disabilities
- to restore function
- to prevent functional decline.

The SF-36 survey includes one multi-item scale measuring each of eight health concepts:

- physical functioning (PF)
- role limitations due to physical health problems (RP)
- bodily pain (BP)
- general health (GH)
- vitality (energy/fatigue) (VT)
- social functioning (SF)
- role limitations due to emotional problems (RE)
- mental health (psychological distress and psychological well-being) (MH).[7]

These eight concepts were chosen to measure behavioral functioning, perceived well-being, social and role disability, and personal evaluations (perceptions) of health in general. An example of a question for each item is shown in Table 15.2.

The SF-36 is a validated instrument. This means it has passed the rigorous process associated with validity studies. Validity studies increase understanding of what a difference or a change in a score means. When enough evidence has been accumulated to show that a scale measures the intended health concept and does not measure other concepts, the scale is said to be validated. Guidelines for validating the SF-36 have been derived from those used to validate psychological and educational measures by the American Psychological Association, the American Educational Research Association, and the National Council on Measurement in Education.[7]

**Table 15.2** Sample items from the SF-36 Health Survey

| Scale | Item | Question |
|---|---|---|
| Physical functioning (RP) | 3i | Walking one block |
| Role functioning (RE, RE) | 4b,5b | Accomplished less than you would like |
| Bodily pain (BP) | 7 | How much bodily pain have you had during the past 4 weeks? |
| General health | I | In general, would you say your health is: excellent, very good, good, fair, poor |
| Vitality (VT) | 9i | Did you feel tired? |
| Social functioning (MH) | 6 | During the past 4 weeks, to what extent has your physical health or with your normal social activities with your family, friends, neighbors, or groups? |
| Mental health (HT) | 9f | Have you felt downhearted or blue? |
| Reported health transition (HT) | 2 | Compared to one year ago, how would you rate your health in general now? |

Source: Ware *et al.*[7]

Scoring the SF-36 is a complex process better left to a computer equipped with the appropriate scoring algorithms. SF-36 items and scales are scored so that the higher score indicates a better health state. For example, functioning scales are scored so that a high score indicates better functioning and the pain scale is scored so that a high score indicates freedom of pain. After data entry, items and scales are scored in three steps:

* item re-coding, for the 10 items that require recoding
* computing scale scores by summing across items in the same scale (raw score scale scores)
* transforming raw scale scores to a 0–100 scale (transformed scale scores).[7]

The SF-36 has widespread use with over 150 topics from acetabular fracture to weight loss under study. It complements the knee-specific tools well and adds reliable QOL data to the TKR patient profile. Kantz *et al.*[13] analyzed the sensitivity and specificity of the SF-36 and the Knee Society's clinical rating system in a study of patients with osteoarthritis and concluded that for assessing knee pain and knee-related limitations in role function, measures that refer explicitly to the knee provide greater specificity. Comprehensive assessment of the health of TKR patients requires both generic and condition specific measures of key health concepts, including physical function, role limitations, and pain.

Hozack *et al.*[14] reported improvement in SF-36 scores in a series of 149 patients with primary total knee replacement. They also found that the patients with primary hip replacement provided even better physical and social scores, better pain relief, and improved energy scores, although the patients who had total knee arthroplasty were older and heavier, thus creating potential for inferior results. It is expected that more and more research studies will continue to demonstrate positive change in SF-36 scores and this will further validate its use.

## Patient satisfaction survey

Patient (customer) service is an important aspect that is becoming more routinely assessed in the healthcare arena. Many factors influence a patient's decision on TKR surgery:

- Where is the best place?
- Who are the most competent surgeons?
- What are their outcomes?

The market is more competitive as increased information and quality reporting on individual practitioners becomes more commonplace. Some patients value ease of access. Their priority is convenience of office location. Other, more sophisticated patients do research on their own to determine physician and hospital reputation for quality care. Quality outcome data can support the marketing department.

The Group Health Association of America[15] developed a simple, 11 question, satisfaction survey designed to ascertain information pertaining to clinic visits. Questions include rating the facility by the ability of the patient to reach office by phone, the amount of time spent with the physician, explanation of care, personal manner, and technical skills.

This information is extremely valuable when one realizes that physicians get a large percentage of patient referrals from other patients. Satisfied and dissatisfied patients should have a mechanism available to communicate their comments and concerns. The care provider should have a way to identify problem areas so corrective or preventive measures can be taken. Validation of satisfactory service is helpful to maintain quality processes. Satisfaction questions should be consistent and offered routinely.

TKR surgeons should discuss expected outcomes with their patients before treatment. This eliminates dissatisfaction related to patients with unrealistic expectations. A question asking if their expectations have been met post procedure can help with subsequent care decisions.

- Is the patient satisfied with the ability to perform activities after TKR surgery?
- Has pain level improved?
- Has their use of pain medication decreased?

## Methods of collection

Collection of TKR data is an ongoing process. Outcomes management relies on the ability to collect, analyze, and interpret information quickly. Information obtained through questionnaires or placed on a form is limited in its use if it can not be entered and retrieved easily. Progress notes written or dictated into the patient record are still the overwhelming method of data collection, but computerized systems have been on the increase.

Outcome management has become a much more efficient process with the increased utilization of computer technology. Computers have turned the once laborious data retrieval task into a more manageable and efficient one. Statistical analysis software can manipulate data and perform multiple calculations with a few simple keystrokes. A growing number of surgeons in practice today have embraced computer technology and welcome the industry's urgency to collect outcome data. These few recognize the peripheral benefits and have devoted the time and resources necessary to design a process tailored to their individual practice.

A commitment to a computerized outcome process is not an easy proposition as there is a multitude of questions to answer:

- What type of computer and which software should I use?
- How much will it cost?
- Is there any support available?
- What is the best way to enter data?
- Who is responsible for entering the most critical aspects?

These questions must be answered on an individual basis as everyone has a unique background with different abilities, needs, and goals.

Many options are currently available. Some hospital centers and group practices have created outcomes units and invested significant resources to improve the data collection process. Scannable forms are used to eliminate timely data processing. The American Academy for Orthopedic Surgeons (AAOS), for example, has instituted the Musculoskeletal Outcomes Data Evaluation and Management System (MODEMS) program. The purpose of this program is to provide participants with a process for directly measuring, recording, storing, and analyzing information about the outcomes of the musculoskeletal care they provide.[16]

Orthopedic and computer consultants have joined forces to provide services to improve data collection, management, and processing. Innovations in computer design continue to make things easier. One innovative practice for example uses a handheld, palm-sized pocket organizer loaded with the orthopedic tools to manage their entire outcomes program (Table 15.3). The 170 data items, identified as relevant are embedded in a preoperative intake customized electronic form. Items include patient demographics, diagnosis, height and weight, medical history, surgical history, source of referral, type of insurance, TKR specific questions, Knee Society clinical rating and roentgenographic scoring system, medication usage, Charnley classification, Lahey Clinic score, and patient satisfaction

**Table 15.3** Outcomes management using a pocket organizer in a TKA office practice

| Patient data | Time collected | Method of collection | Purpose |
|---|---|---|---|
| Demographic | Pre visit | Registration form completed by patient | Insurance verification and chart generation |
| Health history | Initial visit and subsequent visits | Health assessment given and reviewed by practitioner during exam | Appropriate plan of to patient care, track complications |
| Knee Society Clinical Rating Score | Initial visit, 1, 3 month post-op, annually | Completed by practitioner during exam | Clinical and functional assessment |
| Charnley Classification | Initial visit, 1, 3 month post op, annually | Completed by practitioner during exam | Clinical and functional assessment |
| Lahey Clinic Scores | Initial visit, 1, 3 month post op, annually | Completed by practitioner during exam | Clinical and functional assessment |
| Knee Society Radiographic Assessment | Initial visit, 1, 3 month post op, annually | Completed by practitioner during exam | Clinical assessment |
| SF-36 | Pre op, 3 and 6 months post op, and annually | Mailed form completed by patient | Quality of life assessment |
| Patient satisfaction | Bimonthly as per office | At time of visit | Quality improvement |

Outcomes process based on practice of Richard S. Laskin, MD, Hospital for Special Surgery, New York, NY.

questions. All the data is entered with a pen stylus directly to the handheld computer. Data can then be transferred to a desktop personal computer at the touch of a button. Once stored, it can be exported into a program for statistical analysis, or to a word processing program for progress notes or reports. This can eliminate approximately 75% of patient dictation and save valuable time and money. Operative report information is entered this way as well, making the printed record available minutes after surgery. This has speeded up the surgical billing process. The use of this type of computer technology demonstrates that management of voluminous amounts of TKR specific data can be simple, inexpensive and efficient.

## Conclusion

Outcome measurement is deeply ingrained into the fabric of healthcare. The TKR specialist has access to all the elements of a quality system: knee-specific standards of care, validated data collection tools, process development, quality management, and innovative computer technology. The utilization of a comprehensive outcome process is a valuable commodity to the physician practice and is becoming more essential for long-term survival in the volatile healthcare industry.

Improved quality of patient care and continued advancements in the treatment of orthopedic diseases relies on the clinician's ability to track outcomes. Clinical research can be enhanced if a structured environment is in place. Clinicians need to be aware that future clinical practice policy decisions will be made based on outcome statistics. It is in their best interest as well as the patient's best interest to have this information originate from the care providers.

# References

1 Bradham DS: Outcomes research in orthopaedics: history, perspectives, concepts, and future. Arthroscopy: *Journal of Arthroscopic and Related Surgery* **10**(5): 493–501, 1994.

2 Keller RB: Outcomes research in orthopaedics. *Journal of the American Academy of Orthopaedic Surgeons* **1**(2):122–129, 1993.

3 Gartland JJ: Orthopaedic clinical research: deficiencies in experimental design and determinations of outcome. *Journal of Bone and Joint Surgery* [Am] **70**:1357–1364, 1988.

4 National Center for Health Statistics: *Advanced Data No. 301*. 31 August, 1998.

5 Drake BG, Callahan CM, Dittus RS, Wright JG: Global rating systems used in assessing knee arthroplasty outcomes. *Journal of Arthroplasty* **9**(4):409–417, 1994.

6 Kettlekamp DB, Thompson C: Development of a knee scoring scale. *Clinical Orthopaedics and Related Research* **107**:93, 1975.

7 Ware JE, Snow KK, Kosinski MA, Gandek MS: *SF-36 Health Survey, manual and interpretation guide*, 1993.

8 Insall JN, Dorr LD, Scott RD, Scott WN: Rationale of the Knee Society Clinical Rating System. *Clinical Orthopaedics and Related Resarch* **248**:13–14, 1989.

9 Konig A, Scheidler M, Rader C, Eulert J: The need for a dual rating system in total knee arthroplasty. *Clinical Orthopaedics and Related Research* **345**:161–167, 1997.

10 Ewald FC, on behalf of the Knee Society: The Knee Society total knee arthroplasty roentgenographic evaluation and scoring system. *Clinical Orthopaedics and Related Research* **248**:9–12, 1989.

11 Naughton MJ, Shumaker SA: Assessment of health-related quality of life in orthopadic outcome studies, arthroscopy: *Journal of Arthroscopic and Related Surgery* **13**(1):107–113, 1997.

12 Wright JG: Quality of life in orthopaedics. In *Quality of life and pharmacoeconomics in clinical trials*, ed. B Spilker, pp.1039–1044. Lippincott-Raven, Philadelphia, 1996.

13 Kantz ME, Harris WJ, Levitsky K et al.: Methods for assessing condition-specific and generic functional status outcomes after totoal knee replacement. *Medical Care* **30**(Suppl):MS240–MS252, 1992.

14 Hozak WJ, Rothman RH, Albert TJ et al.: *Clinical Orthopaedics and Related Research* **344**:88–93, 1997.

15 Group Health Association of America: Satisfaction survey. GHAA/Davies and Ware, 1991.

16 MODEMS: Musculoskeletal Outcomes Data Evaluation and Management System. American Academy of Orthopaedic Surgeons, Rosedale, IL. www.modems.org, 1999.

# Index